Controversial Topics in Dentistry and Oral and Maxillofacial Surgery

Editor

HARRY DYM

DENTAL CLINICS OF NORTH AMERICA

www.dental.theclinics.com

January 2024 • Volume 68 • Number 1

ELSEVIER

1600 John F. Kennedy Boulevard • Suite 1800 • Philadelphia, Pennsylvania, 19103-2899

http://www.dental.theclinics.com

DENTAL CLINICS OF NORTH AMERICA Volume 68, Number 1
January 2024 ISSN 0011-8532, ISBN: 978-0-443-18308-9

Editor: John Vassallo; j.vassallo@elsevier.com
Developmental Editor: Akshay Samson

Dental Clinics of North America (ISSN 0011-8532) is published quarterly by Elsevier Inc., 360 Park Avenue South, New York, NY 10010-1710. Months of issue are January, April, July, and October. Business and Editorial Offices: 1600 John F. Kennedy Boulevard, Suite 1800, Philadelphia, PA 19103-2899. Periodicals postage paid at New York, NY and additional mailing offices. Subscription prices are $333.00 per year (domestic individuals), $100.00 per year (domestic students/residents), $396.00 per year (Canadian individuals), $100.00 per year (Canadian students/residents) $463.00 per year (international individuals), and $200.00 per year (international students/residents). For institutional access pricing please contact Customer Service via the contact information below. International air speed delivery is included in all *Clinics* subscription prices. All prices are subject to change without notice. **POSTMASTER:** Send address changes to *Dental Clinics of North America*, Elsevier Health Sciences Division, Subscription Customer Service, 3251 Riverport Lane, Maryland Heights, MO 63043. **Customer Service (orders, claims, online, change of address): Elsevier Health Sciences Division, Subscription Customer Service, 3251 Riverport Lane, Maryland Heights, MO 63043. Tel: 1-800-654-2452 (U.S. and Canada). Fax: 314-447-8029. E-mail: journalscustomerservice-usa@elsevier.com (for print support); journalsonlinesupport-usa@elsevier.com (for online support).**

Reprints. For copies of 100 or more, of articles in this publication, please contact the Commercial Reprints Department, Elsevier Inc., 360 Park Avenue South, New York, NY 10010-1710. Tel.: 212-633-3874; Fax: 212-633-3820; E-mail: reprints@elsevier.com.

The *Dental Clinics of North America* is covered in *MEDLINE/PubMed (Index Medicus), Current Contents/Clinical Medicine, ISI/BIOMED* and *Clinahl.*

Contributors

EDITOR

HARRY DYM, DDS, FACS
Chair of Dentistry and Oral and Maxillofacial Surgery, Director of Oral and Maxillofacial Surgery Residency Training Program, The Brooklyn Hospital Center, Brooklyn, New York

AUTHORS

SHELLY ABRAMOWICZ, DMD, MPH
Associate Professor, Division of Oral and Maxillofacial Surgery, Department of Surgery, Emory University School of Medicine, Chief, Oral and Maxillofacial Surgery, Children's Healthcare of Atlanta, Atlanta, Georgia

DAVID RUSSELL ADAMS, DDS, FICD
Associate Professor, Section Head, Oral and Maxillofacial Surgery, University of Utah, School of Dentistry, Salt Lake City, Utah

AMANDA ANDRE, DDS
Oral and Maxillofacial Surgery Resident, The Brooklyn Hospital Center, Brooklyn, New York

MICHAEL BENICHOU, DMD
Oral and Maxillofacial Surgery Resident, The Brooklyn Hospital Center, Brooklyn, New York

MICHAEL H. CHAN, DDS
Director, Oral and Maxillofacial Surgery, Department of Veterans Affairs, New York Harbor Healthcare System (Brooklyn Campus), Senior Attending, Oral and Maxillofacial Surgery, Department of Oral and Maxillofacial Surgery, The Brooklyn Hospital Center, Brooklyn, New York

EARL CLARKSON, DDS, FACS
Director, Oral and Maxillofacial Surgery, Woodhull Medical Center, Attending, Oral and Maxillofacial Surgery, The Brooklyn Hospital Center, Brooklyn, New York

JENNIFER B. COHEN, DDS
General Dentist, Jesse Brown VA Medical Center, Chicago, Illinois; Dental/OMS Service, Chicago, Illinois

CHAD DAMMLING, DDS, MD
Resident, Department of Oral and Maxillofacial Surgery, School of Dentistry, The University of Alabama at Birmingham, Birmingham, Alabama

HARRY DYM, DDS, FACS
Chair of Dentistry and Oral and Maxillofacial Surgery, Director of Oral and Maxillofacial Surgery Residency Training Program, The Brooklyn Hospital Center, Brooklyn, New York

YIJIAO FAN, DDS
Oral and Maxillofacial Surgeon, Private Practice, Flushing, New York

REBECCA FISHER, DMD
Department of Oral and Maxillofacial Surgery, Woodhull Medical Center, Brooklyn, New York

EVAN M. GILMARTIN, BS
Dental Student, School of Dentistry, The University of Alabama at Birmingham, Birmingham, Alabama

REZA HADIOONZADEH, DDS
Resident, Oral and Maxillofacial Surgery, Woodhull Medical Center, Brooklyn, New York

LESLIE ROBIN HALPERN, MD, DDS, PHD, MPH, FACS, FICD
Professor, Section Chief/Program Director, Residency in Oral and Maxillofacial Surgery, New.York Medical College/NYCHHC, Metropolitan Hospital, Valhalla, New York

ZACHARY A. HELLER, DO, DMD
Resident, Department of Oral and Maxillofacial Surgery, Nova Southeastern University College of Dental Medicine, Davie, Florida

MARITZABEL HOGGE, MS, DDS
Director, Associate Professor, Department of Maxillofacial Medicine, Nova Southeastern University College of Dental Medicine, Davie, Florida

RAZA A. HUSSAIN, BDS, DMD, FACS
Acting Chief of Dentistry, Chief of Oral and Maxillofacial Surgery, Jesse Brown VA Medical Center, Dental/OMS Service, Clinical Associate Professor, Department of Oral and Maxillofacial Surgery, University of Illinois Chicago, Chicago, Illinois

JOSEPH KANG, DDS
Chief Resident, Department of Oral and Maxillofacial Surgery, The Brooklyn Hospital Center, Brooklyn, New York

BRIAN KINARD, DMD, MD
Assistant Professor, Department of Oral and Maxillofacial Surgery, School of Dentistry, The University of Alabama at Birmingham, Birmingham, Alabama

JONATHAN MALAKAN, DDS
Resident, Department of Oral and Maxillofacial Surgery, The Brooklyn Hospital Center, Brooklyn, New York

IAN MARK, DMD
Resident, Department of Oral and Maxillofacial Surgery, The Brooklyn Hospital Center, Brooklyn, New York

NABIL MOUSSA, DDS
Fellow, Department of Oral and Maxillofacial Surgery, Anne Arundel Medical Center, Bowie, Maryland

ANH THIEU NGUYEN, DMD
Resident, Department of Oral and Maxillofacial Surgery, The Brooklyn Hospital Center, Brooklyn, New York

ORRETT E. OGLE, DDS
Former Chief and Program Director, Department of Oral and Maxillofacial Surgery, Woodhull Hospital, Brooklyn, New York

BENJAMIN PALLA, DMD, MD
Dental/OMS Service, Department of Oral and Maxillofacial Surgery, University of Illinois Chicago, Chicago, Illinois

SCOTT M. PETERS, DDS
Associate Professor, Oral and Maxillofacial Pathology, Geisinger Medical Center, Wilkes-Barre, Pennsylvania

JASON E. PORTNOF, DMD, MD, FACS, FACD, FICD
Adjunct Associate Professor, Department of Oral and Maxillofacial Surgery, Nova Southeastern University College of Dental Medicine, Davie, Florida, Private Practice, Boca Raton, Florida

MICHAEL R. RAGAN, DMD, JD, LLM
Adjunct Associate Professor, Department of Oral and Maxillofacial Surgery, Nova Southeastern University College of Dental Medicine, Davie, Florida

TAL SASTOW, MS, DMD
Resident, Department of Oral and Maxillofacial Surgery, The Brooklyn Hospital Center, Brooklyn, New York

FEIYI SUN, DDS
Resident, Department of Oral and Maxillofacial Surgery, The Brooklyn Hospital Center, Brooklyn, New York

JAYKRISHNA THAKKAR, DDS
Chief Resident, Department of Oral and Maxillofacial Surgery, The Brooklyn Hospital Center, Brooklyn, New York

EDWARD ZEBOVITZ, DDS
Attending, Oral and Maxillofacial Surgery, Anne Arundel Medical Center, Bowie, Maryland

Contents

> This chapter discusses controversies in diagnosis and management of obstructive sleep apnea (OSA), with particular focus on surgical management to improve quality of life. Though OSA is a complex disorder that affects millions of people worldwide, its management remains controversial among clinicians. Gaps in understanding its pathophysiology, long-term health consequences, diagnostic methods, and treatment strategies exist. While continuous positive airway pressure (CPAP) therapy is considered the gold standard for moderate to severe obstructive sleep apnea (OSA), its adherence rate is often low, and its efficacy in improving outcomes beyond symptom reduction and quality of life improvement is uncertain. As such, surgical intervention may be an alternative for specific patient populations. Additionally, the type of surgical intervention may depend on individual patient needs, anatomic features, as well as preferences.

> Dental procedures can pose a risk of bleeding, and it is not uncommon for dentists to consult prescribing physicians regarding a mutual patient's antiplatelet and anticoagulant medication to prevent excessive bleeding during or after an upcoming procedure. However, there has been a growing controversy in the dental community surrounding the stoppage of these medications prior to dental procedures. Some believe that stopping these medications prior to dental procedures is necessary to reduce the risk of bleeding complications, while others argue that stopping them can increase the risk of stroke or other thromboembolic events. The debate has left many dentists and specialists unsure about the best course of action when it comes to managing bleeding risk during dental procedures. In this article, we will review the antithrombotic medications, indications, mechanism of action, and its effects on the coagulation pathway, laboratory testing and reversal agents. Also, we will explore the controversy surrounding the stoppage of novel anitplatelets (eg,: prasurgrel and ticagrelor), dual-antiplatelets, triple-antiplatelet, vitamin K antagonists (eg,: wafarin, coumadin), and direct oral anticoagulants (eg,: dabigatran, rivaroxaban, xarelto and endoxaban) in dentistry and examine the current evidence and guidelines for managing dental patients undergoing oral surgery.

Short dental implant placement has become a more popular surgical option for the reconstruction of the dentoalveolar region. In this article, we briefly discuss the considerations that the clinician must take into account when considering the use of short dental implants.

A cone beam central tomography (CBCT) scan produces images in orthogonal and non-orthogonal with great spatial resolution. When a dental health care practitioner (DHP) orders a CBCT scan, they should consider if it is truly indicated, as CBCT scans carry up to four times the dosage of radiation compared to panoramic radiographs. Any diagnostic imaging obtained of a patient should include a formal interpretive report commenting on the findings within the imaging. Ordering of limited field of view (FOV) CBCT scans and failing to report on abnormal findings present outside of the region of interest (ROI) is a potential medicolegal issue.

Medication-related osteonecrosis of the jaw (MRONJ) is a most interesting, complex and "elusive" condition seen by the oral health care provider. It is plagued by controversy and although a wealth of research has created clinical treatment databases, there is no "gold standard" algorithm to be applied in a universal fashion. The purpose of this article is to explore several controversies associated with the etiology(s), staging, treatments, and long-term resolution of MRONJ in patients who are treated by the oral health care provider. Controversies for optimizing prevention, and disease control will also be discussed from an interdisciplinary perspective.

The one provider anesthesia model used in oral and maxillofacial surgery (OMS) practices has been a subject of debate due to concerns about patient safety, inadequate attention, and mortality and morbidity rates. Historically, OMS specialists have made significant contributions to modern anesthesia; however, recent changes in Centers for Medicare and Medicaid Services have led to increased scrutiny of the OMS anesthesia model. Proponents argue that the model is safe and effective, thanks to well-trained Dental Anesthesia Assistants and OMS surgeons' extensive experience in dental anesthesia cases.

Antibiotic prophylaxis is the use of antibiotics perioperatively to prevent infections at the surgical site or distant locations. The decision to provide prophylaxis must balance risks of antibiotic resistance, adverse drug reactions, and increased health care costs with the benefit of decreasing infection. This determination has been studied extensively in patients with specific cardiac conditions and prosthetic joints. Prophylactic antibiotics in healthy patients have been shown to reduce the frequency of alveolar osteitis and decrease the failure rates of dental implants.

Periimplant mucositis and periimplantitis are common complications of
dental implant. This article provides a comprehensive overview of the
2017 World Workshop's new definition, clinical and radiographic presentation, pathogenesis, risk factors, and classification of periimplant diseases.
Also, the authors discuss various types of instruments, materials, and
techniques commonly used for treatment of nonsurgical and surgical peri-
implantitis. Lastly, the authors include some controversial topics surrounding this subject.

As the field of implant dentistry continues to evolve, new technologies and
technologies arise that can provide great benefits to the partial or completely edentulous patient. The purpose of this article is to review the history, definition, and rationale of immediate loading of dental implants with
the goal of providing evidence-based recommendations for implementation into clinical practice. Relevant literature is summarized and includes
discussion regarding prerequisites for immediate loading/restoration of
an endosseous implant. Surgical techniques and methodologies to prevent implant failure in immediate-load cases are discussed as well. The
greatest success has been demonstrated with 4 or more mandibular implants. Although there is support in the literature demonstrating successful
outcomes in immediate functional loading of single implants, the opinion of
the author is to opt for a nonfunctional load that does not have any occlusal
contacts when considering immediate loading of a single dental implant.

During the development of multimodal pain management protocols, practitioners need to consider the potential risks each treatment modality inherently carries in order to prevent or diminish harmful outcomes. As an
example, the part dentists played in the early stages of the opioid epidemic
in the United States of America should serve as a cautionary account. By
understanding the roots of this crisis, as practitioners we are better equip-
ped to implement the novel analgesic agents available today to optimize
post-operative pain control while minimizing any risk of addiction and
harm to our communities. It is therefore critical that our colleagues understand the variety of accessible options for pain management to assure that
our profession is able to seek adequate and sustainable relief for our post-
operative patients. This article will go in depth to explain the analgesic
tools practitioners can implement for an effective low-risk protocol, including a combination of NSAIDS and acetaminophen approach, using long-
acting local anesthetics such as Exparel, pregabalin, gabapentin, ketamine, dexmedetomidine, and corticosteroids, and enhanced recovery
after surgery protocols.

DENTAL CLINICS OF NORTH AMERICA

SERIES OF RELATED INTEREST

Atlas of the Oral and Maxillofacial Surgery Clinics
https://www.oralmaxsurgeryatlas.theclinics.com/

Oral and Maxillofacial Surgery Clinics
https://www.oralmaxsurgery.theclinics.com/

THE CLINICS ARE AVAILABLE ONLINE!
Access your subscription at:
www.theclinics.com

Preface

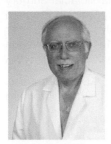

Harry Dym, DDS, FACS
Editor

Much has changed in our profession since I graduated Dental School in 1978. Like the practice of medicine, the profession of Dentistry and Oral Surgery has certainly evolved and mutated (for the better) during the past 45 years. We have moved on from the previous decades where techniques and procedures were handed down through the years based more on tradition than sound scientific principles.

Organized Dentistry, like Medicine, has adopted an evidence-based practice approach prior to making clinical recommendations. Evidence-based Dentistry has been defined by the American Dental Association "as an approach to oral healthcare that requires the judicious integration of systematic assessments of clinically relevant scientific evidence coupled with the dentist's clinical experience."

High-quality research is essential to help develop new treatment and alternative options. This issue, entitled "Controversial Topics in Dentistry and Oral and Maxillofacial Surgery," was written to tackle clinically relevant controversial subjects and help present cogent clear information for the clinician to determine the best possible solution or approach.

I feel strongly that my most able contributors have successfully accomplished the tasks I asked of them, and I congratulate them one and all on a job well done.

This text should not be construed as setting the definitive standard of care for the practice of Oral and Maxillofacial Surgery in the clinical areas that were discussed. The contributors have done an excellent job in presenting various opinions and literature reviews regarding specific treatment modalities. It is up to the reader based upon his or her own clinical experience and interpretation of the literature to arrive at a conclusion to guide their own clinical practice.

The *Dental Clinics of North America* series by Elsevier and its associate publisher, John Vassallo, play an important role in the continuing evolution of evidence-based Dentistry. Dental graduates must become lifelong learners if they wish to practice at a high level of quality Dentistry and Oral Surgery. Evidence-based high-quality textbooks are a critical part of the necessary tools one needs for continuing education, and

Dent Clin N Am 68 (2024) xiii–xiv
https://doi.org/10.1016/j.cden.2023.08.004
0011-8532/24/© 2023 Published by Elsevier Inc.

I appreciate the efforts of my editors, Akshay Samson and Ann Gielou M. Posedio, in bringing this issue to print.

Harry Dym, DDS, FACS
Chair of Dentistry and Oral & Maxillofacial Surgery
Director of Oral & Maxillofacial Surgery Residency Training Program
The Brooklyn Hospital Center
121 Dekalb Avenue
Brooklyn, NY 11201, USA

E-mail address:
hdym@tbh.org

Acknowledgments

The older I become, the more grateful I am for the various people I have encountered in my life. Whatever success I have achieved is mainly due to them, and I am fortunate to be given the opportunity to acknowledge and memorialize them now in print.

The Brooklyn Hospital Center is the oldest hospital in the great borough of Brooklyn, where I have been employed full time for the past 36 years (my entire career). It is an outstanding institution committed to providing high-quality patient-centered care to a wonderful community of patients. The Hospital is capably administered by Ms Lizanne Fontaine, Chairwoman of the Hospital Board of Trustees, and Mr Gary Terrinoni, CEO and President. Both of these outstanding individuals are deeply committed and devoted to the concept of providing high-quality care to a community that, due to socioeconomic reasons, often lacks the opportunity to avail themselves of such sophisticated and vital services. Both of these individuals also understand and value the essential need for quality dental and oral surgical services as part of their commitment to providing complete health care to our community.

I am fortunate to have as attendings in my Department of Dentistry/Oral and Maxillofacial Surgery outstanding dedicated clinicians, who also are committed to resident education, which are the life blood of our profession:

Dr Ricardo Boyce, Vice Chairman of the Department of Dentistry and Program Director of the General Practice Residency Program;

Dr Earl Clarkson, an outstanding oral and maxillofacial surgeon, who is the Associate Chief of the Oral and Maxillofacial Surgery Residency Training Program;

Dr Edward Woodbine, Dr Michael Chan, and Dr Jared Miller, who are integral to our Oral and Maxillofacial Surgery Residency Training program and who perform most of the highly complex maxillofacial surgical procedures;

Dr Reena Clarkson, Chief of the section of Orthodontics;

Dr Shira Weisel, Dr Saad Butt, Dr William Perez, and Dr Gary Klemons, who are attendees in our General Dentistry Residency Training Program.

Special acknowledgment to my Executive Assistant and both Oral and Maxillofacial Surgery and General Practice Residency coordinator, Ms Gloria Stallings. Gloria has been a part of our program for 29 years. Her dedication and commitment to the department grow more with each passing year.

I am also thankful for my Administrator, Mr Javier Velez, and my clerical staff and dental assistants for their hard work, and my capable oral and maxillofacial surgical residents. Also, I am indebted as well to Dr Orrett Ogle, Dr Peter M. Sherman, Dr Elliot Siegel, and Dr Stan Bodner for their continued friendship and advice.

Dent Clin N Am 68 (2024) xv–xvi
https://doi.org/10.1016/j.cden.2023.08.005
0011-8532/24/© 2023 Published by Elsevier Inc.

dental.theclinics.com

Finally, to my wife, Freidy, and my children, Yehoshua, Hindy, Daniel, and Akiva, and their families—all of you have brought and continue to bring me great joy and harmony, and I am deeply proud of you all.

Harry Dym, DDS, FACS
Chair of Dentistry and Oral & Maxillofacial Surgery
Director of Oral & Maxillofacial Surgery Residency Training Program
The Brooklyn Hospital Center
121 Dekalb Avenue
Brooklyn, NY 11201, USA

E-mail address:
hdym@tbh.org

Controversies in Sleep Apnea

Tal Sastow, MS, DMD[a],*, Nabil Moussa, DDS[b,1],
Edward Zebovitz, DDS[b,1]

KEYWORDS

- OSA • obstructive sleep apnea • AHI • MMA • CPAP • PSG • MARPE • DOME

KEY POINTS

- Nocturnal Polysomnography (PSG) is considered the gold standard for diagnosing OSA.
- CPAP is the most commonly used treatment modality for OSA.
- OSA is the most prevalent sleep disorder, with incidence and prevalence on the rise.
- Increasing prevalence of OSA is due to rising obesity rates, aging populations, and increased awareness and detection rates.
- Face-to-face evaluation by a sleep medicine physician is essential for making OSA diagnosis.

INTRODUCTION

Sleep Apnea is a prevalent and multifaceted sleep disorder affecting millions worldwide. In fact, sleep apnea is the most common respiratory disorder of sleep (Faria and colleagues, 2021).[1] This condition is characterized by recurring episodes of partial or complete upper airway obstruction during sleep, resulting in a reduction in oxygen saturation, sleep fragmentation, and arousals. Morbidity frequently associated with OSA includes hypertension, coronary artery disease, obesity, and diabetes. Impacts of OSA on an individual's quality of life can have detrimental effects on their daily activities. Reported negative effects on daily life include sleepiness, impaired memory, attention, and cognitive function. In 2019, a study deduced that the prevalence of obstructive sleep apnea was estimated at 936 million for severe OSA and 425 million for moderate OSA globally.[2] Sleep apnea has been reported to have been the cause of 810,000 collisions and 1400 fatalities from car crashes in the United States.[1] Currently several nonsurgical and surgical therapeutic modalities exist. Conservative measures

[a] Oral and Maxillofacial Surgery, The Brooklyn Hospital Center, 155 Ashland Pl, Brooklyn, NY 11201, USA; [b] Oral and Maxillofacial Surgery, Anne Arundel Medical Center, 4311 Northview Drive, Bowie, MD 20716, USA
[1] Present address: 4311 Northview Drive, Bowie, MD 20716.
* Corresponding author. 155 Ashland Pl, Brooklyn, NY 11201.
E-mail address: talsastow@gmail.com

Dent Clin N Am 68 (2024) 1–20
https://doi.org/10.1016/j.cden.2023.08.003
dental.theclinics.com

include oral mandibular advancement appliances, continuous positive airway pressure (CPAP) and diet modifications. Surgical treatment focus on modifying the soft tissue anatomy of the oropharynx, hypoglossal nerve stimulators or weight loss therapy such as bariatric surgery. Current treatment efforts often involve more than one provider and often providers have conflicting opinions on treatment strategies which may make treatment challenging and controversial. To muddy the water further, OSA is associated with a wide range of vague symptoms and objective parameters used for diagnosis (polysomnography) can be difficult to detect and analyze. It is important to focus on evidence-based treatment. The purpose of this paper is to provide a evidence based review of the current therapeutic treatment options for patients suffering from OSA. A particular focus will be placed on surgical options.

Apnea is defined as a complete pause or cessation of breathing, lasting for several seconds to over a minute, whereas hypopnea is defined as an overall partial reduction in airflow during sleep.[3] It is important to first define and distinguish between the two primary categories of sleep apnea: Obstructive Sleep Apnea (OSA) versus Central Sleep Apnea (CSA). Central Sleep Apnea is less common than OSA but is associated with the higher mortality rates. Per 100 people, in moderate and severe OSA, patients had a mortality rate of 9.36 and 13.11 respectively, compared to 11.47 and 15.59 in CSA.[4] In comparison, CSA can be characterized as a failure of ventilatory motor output via absence of nerve signals to thoracic muscles of inspiration, such as the diaphragm and the intercostal muscles, as well as the genioglossus muscle.[5,6] Central sleep apnea can result from damage to the respiratory centers such as from a stroke or heart failure. Certain medications such as opioids and benzodiazepines can have central apnea-like effects depressing the respiratory drive and suppressing the body's ability to respond to increased levels carbon dioxide.[7] Depending on the underlying cause and specific characteristics of the breathing disturbance, the pathophysiology of CSA can be further categorized as non-hypercapnic or hypercapnic. Non-hypercapnic CSA is marked by ventilatory instability due to high loop gain. In this context, "loop gain" refers to the relationship between the body's respiratory control system and its response to changes in oxygen and carbon dioxide levels. A high loop gain means that the body's response to these changes is exaggerated, leading to excessive fluctuations in breathing during sleep. Non-hypercapnic CSA is often seen in individuals with heart failure and other cardiovascular diseases. Hypercapnic CSA, on the other hand, is primarily a disorder of hypoventilation, meaning that the individual is not breathing enough to adequately remove carbon dioxide from the body. This can result in a buildup of carbon dioxide in the bloodstream, which can have serious health consequences. Hypercapnic CSA is often seen in individuals with chronic obstructive pulmonary disease (COPD) or other respiratory disorders that impair lung function.[8]

Obstructive Sleep Apnea is caused by an anatomic obstruction of the upper airway during sleep, typically due to relaxation of the parapharyngeal muscles and tongue. This obstruction leads to a cessation of breathing with resulting desaturation. In response to the decrease in oxygen saturation, there is a subsequent sympathetic response with catecholamine release triggering a microarousal facilitating a breath. OSA is increasingly prevalent in the population with recent estimates of as many as 1 billion adults between the ages of 30 to 69 worldwide. OSA is often associated with obesity, increasing age, and certain upper airway anatomic features such as enlarged neck circumference (>16 inches for women, >17 inches for men), macroglossia, tonsillar hypertrophy, an enlarged or elongated uvula (>35 mm), retrognathia, a high or arched palate, a Mallampati score of 3 or 4, nasal septum deviation or polyps, mandible to hyoid distance of 17 mm.[9,10]

Of note, it is also important to distinguish OSA from Upper Airway Resistance Syndrome (UARS). Since UARS was first diagnosed in the early 1990's, there has been debate over whether it is merely a part of the same spectrum as OSA and therefore not a distinct diagnosis. However, the current available evidence now supports the argument that suggests that UARS is, in fact, a distinct clinical phenomenon and should not be considered merely as a milder form of OSA.[11] UARS is characterized by repeated increases in the resistance of airflow in the upper airway, which causes a subsequent increase in respiratory effort, causing brief awakenings. These awakenings are known as respiratory effort-related arousals (RERAs) and are identified by a shift in alpha or fast theta frequency on the electroencephalogram (EEG), lasting from 3 to 10 seconds. RERAs differ from apneas or hypopneas, as they do not involve complete cessation of airflow or oxygen desaturation and are typically shorter in duration, comprising only one to three breaths. Additionally, patients with UARS have an apnea-hypopnea index (AHI) of less than five, which, would not meet the criteria for apneas or hypopneas.

Detection and treatment go hand-in-hand when diagnosing and treating OSA. Nocturnal Polysomnography (PSG) is considered the gold standard for diagnosis. It requires an overnight stay in a sleep lab and involves the use of various sensors to monitor brain activity, eye movement, heart rate, and breathing patterns. Essential to PSG studies are measurements via electrocardiograph (ECG), electroencephalogram (EEG), electro-oculogram (EOG), chin and limb electromyogram (EMG), and measurements of airflow signals, respiratory effort signals, oxygen saturation and body position. Though not required for essential PSG, some laboratories will also perform capnography studies to measure hypoventilation.[12] The second method is Home Sleep Apnea Testing (HSAT), which involves the use of a portable device to monitor breathing patterns and blood oxygen levels while the individual sleeps at home. The third method is the use of questionnaires and symptom assessments to identify potential sleep apnea symptoms such as snoring, daytime fatigue, and gasping for air during sleep. The fourth method is physical examination to identify anatomic abnormalities in the airway that may contribute to OSA. The fifth primary method is the use of smartphone apps and wearable devices that monitor sleep patterns and breathing during sleep. These methods can be used alone or in combination to detect OSA. These detection methods are important for identifying OSA and determining the appropriate treatment plan. A meta-analysis compared all currently available detection methods for OSA against PSG, finding PSG as a superior detection method to all, in its accuracy.[13]

With regards to treatment modalities, the most used treatment is Continuous Positive Airway Pressure (CPAP) therapy, achieving approximately 73% improvement in AHI, according the sleep foundation's analysis of available publications.[14,15] which involves wearing a mask over the nose and/or mouth during sleep, delivering a continuous flow of air to keep the airway open. Oral appliances are custom-made devices that position the jaw forward to help keep the airway open. The mechanics are thought to help with improving the diameter of the retroglossal space. Advancing the genial tubercule advances the tongue improving the posterior airway space. Surgery is another option for patients where CPAP and oral appliances are not effective or well-tolerated. Common surgical procedures include uvulopalatopharyngoplasty (UPPP), maxillomanibular advancement surgery, and genioglossus advancement. Additionally, surgical implantation of a nerve stimulation device, namely, the Inspire device, is also a less invasive surgical option. Weight loss is another option as obesity is a major risk factor for OSA, which has been shown to significantly improve AHI and symptoms in some patients. Longitudinal studies demonstrated that a weight gain of

10% over a period of 4 years is correlated with a 32% increase in AHI, and conversely, a reduction in weight of 10% is associated with a 26% decrease in AHI.[16] Lastly, positional therapy can help reduce symptoms of OSA, where sleeping in a different position, such as sleeping on one's side, may prevent the tongue and soft palate from collapsing into the airway.[17]

Despite the availability of several diagnostic and treatment modalities, there are still controversies regarding the optimal approach to diagnosing and treating OSA. A primary discussion surrounds the use of HSAT versus PSG. While HSAT is more convenient and cost-effective, some studies suggest that it may underestimate the severity of OSA compared to PSG. Another controversy surrounds the use of surgical versus non-surgical treatment options for OSA. While surgery may be effective in some patients, there is concern about the potential risks and complications associated with these procedures. Finally, there is controversy regarding the effectiveness of newer treatment modalities, such as hypoglossal nerve stimulation, in comparison to more established treatments like CPAP.[18] Overall, the controversies in diagnosing and treating OSA highlight the need for further research and individualized approaches to patient care and will be further discussed in this chapter.

EPIDEMIOLOGY OF OSA

It is widely posited that OSA poses significant health risks, specifically, linking it to increased risks of hypertension, stroke, myocardial infarction, diabetes, depression, anxiety, and cognitive impairment.[19] In addition, untreated OSA can lead to daytime fatigue, reduced productivity, and an increased risk of car accidents. However, despite the significant increase in the annual research publications attesting to the strong association between OSA and coronary artery disease, hypertension, heart failure and arrhythmias, whether or not OSA lies along the causal pathway to these conditions is not yet proven.[20,21]

Though OSA is already the most prevalent sleep disorder in the world, affecting millions of people worldwide, its incidence and prevalence continue to climb.[2] In North America, it is currently assumed that this is likely due to rising obesity rates, aging populations, and increased awareness and detection rates. Globally, it is estimated that 936 million people worldwide have mild to severe OSA, and 425 million people worldwide have moderate to severe OSA, between the ages of 30 and 69 years of age.[2] The condition is particularly prevalent in Western countries, where sedentary lifestyles and unhealthy diets are contributing to high rates of obesity and other metabolic disorders.[22]

Despite the high prevalence of sleep apnea, there is a general lack of awareness among the public about its serious health consequences. Many individuals who experience symptoms of sleep apnea, such as snoring, daytime fatigue, and gasping for air during sleep, may not recognize these as potential signs of a sleep disorder.[1] This perception is concerning as it may prevent individuals from seeking medical consultation, delaying diagnosis and treatment of OSA. As such, the timely and effective treatment of OSA is crucial for improving patients' health outcomes and quality of life, in addition to making a substantial socioeconomic impact.

CONTROVERSIES OF DIAGNOSIS

The World Sleep Society (WSS) and the American Academy of Sleep Medicine (AASM) provided recommendations and subsequent caveats to those recommendations for detecting OSA in clinical practice. In general, according to both organizations, clinical testing for OSA should be performed along with a thorough diagnostic test for OSA in adult patients who are suspicious for OSA based on clinical exam. The WSS advises that medical supervision of the diagnostic and treatment process are crucial, and clinicians must be aware of the advantages and limitations of HSATs and limited-channel sleep tests. The WSS also recommends that clinicians reassess the clinical assessment before further testing and prioritize PSG where available. However, if PSG is not an option, a higher-level limited channel test should be performed.[23] Testing may include or be limited to any or all the following: PSG (Type 1 testing), unattended HSAT (Type 2 testing), or cardiorespiratory polygraphy (Type 3 testing). The WSS recommends that medical professionals oversee the diagnostic and treatment process and have a clear understanding of the advantages and limitations of HSAT and limited channel sleep tests. They also advise caution when using limited, single-channel Type 4 tests (such as oximetry) as this requires a high level of clinical proficiency to determine the appropriate testing group and interpret the results (**Table 1**).

Due to the high prevalence of OSA, there is potential for substantial monetary strain on healthcare systems at large linked to conducting PSG for all patients suspicious for OSA. Additionally, in certain regions, in-laboratory testing may not be readily available. HSAT, despite its drawbacks, is a substitute method for diagnosing OSA in adults and may be less expensive and more practical in certain populations. However, HSAT may present certain drawbacks due to differences in which physiologic parameters are being measured and the availability of healthcare personnel to make sensor adjustments overnight as needed. The type and quantity of sensors utilized by HSAT devices can also vary significantly. Presently, sleep studies are classified as Type I, II, III, and IV, with unattended studies being categorized under Types II, III, and IV. Type II studies and PSGs utilized the same sensors, with the difference being that the patient is left unattended in type II studies (**Table 2**). In Type III studies, sensors will measure a restricted number of cardiopulmonary parameters, including at least two respiratory variables, such as effort to breathe and airflow, a cardiac variable, such as heart

Table 1
Primary detection methods of sleep apnea

Primary Detection Methods	Description
1. Nocturnal Polysomnography	Comprehensive sleep study that measures various physiologic variables during sleep, including airflow, respiratory effort, oxygen saturation, and brain wave activity. Considered gold standard for OSA Diagnosis.
2. Home Sleep Apnea Testing	Portable devices that monitor breathing patterns, oxygen levels, and heart rate during sleep. Less expensive and more convenient than PSG, but it may not be as accurate in detecting mild or positional OSA.
3. WatchPAT	Portable diagnostic device that measures peripheral arterial tone, heart rate, oxygen saturation, and body position to detect OSA. It is a simplified version of HSAT.
4. Clinical evaluation	Evaluate a patient's symptoms, medical history, and physical exam. However, clinical evaluation alone is not as reliable as NPSG or HSAT.
5. Questionnaires	Patients may be asked to fill out questionnaires, such as the Epworth Sleepiness Scale or the Berlin Questionnaire, to assess their risk for OSA. These questionnaires are not diagnostic tools but may be useful for identifying patients who need further evaluation.

Table 2 Sleep study types, excluding SCOPER classification system			
Sleep Study Types	Monitoring Parameters	Advantages	Disadvantages
Type I	Full PSG monitoring sensors	High diagnostic accuracy	Costly, time-consuming, requires trained staff
Type II	Same monitoring sensors as Type I but unattended	Performed outside sleep laboratory, less expensive	Limited monitoring parameters, lack of real-time monitoring, inability to initiate CPAP
Type III	Limited cardiopulmonary parameters: 2 respiratory variables, O2 saturation, 1 cardiac variable	Easy to use, portable	No real-time monitoring, limited monitoring parameters, No CPAP
Type IV	Measures 1–2 parameters, typically oxygen saturation and heart rate, or in some cases, just airflow	Inexpensive, easy to use, portable	Limited monitoring parameters, lack of real-time monitoring, inability to initiate CPAP

rate, and oxygen saturation. Lastly, Type IV studies, which are the most restricted studies, are limited to measuring as few as 1 or 2 variables, such as heart rate and oxygen saturation, and in certain instances, merely a patient's airflow and nothing else.[23]

Compared to attended studies, the utilization of HSAT devices may heighten the risk of technical failures due to the absence of real-time monitoring by medical personnel and may also have intrinsic limitations stemming from the lack of capability of most devices to distinguish between the sleep state and waking states. Additionally, it is important to note that CPAP cannot be initiated with HSAT, in contrast to PSG, where CPAP can be administered if and when it is necessitated. Additionally, HSAT is associated with substantial measurement errors when compared to PSG since standard sleep staging channels, such as EEG, EOG, and EMG, are not typically monitored in HSAT. Due to this limitation, hypopneas that are only associated with cortical arousals cannot be detected. Also, from a logistical standpoint, measurement errors can arise due to sensor dislodgement and poor-quality signal during HSAT, which would not be noticed due to the lack of real-time personnel monitoring. These factors may lead to the underestimation of the actual Apnea-Hypopnea Index (AHI), an index used to indicate the severity of sleep apnea, and may necessitate repeat studies due to faulty data.[23]

Importantly, included in the battery of essential measurements of PSG, Electromyograms (EMGs) can be categorized into different types based on their purpose or technique. Needle EMG is a diagnostic test that involves inserting a needle electrode into a muscle to measure its electrical activity. Surface EMG is a non-invasive test that involves placing surface electrodes on the skin to measure the electrical activity of the muscles underneath. Single-fiber EMG is a diagnostic test that involves inserting a very fine needle electrode into a muscle to measure the electrical activity of individual muscle fibers. Repetitive nerve stimulation EMG is a diagnostic test that involves stimulating a nerve repeatedly and measuring the resulting muscle responses with surface electrodes. EMG can provide valuable information about muscle activity during different stages of sleep. During rapid eye movement (REM) sleep, muscle tone is typically relaxed, and the EMG activity is low, except for bursts of phasic activity during rapid eye movements. Alpha, beta, delta, and k-complex spindles can also be observed during sleep using EMG. Alpha activity is most observed during relaxed wakefulness and can also be seen during the transition to sleep. Beta activity is associated with wakefulness and is characterized by fast, low-voltage oscillations. Delta activity is associated with deep sleep and is characterized by slow, high-voltage oscillations. K-complexes are large, high-amplitude waves that are typically seen during non-rapid eye movement (NREM) sleep.[24,25] Sleep EEG characteristics associated with OSA include increased EEG power in certain frequency bands. These changes in EEG activity can indicate states of poor sleep quality in OSA patients. Ongoing studies are investigating EEG microstates that may serve as biomarkers to indicate OSA in patients.[26]

The AASM further conducted a review and analysis of all presently accepted, prominent OSA screening questionnaires and predictive models, including STOP-BANG and Epworth Sleepiness Scale (ESS). The STOP-BANG questionnaire is a widely-used screening tool used to assess the likelihood of a patient having obstructive sleep apnea (OSA). It consists of eight questions that ask about snoring, tiredness during the day, observed apneas, high blood pressure, body mass index (BMI), age, neck circumference, and gender. The ESS is a self-administered questionnaire that is also used to identify OSA, however, unlike STOP-BANG, ESS does not include metrics such as BMI, age, gender, and neck circumference. Compared to other screening tools for OSA, such as the ESS and the Berlin Questionnaire, the STOP-BANG questionnaire is more sensitive and specific. It has a higher positive predictive value for OSA and can accurately identify patients who are at a high risk of having OSA.[27]

The review then went on to compare STOP-BANG and ESS against PSG and HSAT regarding their diagnostic value. This review concluded that, by and large, clinical questionnaires, morphometric models, and clinical prediction rules paled in comparison in diagnostic power versus PSG or even HSAT. Although sensitivity levels were relatively high for these alternate predictive screening methods, they are not robust enough to effectively rule out OSA. Meanwhile, the low specificity led to the AASM's position that PSG or HSAT are required to make a definitive diagnosis of OSA, regardless of predictive screening tool results.[13]

Importantly, it is necessary to review the utility of radiological study of the airway to assist in diagnosis of OSA. 3D computed tomography (CT) imaging of the upper airway can help identify anatomic variations that may cause obstructions and can quantify anatomic dimensions of the airway that may be helpful in predicting at-risk patients for OSA. Presently, cone-beam computer tomography (CBCT), which is now routinely used in dental offices, has become a helpful tool in screening for patients who may be at risk for OSA. These radiographic tools can aid in the study of anatomic landmarks such as the mandibular plane to hyoid (MP-H) distance (15.4 ± 3 mm),[28] thickness of the soft palate, the diameter and area of the posterior airway space (PAS), as well as the volume of the tongue.[29,30]

Drug-induced sleep endoscopy (DISE) is another well-established diagnostic tool that has been increasingly utilized in clinical practice for evaluation of the upper airway. Specifically, DISE provides a dynamic assessment of the collapsibility of the upper airway and is performed under conscious sedation. The identification and characterization of specific sites of obstruction and the degree and pattern of collapse have important implications for the selection and planning of therapeutic interventions. This is particularly true in cases where CPAP or other conservative treatments have failed to provide adequate relief. The recorded findings of DISE are comprehensive and include documentation of the level, pattern, and degree of collapse observed, providing clinicians with valuable information to guide individualized treatment strategies for their patients. The precise characterization of airway obstruction through DISE may also aid in the development of new therapeutic modalities and further enhance the management of patients with sleep-disordered breathing.[31] Circumferential and anteroposterior (AP) collapse are two common types of airway collapse that occur in patients with sleep apnea. Circumferential collapse refers to the collapse of the upper airway in a circular or circumferential manner, typically involving the collapse of soft tissues such as the lateral walls of the pharynx, the tonsils, the base of the tongue, or the lateral pharyngeal walls. AP collapse refers to the collapse of the upper airway in an anteroposterior direction, often involving the posterior part of the tongue, the soft palate, or the base of the tongue. Treatment approaches for circumferential and AP collapse in sleep apnea aim to address the underlying causes of airway obstruction and may include CPAP therapy, oral appliances, weight loss, positional therapy, and surgical interventions. The specific treatment approach depends on the severity of the airway collapse and individual patient characteristics.

The Muller maneuver is an additional diagnostic technique commonly utilized to evaluate upper airway obstruction in patients with sleep apnea. This maneuver involves having the patient inhale to the maximum capacity and then exhale forcefully while the nose and mouth are closed. The resulting negative pressure in the upper airway can potentially aggravate any existing obstructions and cause a collapse of the airway, thereby reproducing the features of an apneic event. The Muller maneuver is a valuable tool for pinpointing the specific sites of airway obstruction and determining the extent of collapsibility, which can assist in determining the most appropriate treatment strategies for managing sleep apnea. However, when compared to DISE, there was a discrepancy between the incidence of severe retrolingual airway collapse in patients with OSA. Further research is needed to determine the source of this discrepancy (Soares and colleagues, 2013).[32]

It is important to define and delineate the role of Oral Surgeons and Dentist in diagnosis of OSA. Clarification has been provided via the publication of joint policy and practice guidelines by the AASM and the American Academy of Dental Sleep Medicine (AADSM), as well as a treatment protocol outlined by the AADSM. According to these guidelines and protocol, it is essential that patients receive a face-to-face evaluation by a sleep medicine physician to obtain a definitive diagnosis of OSA. While dentists certified by the American Board of Dental Sleep Medicine (ABDSM) may play a valuable role in the overall management of patients with OSA, they are not qualified to diagnose the condition themselves and must been evaluated by medical sleep specialists for definitive diagnosis.[33]

CONTROVERSIES OF MANAGEMENT

Several key issues lie at the center of ongoing debates regarding the management of OSA. These include uncertainty over the most appropriate initial therapy for mild to moderate OSA, with some advocating for CPAP as first-line treatment, and others suggesting alternative approaches such as oral appliances. Additionally, the role of surgery in managing severe OSA in patients who are intolerant or non-compliant with CPAP remains a topic of debate. Optimal follow-up protocols for patients undergoing OSA treatment, including the frequency and type of monitoring required, have yet to be agreed upon. Finally, it is increasingly recognized that individualized treatment plans that consider patient preferences, co-existing medical conditions, and other factors are important for achieving successful outcomes in OSA management[34] (Table 3).

Table 3
List of treatment modalities and subtypes

Treatment Modality	Types
Positive Air Pressure (PAP)	(1) Continuous PAP (2) Bi-level PAP (Bi-PAP)
Oral Appliance	(1) Tongue-retaining (2) Mandibular advancement
Surgery	(1) Phase I (nasal, palatal, tongue) (2) Phase II (maxillomandibular advancement)
Adjunctive	(1) Weight loss (medical, bariatric surgery) (2) Positional therapy (3) vNasal expiratory PAP (4) Noninvasive oral pressure therapy

FIRST-LINE MANAGEMENT

In contrast to other guidelines, according to the American Academy of Dental Sleep Medicine, it is reasonable to consider alternatives to CPAP therapy as a first-line treatment modality depending on the circumstances. For patients diagnosed with OSA, Oral Appliance Therapy (OAT) may be considered or recommended as a secondary option after other treatments, such as CPAP, have been unsuccessful. However, clinicians may even opt for referral for OAT as the first-line treatment. In a randomized crossover open label study, the efficacy of CPAP and MAD were compared over the course of 1 month of optimal treatment of OSA with CPAP, with optimal treatment being defined as achieving the greatest possible compliance and highest efficacy with each treatment under standard clinical conditions and practices. The study found that the two modalities were comparable in improving health outcomes for patients with OSA. In fact, the results showed that CPAP was more efficacious than MAD in reducing Apnea-Hypopnea Index (AHI) events (CPAP AHI, 4.5 ± 6.6/h; MAD AHI, 11.1 ± 12.1/h; $P < .01$), though compliance was greater with MAD (MAD, 6.50 ± 1.3 h per night vs CPAP, 5.20 ± 2 h per night; $P < .00001$).[35] OAT has been shown to have utility for patients with mild, moderate, and even severe OSA. Additionally, patients generally prefer OAT over CPAP therapy and are more likely to comply with treatment.[36] This also strongly suggests that patient preferences should be considered when recommending OSA therapy, given that patient compliance is instrumental in the treatment of OSA. However, it is worth noting that reported complaints are common for pain and/or discomfort in teeth, facial muscles, temporo-mandibular joint (TMJ), tongue, or other oral structures.[37]

At present, the use of CPAP therapy is widely accepted as the gold standard for treating Obstructive Sleep Apnea (OSA). However, the practicality of CPAP therapy and its impact on patient compliance must not be overlooked, as they can affect the success of OSA therapy. In a 2013 study by Vanderveken, it was found that OAT was as effective as CPAP therapy in reducing the AHI and improving subjective sleep quality.[36] They found that mean AHI (apnea-hypopnea index) decreased significantly from 18.4 ± 11.5 at baseline to 7.0 ± 6.5/h sleep with OA (oral appliance therapy), with a P-value of less than 0.001. The study also reported an OA efficacy of $56.0 \pm 38.2\%$ based on a sample size of 43 patients. This suggests that OA is an effective treatment for OSA, as it resulted in a significant reduction in AHI for most patients in the study. Subsequently, A previous study reported that patients with moderate OSA (defined as AHI between 15 and 30) who used CPAP (continuous positive airway pressure) for 4 hours per night saw a reduction in AHI ranging from 33.3% to 48.3%, with AHI scores ranging from 0 to 5. This suggests that CPAP is also an effective treatment for OSA, though it may be less effective than OA for some patients.[38,39]

Patients using OAT also reported fewer side effects than those using CPAP therapy. The study attributed these findings to differences in patient compliance, with patients using an oral appliance complying with the therapy 82% of the time, compared to considerably lower compliance rates for CPAP therapy. Over a period of 2 decades, from 1994 through 2015, CPAP compliance rates were found to be at a rate of 65.9%, with no trend of improvement in the compliance rate of CPAP over the course of that timeframe.[40] Furthermore, compliance appears not to be a static metric. In a 2015 paper by BaHammam et al., it was observed that adherence to CPAP sharply declined over the course of 10 months, with only one-third of OSA patients exhibiting good adherence even after receiving an educational intervention reinforcing compliance.[18] Long-term compliance with positive airway pressure therapy for OSA can vary widely, with rates ranging from 46% to 85%. According to a study published in the Journal of Sleep Medicine, in 2018, that measured CPAP compliance both with in-lab PSG and at home PSG monitoring, the mean CPAP use compliance was over 5 hours per night (5.8 ± 1.4 hours for at home PSG; 5.6 ± 1.3 hours for in-lab PSG), in more than 70% of days.[41] Patients often cite multiple impediments to complying with CPAP therapy, such as nasal discomfort, congestion, mask leaks, and claustrophobia, which can make therapy difficult to tolerate over extended periods.[42]

To complicate matters further, a randomized-controlled trial published in 2013 suggested that there was, in fact, no significant difference in compliance between CPAP and OAT.[35] However, the findings of this study did indicate that CPAP was more effective in reducing the AHI and resulted in higher levels of oxygen saturation in comparison to OAT. Additionally, CPAP was found to be more successful in treating patients with severe OSA. Nevertheless, oral appliance therapy remains a feasible alternative to CPAP, particularly when treating mild to moderate OSA. In patients with severe OSA who do not respond well to CPAP or have failed CPAP treatment attempts, oral appliances may be considered as a viable long-term option.

SURGICAL MANAGEMENT

In 2010, the American Academy of Sleep Medicine published its guidelines for how to treat OSA with surgical intervention. However, it failed to consider when and in what scenarios it is appropriate and beneficial to treat with various surgical interventions.[43] In 2021, The Journal of Sleep Medicine (JOSM) published a new proposed guideline to supplant the AASM's 2010 guideline by incorporating assertions for exactly when to opt for surgery and which surgical intervention is appropriate and why.[44]

As previously discussed, although CPAP is considered the most effective treatment for OSA when adhered to, some patients may have difficulties adhering to therapy or are unable to obtain optimal results with CPAP. As a result, although surgery may be considered a less effective treatment option, it could ultimately be a more effective solution in the long term due to its independence from compliance issues. The purpose of the JOSM's present guideline is to formulate a guideline that also incorporates patient-specific needs and preferences that evaluates the benefits, costs, risks, and potential adverse effects of different medical and surgical treatments. This guideline refers to existing evidence to endorse suggestions for considering surgical intervention based on the following 3 clinical situations: 1) Patients who are unable or unwilling to tolerate CPAP therapy; 2) Patients who exhibit ongoing inadequate CPAP adherence resulting from side effects associated with increased pressure; 3) Patients anatomic abnormalities of the upper airway that may be treatable with surgical intervention as a first-line approach to managing OSA.

Though many studies and reviews indicate the possible benefits of surgery for treatment of OSA in certain scenarios, controversy persists. The Annals of Internal Medicine offered a guideline in 2013 with regards to recommendations for surgical treatment of OSA. After their literature review of studies comparing control treatments to surgical interventions (UPPP, laser-assisted UPPP, radiofrequency ablation of inferior nasal turbinates, various combinations of pharyngoplasty, tonsillectomy, adenoidectomy, and genioglossal advancement septoplasty), there was insufficient data to support the superiority of surgical intervention as compared to control treatments.[45] As a follow-up to these guidelines, in 2019, Patel and colleagues published a review also in the Annals of Internal Medicine, expanding and commenting upon the Journal's previous recommendations. Their findings suggest that the role of surgical intervention in treating OSA is limited to certain patient populations with anatomic abnormalities that make it difficult to tolerate CPAP. In these cases, nasal procedures such as septoplasty or turbinate reduction can help increase tolerability in these patients. However, in the general OSA population, most surgeries to decrease upper airway collapsibility do not significantly reduce OSA severity or symptoms. For example, UPPP is a commonly known procedure for treating OSA, however, in the general OSA population it has been shown to have limited benefits, as fewer than half of patients experience a significant reduction in OSA severity over the long term. In contrast, there is some hope to be gleaned from the use of maxillomandibular advancement (MMA) in treating OSA. Though a highly invasive procedure with prolonged postoperative recovery, MMA has been shown to have a cure rate of over 90% for OSA, particularly in non-obese patients with retrognathia. Another emergent treatment modality is hypoglossal nerve stimulation, which has gained popularity due to its minimally invasive nature. However, though it does display high success rates in selected patients, it is recommended only for a patient with a body mass index (BMI) less than 32 kg/m2, in whom airway collapse in an anteroposterior direction can be seen under drug-induced sleep endoscopy (DISE).[10]

In a review published in 2009 by Powell of Stanford University, the data on the most performed surgical procedures for treating sleep apnea were reviewed. A protocol was developed for determining the appropriate surgical approach, which divided surgical procedures into 2 phases: Phase I, consisting of soft tissue procedures such as tonsillectomy, UPPP, and genioglossus advancement, and Phase II, consisting of the hard tissue procedure of Maxillomandibular Advancement (MMA). Phase I was further broken down by Dr. Fujita into 3 categories based on the level of upper airway obstruction: Type I, where the obstruction is at the retropalatal level, Fujita Type II, where the obstruction is at both the retropalatal and retrolingual levels, and Fujita Type III, where the obstruction is only at the retrolingual level. According to their findings, when Type I obstruction patients underwent UPPP soft tissue reconstruction surgery, a cure rate ranging from 80% to 90% was achieved. However, conversely, in patients with either Type II or Type III obstructions, that cure rate dropped to rates of only 5% to 30%. These data were compared to MMA surgery, which is a surgery of hard tissue. They found that Phase II MMA surgery achieved documented cure rates of 90% or greater. This is in comparison to the average cure rates of Phase I soft tissue surgeries in general of 42% to 75%.[46] Overall, surgical intervention should be tailored to specific patient-centric populations and should be carefully considered based on individual patient needs and characteristics.

A prominent multicenter randomized controlled trial studying Sleep Apnea Multilevel Surgery (SAMS) was conducted in 2019, with analysis and conclusions published in the Journal of the American Medical Association in 2020. In this initial investigation, adults suffering from moderate to severe OSA, who did not respond to traditional treatment such as CPAP or OAT, underwent a combination of palatal and tongue surgery. These patients exhibited a decrease in the occurrence of apnea and hypopnea events, as well as an improvement in self-reported sleepiness at the 6-month follow-up compared to those receiving conservative medical management. However, in a follow-up response to this publication by MacKay et al. in 2021, the 6-month follow-up was heavily criticized as being insufficient to monitor long-term success of surgical intervention. Additionally, this reply noted that long-term potential improvements in cardiovascular health and overall benefit to mortality in the long-term were not assessed. It goes on to note that the analysis of long-term follow-up of this clinical trial is still ongoing and will be complete in the near future. However, it does provide an encouraging update, stating that surrogate measures to cardiovascular health did improve over the long-term course of the study, such as AHI, 4% oxygen desaturation index, and sleep time with oxygen desaturation less than 90%.[47] The response concludes that given the present data, surgical procedures akin to those being studied in the trial may pose a very significant benefit to the estimated 50% of OSA patients who cannot tolerate conservative management, such as CPAP. All parties agree upon the assertion that further investigation is necessary to validate these outcomes across diverse patient populations and assess the clinical practicality, long-term effectiveness, and safety of multilevel upper airway surgery as a treatment option for OSA.

In a multicenter prospective cohort study published in 2019, the authors concurred with the findings for the SAMS study, primarily further specifically investigating the efficacy of MMA surgery. They attest to the safety and excellent success rate of MMA, concluding that it can lead to marked improvements in daytime sleepiness, quality of life (QOL), sleep-disordered breathing, and neurocognitive performance, as well as improvements in cardiovascular health, specifically blood pressure. With regards to daytime sleepiness, the authors compared results of patients' scores on the Epworth Sleepiness Scale (ESS), which is a self-reported questionnaire that measures daytime sleepiness. They found a significant reduction in patients' documented ESS score, from 13.3 to 4.9, with scores above 10 being classified as having excessive daytime sleepiness. 73% of these patients reported pathologic levels of daytime sleepiness prior to MMA, which sharply decreased to a mere 6.6% still reporting excessive levels of sleepiness. Similarly, when evaluating sleep-specific QOL metrics, 66.7% of patients reported normal QOL post-operatively, compared to only 10% pre-operatively. With regards to cardiovascular health as it pertains to blood pressure, the data suggests that there is a decrease in both mean systolic blood pressure (SBP) and mean diastolic blood pressure (DBP). Specifically, the mean SBP decreased by 3.7 mm Hg with a 95% confidence interval ranging from a decrease of 9.46 mm Hg to an increase of 2.06 mm Hg. Similarly, the mean DBP has decreased by 3.6 mm Hg with a 95% confidence interval ranging from a decrease of 6.50 mm Hg to a decrease of 0.70 mm Hg.[48]

An alternate and relatively new treatment modality is the Inspire implantable nerve stimulation device for treatment of OSA. It is a less invasive surgical option that may be recommended in situations where CPAP and/or OAT have failed.[49] The Inspire device works by sending electrical impulses to the hypoglossal nerve during sleep. The hypoglossal nerve controls the tongue's movement, and electrical stimulation of this nerve can prevent upper airway collapse during sleep. The Inspire system consists of three components: a small generator, a breathing sensor, and a stimulation lead. The generator is implanted in the chest wall, and the stimulation lead is placed near the hypoglossal nerve. The breathing sensor is placed under the skin between the ribs and monitors the patient's breathing during sleep.[50] In a 5-year retrospective analysis of patients who underwent surgical implantation of hypoglossal nerve stimulator devices, at patients' 5-year PSG exam, it was observed that 75% of participants achieved successful results, defined as a decrease in AHI of more than 50% and an AHI less than 20. Additionally, 44% and 78% of participants had AHIs less than 5 and 15, respectively at the 5-year mark. The proportion of participants with a normal ESS score of less than 10 rose from 33% at the start of the study to 78% after 5 years.[51] Furthermore, in the STAR study published in 2014 in the New England Journal of Medicine, the surgical outcomes were measured for patients who underwent implantation of hypoglossal nerve stimulation devices, such as the Inspire device. At the 12 month follow up interval, patients showed a decrease in AHI from 29.3 events/hr to a mere 9 events/hr, a 68% decrease.[52] The 5-year outcomes from the STAR study showed 75% of participants meeting the surgical definition of success, which was a reduction in AHI greater than 50% from baseline and an AHI of less than 20 events per hour, amounting to a 63% overall success rate at 5 years.[53]

An emerging and relatively new treatment modality for OSA is Distraction Osteogenesis Maxillary Expansion (DOME). This technique was developed by Drs. Stanley Liu and Audrey Yoon at Stanford University, specifically for the treatment of adult OSA patients with normal occlusion, narrow maxillae and high-arched palates. This phenotype is typically also associated with increased nasal resistance and posterior displacement of the tongue. DOME minimizes the need for extensive invasive surgery, while ensuring effective expansion of the adult maxilla. The procedure consists of the following steps: First, the maxillary expander with mini-implants is custom-fabricated to fit the narrow palatal vault. The implants and expander may be placed in an outpatient setting under local anesthesia. Next, a maxillary Lefort level I osteotomy is performed to separate the maxilla at the mid-palatal suture. Subsequent to the placement of the expander, patients themselves must turn the expander daily, achieving a gradual expansion of the nasal floor, at approximately 0.25 mm increments, with a final nasal floor expansion goal of 8 mm to 10 mm within 1 month. Finally, after completion of expansion, orthodontic treatment is initiated to close the diastema between the maxillary incisors. In their prospective cohort study, the authors observed significant improvements in measures such as the Epworth Sleepiness Scale (−36.59% change), Nose Obstruction Symptom Evaluation (−67.52% change), apnea-hypopnea index (−54.06% change), oxygen desaturation index (−62.17% change), and nasal airflow resistance (−28.57% change left nostril, and in −35.71% right nostril). Though these data are encouraging, the authors suggest that further long-term studies are needed to evaluate the sustained improvement in both objective and subjective indicators of OSA in this specific patient group.[54]

While CPAP therapy remains the most effective treatment for OSA, surgical interventions have emerged as a viable alternative for certain patient populations. The proposed 2021 guideline by the JOSM takes into consideration patient-specific needs and preferences and evaluates the benefits, costs, risks, and potential adverse effects of different medical and surgical treatments. However, despite the various surgical interventions available, controversy exists as to their effectiveness. While nasal procedures such as septoplasty or turbinate reduction have been shown to increase CPAP tolerability in certain patient populations, most surgeries to decrease upper airway collapsibility do not significantly reduce OSA severity or symptoms. Surgical interventions should be tailored to specific patient-centric populations and should be carefully considered based on individual patient needs and characteristics. Maxillomandibular advancement (MMA) and hypoglossal nerve stimulation have shown promising results but are highly invasive and recommended only for select patient populations. Ultimately, the decision to pursue surgical intervention should be made on a case-by-case basis with a comprehensive evaluation of the risks and benefits involved.[44]

ADJUNCTIVE THERAPY

Microimplant-assisted Maxillary Expansion (MARPE) is a procedure closely related to DOME, sharing similar principles and objectives. However, MARPE differs from DOME in that it is far less invasive, as it does not involve surgical osteotomy, and it is specifically appropriate for non-obese young adults with a maxillary transverse deficiency. MARPE aims to widen the mid-face and enhance the dimensions of the nasal and oral cavities. By doing so, it has the potential to alleviate airflow resistance and play a significant role in the treatment of obstructive sleep apnea (OSA) in certain patients. The MARPE procedure consists of inserting small screws, known as mini-implants, into the palate along with a customized expander appliance. These mini-implants serve as anchors and enable controlled expansion of the upper jaw by applying gradual outward pressure. This expansion widens the mid-face, nasal cavity, and oral cavity, thereby reducing airflow resistance and potentially enhancing breathing and sleep quality in individuals with OSA. As found in a multi-center prospective controlled trial, not only is the success rate of achieving palatal expansion very high, ranging from 87% to 100%, but positive and significant OSA results were also achieved. Participants who underwent MARPE experienced significant improvements in daytime sleepiness and quality of life related to obstructive sleep apnea (OSA), as measured by validated questionnaires. The intervention group also showed statistically significant enhancements in sleep test parameters, including a 65.3% reduction in AHI, improvements in mean oxygen saturation, snoring duration, and the bruxism to apnea index. Approximately 35.7% of the participants in the intervention group achieved an AHI of less than 5, indicating a positive outcome.[55,56]

Apart from the mainstay treatment modalities for OSA as already discussed, such as CPAP, OAT, and upper-airway-oriented surgical intervention, adjunctive therapies also exist, particularly as it pertains to a patient's weight and BMI. Obesity represents a significant risk factor for the development of OSA. In obese adults, the prevalence of OSA ranges from 42% to 48% in males and from 8% to 38% in females. It has been shown that weight loss significantly impacts treating OSA as it pertains to AHI metrics.[57] Observational studies have shown that significant weight loss, regardless of the weight-loss treatment, whether via bariatric surgery, lifestyle changes, or medical management, can substantially reduce OSA symptoms in approximately 60% to 80% of patients.[58] Important to note, that the study by Buchwald and colleagues assert that there was an indistinguishable difference between weight loss from bariatric surgery versus weight loss from lifestyle changes and medical management regarding the effect on OSA symptomatology. This, as well as future updates of this topic, bolster and corroborate the assertion that weight loss, regardless of the means to achieve this weight loss, is a primary treatment modality for the obese patient.[59]

According to Kent and colleagues in their paper published in the Journal of Clinical Sleep Medicine in 2021, they strongly recommend referring a patient for bariatric surgical consultation as a means for weight reduction in hopes to treat OSA. As part of a patient-centered discussion on alternative treatment options, the paper suggests that clinicians consider referring adults with OSA and obesity (BMI $\geq$35 kg/m2, Class II/III) who are intolerant or unwilling to use CPAP therapy. Given that weight loss has been proven to help treat OSA, and that bariatric surgery has been proven the most effective means for weight loss in patients of BMI ≥35 kg/m2, Class II/III, bariatric surgery is strongly recommended as a treatment option for patients of this category.[44]

DISCUSSION

Sleep apnea is a complex disorder that affects a significant portion of the population, and its management remains a controversial topic among clinicians. There are still many gaps in our understanding of its pathophysiology, long-term health consequences, optimal diagnostic modalities, and optimal treatment strategies. Management of the disorder remains a controversial topic among clinicians, with the use of CPAP therapy being one of the primary areas of contention. While CPAP is considered the gold standard treatment for moderate to severe OSA, its adherence rate is often low, and its efficacy in improving clinical outcomes beyond reducing symptoms and improving quality of life is not well-established.

Another contentious issue in OSA management is the use of OAT as an alternative to CPAP therapy. While OAT is less invasive than CPAP and may be more acceptable to some patients, the extent to which it is effective in reducing AHI and improving health outcomes is still debated. Furthermore, the optimal selection of patients for OAT and its long-term safety are not well-understood. The controversies in OSA management also extend to surgical interventions, positional therapy, and the management of co-morbid conditions such as obesity and cardiovascular disease.

Given these controversies, personalized OSA management that considers patients' preferences, comorbidities, and disease severity is crucial. Clinicians should engage in shared decision-making with patients to select the most appropriate treatment modality. Regular monitoring of treatmeœnt adherence and clinical outcomes is necessary to ensure optimal management. Future research should focus on identifying biomarkers and phenotypes that can predict patients' response to different treatment modalities and developing innovative therapeutic approaches that target the underlying pathophysiology of the disorder.

Though CPAP is presently the first-line therapy for treating OSA, there remains definitive consensus regarding the superiority of CPAP versus OAT. Though, in theory, CPAP shows greater efficacy, its compliance has been show to be significantly less OAT. The American Academy of Sleep Medicine currently recommends CPAP as the first line and gold-standard therapy for treating OSA, but it bases its recommendations solely on a comparison between CPAP versus no treatment at all. Further reviews of all treatment modalities when compared to each other are certainly still needed to establish what the most efficacious first-line therapy is, considering compliance and adherence as integral to that determination.

While CPAP therapy remains the most effective treatment for OSA, surgical interventions have emerged as a viable alternative for certain patient populations. The proposed 2021 guideline by the JOSM takes into consideration patient-specific needs and preferences and evaluates the benefits, costs, risks, and potential adverse effects of different medical and surgical treatments. Surgical interventions should be tailored to specific patient-centric populations and should be carefully considered based on individual patient needs and characteristics.

OSA management and diagnosis remain complex and contentious issues with many unanswered questions. A personalized approach that emphasizes shared decision-making and regular monitoring of treatment outcomes is essential for optimal patient care. Collaboration between sleep specialists, primary care physicians, and patients is also necessary to improve sleep apnea awareness, diagnosis, and management. Further research is necessary to identify biomarkers and phenotypes that can predict patients' response to different treatment modalities and develop innovative therapeutic approaches. Ultimately, the decision to pursue a specific treatment modality should be made on a case-by-case basis, considering the individual patient's needs, preferences, and characteristics.

With regards to conservative treatment, there remains no clear consensus regarding CPAP versus OAT as a first-line therapy. By and large, this controversy stems from the issue of compliance and lack of adherence to therapies. Most studies show that compliance with OAT is greater than with CPAP. However, many reviews and guidelines are limited in their scope as they only base their recommendations on comparing the utilization of CPAP therapy to treat OSA compared to no treatment at all. This is presently the case for the American Academy of Sleep Medicine, which currently asserts CPAP to be the first-line and gold-standard therapy for treating OSA. This guideline explicitly stated that it did not base its recommendations on a comparison between CPAP versus OAT, rather, it is solely based on the comparison between CPAP versus no treatment at all. Further reviews of all treatment modalities when compared to each other are certainly still needed to establish what the most efficacious first-line therapy is, considering compliance and adherence as integral to that determination.

SUMMARY

The management of obstructive sleep apnea (OSA) presents a complex and evolving landscape of diagnostic and therapeutic options. This paper has provided an evidence-based review of current therapeutic treatments for patients suffering from OSA, with a particular focus on surgical interventions. Despite the challenges and controversies surrounding OSA diagnosis and treatment, surgery remains a valuable and promising avenue for patients who do not respond to or tolerate conservative measures. Surgical procedures such as uvulopalatopharyngoplasty (UPPP), maxillomandibular advancement surgery, genioglossus advancement, and the use of nerve stimulation devices offer viable alternatives for patients seeking long-term resolution of their sleep apnea symptoms. Moreover, weight loss interventions and positional therapy demonstrate their efficacy in improving OSA severity and associated symptoms. However, the selection of the most appropriate treatment approach should be guided by careful consideration of individual patient characteristics, preferences, and potential risks and benefits associated with each modality. The ongoing controversies and debates in the field underscore the need for continued research, collaborative efforts, and personalized care to optimize outcomes and enhance the quality of life for individuals affected by OSA. By advancing our understanding and refining our approaches, we can strive toward more effective and tailored interventions to alleviate the burden of sleep apnea on individuals and society as a whole.

DISCLOSURES

The authors have nothing to disclose.

CLINICS CARE POINTS

- Surgical intervention may be considered in patients who cannot tolerate CPAP therapy or have ongoing inadequate adherence.
- Obesity is a significant risk factor for OSA. Weight loss interventions, including lifestyle modifications and bariatric surgery, can improve OSA severity and associated symptoms.

- Regular monitoring of treatment adherence and clinical outcomes is essential to ensure optimal management of OSA
- A multidisciplinary approach between sleep specialists, primary care physicians, and patients is necessary to improve sleep apnea awareness, diagnosis, and management.
- Individual patient preferences, co-existing medical conditions, and other factors should be taken into account when determining the most suitable treatment plan for OSA

REFERENCES

1. Faria A, Allen AH, Fox N, et al. The public health burden of obstructive sleep apnea. Sleep Sci 2021;14(3):257–65.
2. Benjafield AV, Ayas NT, Eastwood PR, et al. Estimation of the global prevalence and burden of obstructive sleep apnoea: a literature-based analysis. Lancet Respir Med 2019;7(8):687–98.
3. Yaggi HK, Strohl KP. Adult Obstructive Sleep Apnea/Hypopnea Syndrome: Definitions, Risk Factors, and Pathogenesis. Clin Chest Med 2010;31(2):179–86.
4. Oldenburg O, Wellmann B, Buchholz A, et al. Nocturnal hypoxaemia is associated with increased mortality in stable heart failure patients. Eur Heart J 2016; 37(21):1695–703.
5. Fraigne JJ, Orem JM. Phasic motor activity of respiratory and non-respiratory muscles in REM sleep. Sleep 2011;34(4):425–34.
6. Javaheri S, Badr MS. Central sleep apnea: pathophysiologic classification. Sleep 2022;46(3).
7. Jullian-Desayes I, Revol B, Chareyre E, et al. Impact of concomitant medications on obstructive sleep apnoea. Br J Clin Pharmacol 2017;83(4):688–708.
8. Hernandez AB, Patil SP. Pathophysiology of central sleep apneas. Sleep Breath 2016;20(2):467–82.
9. Daghistani KJ. Conditions of the uvula: a 14 years experience. Auris Nasus Larynx 2000;27(3):261–4.
10. Patel SR. Obstructive Sleep Apnea. Ann Intern Med 2019;171(11):ITC81–96.
11. Tobias L, Won C. Upper Airway Resistance Syndrome Represents a Distinct Entity from Obstructive Sleep Apnea Syndrome. Journal of Dental Sleep Medicine 2016;3(1):21–4.
12. Rundo JV, Downey R. Polysomnography. Handb Clin Neurol 2019;160:381–92.
13. Kapur VK, Auckley DH, Chowdhuri S, et al. Clinical Practice Guideline for Diagnostic Testing for Adult Obstructive Sleep Apnea: An American Academy of Sleep Medicine Clinical Practice Guideline. J Clin Sleep Med 2017;13(3):479–504.
14. Boyd SB, Upender R, Walters AS, et al. Effective Apnea-Hypopnea Index ("Effective AHI"): A New Measure of Effectiveness for Positive Airway Pressure Therapy. Sleep 2016;39(11):1961–72.
15. Pavwoski P, Shelgikar AV. Treatment options for obstructive sleep apnea. Neurol Clin Pract 2017;7(1):77–85.
16. St-Onge MP, Tasali E. Weight Loss Is Integral to Obstructive Sleep Apnea Management. Ten-Year Follow-up in Sleep AHEAD. Am J Respir Crit Care Med 2021;203(2):161–2.
17. Paidi G, Beesetty A, Jean M, et al. The Management of Obstructive Sleep Apnea in Primary Care. Cureus 2022;14(7):e26805.
18. BaHammam AS, Alassiri SS, Al-Adab AH, et al. Long-term compliance with continuous positive airway pressure in Saudi patients with obstructive sleep apnea. A prospective cohort study. Saudi Med J 2015;36(8):911–9.

19. Kendzerska T, Gershon AS, Hawker G, et al. Obstructive sleep apnea and risk of cardiovascular events and all-cause mortality: a decade-long historical cohort study. PLoS Med 2014;11(2):e1001599.
20. Tietjens JR, Claman D, Kezirian EJ, et al. Obstructive Sleep Apnea in Cardiovascular Disease: A Review of the Literature and Proposed Multidisciplinary Clinical Management Strategy. J Am Heart Assoc 2019;8(1):e010440.
21. Yeghiazarians Y, Jneid H, Tietjens JR, et al. Obstructive Sleep Apnea and Cardiovascular Disease: A Scientific Statement From the American Heart Association. Circulation 2021;144(3):e56–67.
22. Peppard PE, Young T, Barnet JH, et al. Increased prevalence of sleep-disordered breathing in adults. Am J Epidemiol 2013;177(9):1006–14.
23. Hamilton GS, Gupta R, Vizcarra D, et al. Endorsement of: "clinical practice guideline for diagnostic testing for adult obstructive sleep apnea: an American academy of sleep medicine clinical practice guideline" by the World Sleep Society. Sleep Med 2021;79:152–4.
24. Patel AK, Reddy V, Shumway KR, et al. Physiology, Sleep Stages. In: StatPearls. StatPearls publishing copyright © 2023, StatPearls Publishing LLC; 2023.
25. Stålberg E, van Dijk H, Falck B, et al. Standards for quantification of EMG and neurography. Clinical neurophysiology 2019;130(9):1688–729.
26. Xiong X, Ren Y, Gao S, et al. EEG microstate in obstructive sleep apnea patients. Sci Rep 2021;11(1):17178.
27. Vana KD, Silva GE, Goldberg R. Predictive abilities of the STOP-Bang and Epworth Sleepiness Scale in identifying sleep clinic patients at high risk for obstructive sleep apnea. Res Nurs Health 2013;36(1):84–94.
28. Kumari P, Roy SK, Roy ID, et al. Changes in posterior airway space and mandibular plane hyoid distance following mandibular advancement DO. Ann Maxillofac Surg 2016;6(2):182–9.
29. Barrera JE, Pau CY, Forest VI, et al. Anatomic measures of upper airway structures in obstructive sleep apnea. World J Otorhinolaryngol Head Neck Surg 2017;3(2):85–91.
30. Steffy DD, Tang CS. Radiographic Evaluation of Sleep-Disordered Breathing. Radiol Clin 2018;56(1):177–85.
31. Lan M-C, Liu SY-C, Lan M-Y, et al. Role of drug-induced sleep endoscopy in evaluation of positional vs non-positional OSA. J Otolaryngol 2020;49(1):83.
32. Soares D, Folbe AJ, Yoo G, et al. Drug-induced sleep endoscopy vs awake Müller's maneuver in the diagnosis of severe upper airway obstruction. Otolaryngol Head Neck Surg 2013;148(1):151–6.
33. Quan SF, Schmidt-Nowara W. The Role of Dentists in the Diagnosis and Treatment of Obstructive Sleep Apnea: Consensus and Controversy. J Clin Sleep Med 2017;13(10):1117–9.
34. Epstein LJ, Kristo D, Strollo PJ Jr, et al. Clinical guideline for the evaluation, management and long-term care of obstructive sleep apnea in adults. J Clin Sleep Med 2009;5(3):263–76.
35. Phillips CL, Grunstein RR, Darendeliler MA, et al. Health Outcomes of Continuous Positive Airway Pressure versus Oral Appliance Treatment for Obstructive Sleep Apnea: A Randomized Controlled Trial. Am J Respir Crit Care Med 2013;187(8):879–87.
36. Vanderveken OM, Dieltjens M, Wouters K, et al. Objective measurement of compliance during oral appliance therapy for sleep-disordered breathing. Thorax 2013;68(1):91–6.

37. Sheats RD. Management of side effects of oral appliance therapy for sleep-disordered breathing: summary of American Academy of Dental Sleep Medicine recommendations. J Clin Sleep Med 2020;16(5):835.
38. de Almeida FR. Complexity and efficacy of mandibular advancement splints: understanding their mode of action. J Clin Sleep Med 2011;7(5):447–8.
39. Ravesloot MJ, de Vries N. Reliable calculation of the efficacy of non-surgical and surgical treatment of obstructive sleep apnea revisited. Sleep 2011;34(1):105–10.
40. Rotenberg BW, Murariu D, Pang KP. Trends in CPAP adherence over twenty years of data collection: a flattened curve. J Otolaryngol Head Neck Surg 2016; 45(1):43.
41. Andrade L, Paiva T. Ambulatory Versus Laboratory Polysomnography in Obstructive Sleep Apnea: Comparative Assessment of Quality, Clinical Efficacy, Treatment Compliance, and Quality of Life. J Clin Sleep Med 2018;14(08):1323–31.
42. Donovan LM, Boeder S, Malhotra A, et al. New developments in the use of positive airway pressure for obstructive sleep apnea. J Thorac Dis 2015;7(8): 1323–42.
43. Aurora RN, Casey KR, Kristo D, et al. Practice parameters for the surgical modifications of the upper airway for obstructive sleep apnea in adults. Sleep 2010; 33(10):1408–13.
44. Kent D, Stanley J, Aurora RN, et al. Referral of adults with obstructive sleep apnea for surgical consultation: an American Academy of Sleep Medicine clinical practice guideline. J Clin Sleep Med 2021;17(12):2499–505.
45. Qaseem A, Holty JE, Owens DK, et al. Management of obstructive sleep apnea in adults: A clinical practice guideline from the American College of Physicians. Ann Intern Med 2013;159(7):471–83.
46. Powell NB. Contemporary surgery for obstructive sleep apnea syndrome. Clin Exp Otorhinolaryngol 2009;2(3):107–14.
47. MacKay S, McEvoy RD, Weaver EM. The Effect of Surgical Treatment on Obstructive Sleep Apnea-Reply. JAMA 2021;325(8):789–90.
48. Boyd SB, Chigurupati R, Cillo JE Jr, et al. Maxillomandibular Advancement Improves Multiple Health-Related and Functional Outcomes in Patients With Obstructive Sleep Apnea: A Multicenter Study. J Oral Maxillofac Surg 2019; 77(2):352–70.
49. Heiser C, Vries Nd. Upper Airway Stimulation in Obstructive Sleep Apnea: Best Practices in Evaluation and Surgical Management, 1st ed., 2022.
50. Heiser C, Knopf A, Bas M, et al. Selective upper airway stimulation for obstructive sleep apnea: a single center clinical experience. Eur Arch Oto-Rhino-Laryngol 2017;274(3):1727–34.
51. Woodson BT, Strohl KP, Soose RJ, et al. Upper airway stimulation for obstructive sleep apnea: 5-year outcomes. Otolaryngology-head and neck surgery 2018; 159(1):194–202.
52. Strollo PJ Jr, Soose RJ, Maurer JT, et al. Upper-airway stimulation for obstructive sleep apnea. N Engl J Med 2014;370(2):139–49.
53. Mashaqi S, Patel SI, Combs D, et al. The Hypoglossal Nerve Stimulation as a Novel Therapy for Treating Obstructive Sleep Apnea-A Literature Review. Int J Environ Res Publ Health 2021;18(4).
54. Liu SY-C, Guilleminault C, Huon L-K, et al. Distraction Osteogenesis Maxillary Expansion (DOME) for Adult Obstructive Sleep Apnea Patients with High Arched Palate. Otolaryngology-head and neck surgery 2017;157(2):345–8.
55. Brunetto DP, Moschik CE, Dominguez-Mompell R, et al. Mini-implant assisted rapid palatal expansion (MARPE) effects on adult obstructive sleep apnea

(OSA) and quality of life: a multi-center prospective controlled trial. Prog Orthod 2022;23(1):3.

56. Ventura V, Botelho J, Machado V, et al. Miniscrew-Assisted Rapid Palatal Expansion (MARPE): An Umbrella Review. J Clin Med 2022;11(5).

57. Dixon JB, Schachter LM, O'Brien PE, et al. Surgical vs conventional therapy for weight loss treatment of obstructive sleep apnea: a randomized controlled trial. JAMA 2012;308(11):1142–9.

58. Buchwald H, Avidor Y, Braunwald E, et al. Bariatric surgery: a systematic review and meta-analysis. JAMA 2004;292(14):1724–37.

59. Chang SH, Stoll CR, Song J, et al. The effectiveness and risks of bariatric surgery: an updated systematic review and meta-analysis, 2003-2012. JAMA Surg 2014; 149(3):275–87.

Controversies in Stoppage of Antiplatelet and Anticoagulant Medications Prior to Oral Surgery

Michael H. Chan, DDS[a,b,*], Feiyi Sun, DDS[c], Jonathan Malakan, DDS[c]

KEYWORDS

- DOAC dental management • Antiplatelet dental management • Dental extractions
- Bleeding risk assessment • Factor Xa inhibitor • Thrombin inhibitor
- Dual antiplatelet therapy dental management • Oral surgery

KEY POINTS

- No consensus on bleeding risk nor standardization on dental procedures exists for patients on antithrombotic.
- Newer generation of DOACs are faster acting and have better pharmacokinetics allowing more flexible perioperative management.
- Newer generation antiplatelet (eg, prasugrel and ticagrelor) behave very similar when compared to older generation (clopidogrel) for low-risk procedures.
- A clear understanding of drug mechanisms allows the practitioner to properly manage a patient perioperatively.

INTRODUCTION

One of the primary concerns regarding the discontinuation of antithrombotics (eg,; antiplatelet and anticoagulant) therapy is the heightened risk of thromboembolic events, such as myocardial infarction or stroke. Patients receiving these medications frequently present underlying medical conditions, including atrial fibrillation, deep vein thrombosis, or prior myocardial infarction, which predispose them to such adverse outcomes. Conversely, the incidence of bleeding complications during dental

[a] Oral & Maxillofacial Surgery, Department of Veterans Affairs, New York Harbor Healthcare System (Brooklyn Campus), 800 Poly Place (Bk-160), Brooklyn, NY 11209, USA; [b] Oral & Maxillofacial Surgery, Department of Oral and Maxillofacial Surgery, The Brooklyn Hospital Center, 121 DeKalb Avenue (Box-187), Brooklyn, NY 11201, USA; [c] Oral & Maxillofacial Surgery, Department of Oral and Maxillofacial Surgery, The Brooklyn Hospital Center, 121 DeKalb Avenue, Brooklyn, NY 11201, USA
* Corresponding author. 800 Poly Place (BK-160), Brooklyn, NY 11209.
E-mail address: chanoms@yahoo.com

Dent Clin N Am 68 (2024) 21–45
https://doi.org/10.1016/j.cden.2023.07.001
0011-8532/24/Published by Elsevier Inc.

dental.theclinics.com

procedures can be significant and necessitate emergency intervention. As the elderly population expands, it is anticipated that a greater number of patients will be on these antithrombotic agents. The older generations (aspirin, clopidogrel and warfarin) have been a workhorse for cardiologists and neurologists. However, a newer generation of direct oral anticoagulants (DOACs) namely dabigatran, rivaroxaban, apixaban and edoxaban and P2Y 12 inhibitors (prasugrel and ticagrelor) have emerged on the market due to its improved properties. In 2020, approximately 4.3 million people are taking clopidogrel and 4.7 million are on aspirin in the United States while the number of patients taking warfarin, rivaroxaban, apixaban are 2.4 million, 2.1 million, 3.3 million, respectively.[1] Finding the balance between managing bleeding risk and preventing thromboembolic events is a complex issue that requires careful consideration of each patient's individual medical history, bleeding risks and the specific dental procedure being performed.

VASCULAR INJURY (SECONDARY HEMOSTASIS: COAGULATION CASCADE)

The initial response to tissue damage during surgery is for platelets to accumulate and form a platelet plug at the site of injury. Simultaneously, the coagulation cascade begins, utilizing plasma clotting factors, proteins from membranes of injured cells (tissue factor), and circulating platelets. Two clotting pathways are involved, the intrinsic pathway begins with exposure to endothelial collagen, and the extrinsic pathway occurs after damage to endothelial cells causing a release of tissue factor.[2] Each pathway results in different clotting factors being activated until the common pathway is reached, finally converting soluble fibrinogen into fibrin threads that are insoluble[3] (**Fig. 1**). The antithrombotic medications discussed in this section each influence a different part of the coagulation cascade.

ANTICOAGULANT MEDICATIONS

We will discuss the commonly encountered outpatient anticoagulants: Warfarin, Dabigatran, Rivaroxaban, Apixaban, and Edoxaban (**Table 1**).

Vitamin K Antagonist

Warfarin, a coumarin derivative, blocks a vitamin K-dependent step in the production of clotting factors, specifically via the inhibition of subunit 1 of the multiunit vitamin K epoxide reductase complex 1 (VKORC1). The result is the depletion of hepatic vitamin K reserves and the impairment of factor II (prothrombin), VII, IX, and X essential for normal coagulation. The effect of warfarin is determined by laboratory tests measuring prothrombin time (PT) and using the standardized international normalized ratio (INR). The initial anticoagulant effect is seen as soon as 24 to 72 hours.[4]

Warfarin is metabolized by the hepatic system, principally via the CYP2C9 pathway. It exhibits a half-life of 20 to 60 hours, which is highly variable among individuals. Most patients will typically begin on an oral daily dose of 5 mg. Once patients are at a therapeutic INR level appropriate for medical their condition (2–3 or 2.5–3.5), dosages will be adjusted between a range of 2 to 10 mg. INR is checked weekly if out of range, and monthly if in range.[5]

Direct Oral Anticoagulant

Dabigatran etexilate (Pradaxa) obtained FDA approval in 2010 as the first DOAC medication. It is a direct thrombin inhibitor (DTI) prescribed orally for prevention and treatment of venous thromboembolism and nonvalvular atrial fibrillation. It is metabolized into its active form primarily by plasma and hepatic esterase. Due to its clearance

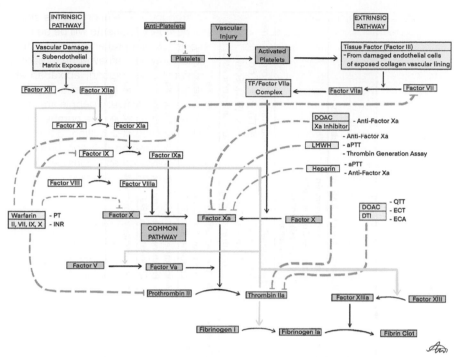

Fig. 1. The coagulation cascade. (Image courtesy of Maya Nunez.) Anti-FXa test, Anti-Factor Xa test; aPTT, Partial thromboplastin time; DOAC, Direct oral anticoagulant; DTI, Direct thrombin inhibitor; ECA, Ecarin chromagenic assay; ECT, Ecarin clotting time; II,VII,IX,X, Factors II,VII,IX,X; INR, International normalized ratio; LMWH, Low-molecular weight heparin; PT, Prothrombin time; QTT, Quantitative thrombin test; TF, Tissue factor.

being primarily through the renal system, guidelines for usage are recommended and provided. For patients with renal impairment being treated for deep vein thrombosis (DVT) or pulmonary embolism (PE), use of dabigatran is avoided. For the prevention of stroke, patients with a creatinine clearance less than 15 mL/minute, use is also avoided. There are no dosing indications for patients with hepatic impairment.[6] The onset is rapid with half-life elimination in adults is about 12 to 17 hours. 150 mg BID is the typical dosage used for atrial fibrillation and treatment of DVT/PE.

Rivaroxaban (Xarelto) is a factor Xa inhibitor indicated for use with patients with non-valvular atrial fibrillation, stable coronary artery disease, and treatment/prophylaxis of DVT/PE. It is also used off-label for acute coronary syndrome (ACS) and heparin-induced thrombocytopenia. Rivaroxaban functions by inhibiting platelet activation and fibrin clot formation via direct and reversible inhibition of factor Xa, found in the intrinsic and extrinsic pathways. Factor Xa is responsible for the conversion of pro-thrombin to thrombin via prothrombinase. Rivaroxaban therefore indirectly inhibits platelet aggregation by blocking the conversion of prothrombinase to thrombin.[7] Rivaroxaban also has a rapid onset but a shorter half-life of 5 to 9 hours (11–13 hours for elderly) and is metabolized by the hepatic system. In patients with mild hepatic impairment, there is no dosage adjustment however, with moderate to severe impairment, use is avoided. In patients with severe renal impairment, creatinine clearance less than 30 mL/minute, use is generally avoided with only some exceptions where a reduction in dosing is advised.[7]

Table 1
Common anticoagulant medications and corresponding properties[5–8,10,15,16]

Drug/Regimen	Mechanism of Action	Onset/Peak	Half-Life	Reversal Agents/Antidote	Lab Tests
Warfarin/QD	Vitamin K Antagonist	1–3 days/5–7 d	20–60 h (mean = 40 h)	Vitamin K, Prothrombin Complex Concentrates (PCC), Fresh Frozen Plasma (FFP)	PT/INR
Dabigatran (Pradaxa®)/BID	Direct Thrombin Inhibitor (DTI)	Rapid/1 h	12–17 h	Idarucizumab (Praxabind®), Prothrombin Complex Concentrates (PCC)	Quantative Thrombin Time (QTT), Ecarin clotting Time (ECT), Ecarin Chromogenic Assay (ECA)
Rivaroxaban (Xarelto®)/QD	Factor Xa Inhibitor	Rapid/2–4 h	5–9 h (11–13 h elderly)	Andexanet-alfa (AndexXa), Prothrombin Complex Concentrates (PCC)	Anti-factor Xa Chromogenic Assay
Apixaban (Eliquis®)/BID	Factor Xa Inhibitor	Rapid/1–2 h	12 h	Andexanet-alfa (AndexXa), Prothrombin Complex Concentrates (PCC)	Anti-factor Xa Chromogenic Assay
Edoxaban (Savaysa® /Lixiana®)/QD	Factor Xa Inhibitor	Rapid/1–2 h	10–14 h	None officially approved	Anti-factor Xa Chromogenic Assay

Abbreviation: hr, = hour(s).

Apixaban (Eliquis) is another factor Xa inhibitor labeled for use in patients with DVT, nonvalvular atrial fibrillation, postoperative DVT prophylaxis following hip and knee replacement surgery and for treatment of PE. Depending on the reason for use, dosage can be modified. Regarding decreased kidney function, even patients on dialysis for ESRD, no modification is required unless the patient is taking apixaban for nonvalvular atrial fibrillation. Such patients are recommended to reduce their dose to 2.5 mg twice daily *if* they are above 80 year old and weigh below 60 kg. As for hepatic impairment, use is not recommended only for patients with severe hepatic impairment (Child-Pugh class C).[8]

Edoxaban (Sold under the brand name Savaysa in the US, and Lixiana in Canada) is a factor Xa and prothrombinase inhibitor indicated for use in patients with nonvalvular atrial fibrillation and for treatment of venous thromboembolism. It exhibits a half-life of 10 to 14 hours and reaches peak effect after 1 to 2 hours. The absorption of this medication is not affected by the consumption of food. It is generally given in doses of 30 or 60 mg but also available as a 15 mg dose. It is excreted by the renal system and is a substrate for P-glycoprotein. It has a boxed warning against use in patients with a high CrCl (>95 mL/minute) due to increase drug clearance and decreased efficacy, and not advised in patients with a CrCl (<15 mL/minute) (Bohula 2016). Routine monitoring of coagulation times is not needed and there is no established therapeutic range.[9] For patients with moderate and severe hepatic impairment (Child-Pugh class B or C), use is not recommended.[10]

REVERSAL AGENTS

Any of these medications may increase the risk of bleeding especially in patients taking concomitant drugs that affect hemostasis, therefore use should be discontinued immediately in cases of life-threatening bleed.

Reversal, if needed, can be done with prothrombin complex concentrates (PCCs), vitamin K, or fresh frozen plasma as an alternative. PCCs, along with vitamin K administered via IV, is the preferred approach to emergency reversal of anticoagulation from warfarin.[4]

Idarucizumab (Praxabind) is the reversal agent for dabigatran while andexanet-alfa (AndexXa) is reserved for rivaroxaban and apixaban. A phase 2 pharmokinetics study demonstrated andexanet-alfa decreases anti-factor Xa activity by 82% compared to 93% in rivaroxaban treated patients, which is still significantly higher than placebo.[11] PCC is an alternative solution that can be used against anti-thrombin II and factor Xa inhibitors.

The reversal strategies in the setting of major bleeding for patients on antiplatelets remain controversial. Platelet transfusion is proven to have inconsistent results in controlling post-operative hematoma expansion, and higher doses (greater than single unit) carry risks such as lung injury, volume overload, and hemolytic reactions. Desmopressin (DDAVP) promotes platelet adhesion by stimulating factor VIII and von Willebrand factor (vWF), making it a better option when countering platelet dysfunction in emergency situations such as intracranial hemorrhage. Despite limited data, intravenous administrating of antifibrinolytic agents such as tranexamic acid (TXA) and epsilon-aminocaproic acid (EACA) has been reported to reduce mortality secondary to uncontrolled hemorrhage.[12]

LABORATORY TESTING

Prior to the initiation of all DOACs; CBC, aPTT, PT, serum creatinine, and liver function tests should be performed (see **Table 1**). Typically, direct oral anticoagulant medications do not require dose adjustment due to laboratory test results; however, the measurement of the anticoagulant effect may prove useful in certain situations. Quantitative thrombin time, ecarin tests and anti-factor Xa (anti-FXa) assays have been developed to assess plasma DOAC concentration.

Quantitative thrombin time and ecarin clotting time are 2 tests that can measure Dabigatran's concentration and level of activity.

Quantitative thrombin time (QTT) can calculate how much time it takes to formulate a clot measured in seconds. The longer the clotting time, the more effective the anticoagulant.

Ecarin clotting time (ECT) measures how much "meizothrombin"(an intermediate proteolytic enzyme) is produced in turn the activation from prothrombin to thrombin and the time to fabricate a clot. Normal ECT is 22.6 - 29.0 seconds. The presence of Dabigatran will block the action of "meizothrombin" and disabling the conversion to thrombin thus prolonging the ECT time.

Ecarin chromogenic assay is another test that can determine clotting efficiency. It has the same mechanism as ecarin clotting time but uses a specific chromogenic substrate to calculate the remaining meizothrombin level. A higher meizothrombin level suggests a lower plasma concentration of Dabigatran remaining.

The anti-factor Xa assay is a chromogenic test that measures the ability of plasma to inhibit factor Xa. The test is carried out by mixing suitable amounts of patient plasma with excess factor Xa. The residual factor Xa is then measured by a chromogenic substrate. The smaller the residual factor Xa, the greater the inhibitor concentration of the anticoagulant.[13]

Typically, these tests are not widely available and are generally not necessary for healthy patients undergoing dental procedures. However, when testing is deemed necessary, it is advised to consult a local lab to inquire if testing is available.[14]

ANTIPLATELET MEDICATIONS

In addition to anticoagulants, antiplatelet medications are also used to decrease the risk of thromboembolism (**Table 2**). In a normal circulation with intact vasculature, platelets do not biochemically interact with one another. However, at the sites of vascular damage, platelet plugs are formed to provide an initial hemostasis response that takes place just before the start of the coagulation cascade. Aspirin, ticlopidine, clopidogrel, prasugrel, and ticagrelor will be discussed here.

VASCULAR INJURY (PRIMARY HEMOSTASIS: PLATELET PLUG FORMATION)

During vascular injury, the subendothelial matrix, which has abundant adhesive ligands such as the von Willebrand factor (vWF), is exposed. Platelet membrane glycoprotein Ib (GpIb) binds to vWF at the site of injury, causing platelets to undergo conformational changes that make them extremely adhesive to endothelium (**Fig. 2**). Meanwhile, molecules such as adenosine diphosphate (ADP), thromboxane A2 (TxA2), and fibrinogen are released from platelets. ADP binds to the P2Y12 receptor on platelet surface to induce the glycoprotein IIb/IIIa (GpIIb/IIIa) receptor complex, which in turn assists in platelet aggregation via fibrinogen binding. More specifically, the GPIIb/IIIa complex undergoes a conformational change and is converted from a low-affinity to a high-affinity fibrinogen receptor in the setting of platelets activation by ADP. TxA2, a prostaglandin metabolite produced by activated platelets, decreases blood flow at the site of endothelial injury and further promotes platelet aggregation before coagulation cascade, or secondary hemostasis, takes place.[17,18]

Table 2
Common antiplatelet medications and corresponding properties

Drug/Class	Mechanism of Action	Onset/Peak	Half-Life	Reversal Agents/Antidote	Lab Test
Aspirin (Bayer®)/(Non-steroidal anti-inflammatory)	Irreversible COX-1 COX-2 inhibitor	Non-enteric coated = <1 h/1–2 h Enteric coated = 3–4 hours/4 h	Lower dose = 20 min Higher dose = 3 h	Controversial Consider DDAVP, TXA, EACA, or platelet transfusion for life threatening bleeding	N/A
Ticlopidine (Ticlid®)/(First generation -Thienopyridine)	P2Y12 inhibitor	6 h/3–5 d	13 h	Controversial Consider DDAVP, TXA, EACA, or platelet transfusion for life threatening bleeding	N/A
Clopidogrel (Plavix®)/ (Second generation -Thienopyridine)	P2Y12 inhibitor	2 hours/45 min	6 h	Controversial Consider DDAVP, TXA, EACA, or platelet transfusion for life threatening bleeding	N/A
Prasugrel (Effient®)/(Third generation -Thienopyridine)	P2Y12 inhibitor	30 min/4 h	7 h	Controversial Consider DDAVP, TXA, EACA, or platelet transfusion for life threatening bleeding	N/A
Ticagrelor (Brilinta®)/(Non-thienopyridine)	P2Y12 inhibitor	30 min/2 h	9 h	Controversial Consider DDAVP, TXA, EACA, or platelet transfusion for life threatening bleeding	N/A

Abbreviations: DDAVP, demopressin; EACA, Epsilon-aminocaproic acid; TXA, tranexamic acid.
Data from Refs.[12,20,22,24]

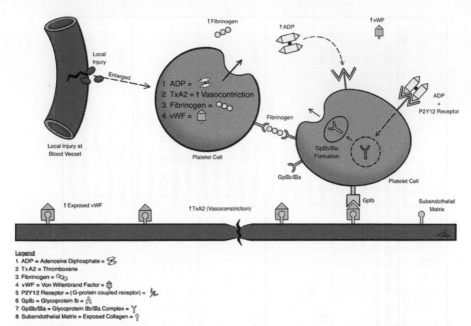

Fig. 2. Platelet adhesion, activation, and aggregation in primary hemostasis within the vascular wall (platelet plug formation). Upon vascular injury, platelets with GpIb bind to exposed vWF on subendothelial matrix. Then ADP, TxA2, and fibrinogen get released from platelets. ADP combines with P2Y12 receptors to form the GpIIb/IIIa complex and with fibrinogen acts as a liaison to form platelet adhesion with one another. Meanwhile, TxA2 production ensures vasoconstriction to decrease blood flow to aid in hemostasis (Image courtesy of Maya Nunez.).[19]

CYCLOOXYGENASE INHIBITORS

Aspirin, acetylsalicylic acid, works by irreversibly inhibiting cyclooxygenase - 1 and 2 (COX-1 and 2) enzymes, preventing the formation of thromboxane A2, a prostaglandin derivative, which is essential in platelet aggregation. In addition, aspirin has antipyretic, analgesic, and anti-inflammatory properties.[20] Nonenteric-coated aspirin has an immediate onset of action that is usually less than 1 hour, reaching a peak effect in 1 to 2 hours, while the enteric-coated one takes effect in 3 to 4 hours, reaching its peak effect in around 4 hours.[20,21] Aspirin is hydrolyzed to salicylate by esterases in GI mucosa, red blood cells, synovial fluid, and blood, and salicylate is further metabolized via hepatic conjugation. It has a dose-dependent elimination half-life ranging from 20 minutes in lower doses (less than 100 mg) to 3 hours in higher doses (greater than 300 mg). It is exclusively excreted through urine as salicyluric acid and salicylic acid. When used as an antiplatelet, there is no dosing adjustment necessary for patients with renal impairment. When used for analgesics and anti-inflammatory purposes, aspirin should be avoided in patients whose creatinine clearance is less than 10 mL per minute.[21] It should also be avoided in patients with severe hepatic impairment. It is contraindicated in patients with GI ulcers and asthma, as the subsequent depletion of prostaglandins causes decrease gastric mucosa protection and the increase leukotrienes can trigger bronchospasm. When aspirin is desired for its antiplatelet use, GI intolerance should be observed.[21]

P2Y12 INHIBITORS

Other than aspirin, platelet inhibitors can be further divided into thienopyridines and non-thienopyridines class, both of which work by inhibiting the P2Y12 receptors, ultimately preventing platelet aggregation.[22] Ticlopidine (Ticlid) is a first generation thienopyridine that works by being metabolized into an unidentified metabolite that blocks ADP, which in turn, prevents the GPIIb/IIIa receptor complex activation and reduces platelet aggregation.[22] This medication has an onset of action of 6 hours, reaching its peak effect in 3 to 5 days. It has an elimination half-life of 13 hours and is excreted via urine and feces. Ticlopidine does not require dosing adjustment among patients with renal impairment but should be avoided in those with severe hepatic impairment. It has black box warnings of life-threatening hematologic events including neutropenia, agranulocytosis, thrombocytopenia purpura (TTP), and aplastic anemia.[23] Due to its bone marrow toxicity, ticlopidine was no longer a commonly prescribed thienopyridine.[24]

Clopidogrel (Plavix), a second generation thienopyridine, requires a 2-step metabolic activation via hepatic cytochrome P450 (CYP) prior to producing the active metabolite that inhibits the P2Y12 receptor. Most of the pro-drug undergo esterase-mediated hydrolysis to an inactive carboxylic acid derivate before intestinal absorption, therefore leading to a delayed therapeutic level and a suboptimal inhibition of platelet aggregation.[22] Platelets that are blocked by clopidogrel usually resume their baseline function 5 days after discontinuing the medication. A dose-dependent onset of action can be detected 2 hours after a single dose of 75 mg clopidogrel orally, and the peak serum level can be reached 45 minutes after administration. The parent drug has an elimination half-life of 6 hours.[25] Because clopidogrel requires a fully functional CYP2C19 gene to be bio-transformed into an active metabolite, patients with defective or mutated alleles will have suboptimal platelet aggregation and therefore contraindicated.[22]

Prasugrel (Effient) is a third generation thienopyridine that shares the same mechanism of action as clopidogrel and ticlopidine. Unlike clopidogrel, prasugrel is rapidly hydrolyzed in the gastro-intestinal system into an intermediate metabolite, which is then converted to an active metabolite via a single-step hepatic activation with CYP.[22] It has a dose-dependent onset of action that takes less than 30 minutes, reaching its peak effect around 4 hours after administration. Its duration of effect lasts 5 to 9 days after discontinuation. The elimination half-life of prasugrel is around 7 hours, and the major excretion route is through urine.[26] There is no dosing adjustment necessary for patients with hepatic and renal impairment. Its black boxing warnings include significant, sometimes fatal, bleeding, and it is contraindicated in patients with active pathologic bleeding or a history of transient ischemic attack or stroke. Its use is also advised against in patients who are greater than 75 year old due to the increased risk of fatal and intracranial bleeding.[26] Hemoglobin and hematocrit should be monitored periodically. Compared to the previous thienopyridine generation, prasugrel is more superior due to its single step hepatic activation that results in a faster onset, its initial hydrolyzation that leads to a much less inactivated fraction, as well as its better therapeutic stability in patients even with genetic CYP variant.[22]

Ticagrelor (Brilinta) is a non-thienopyridine that functions by binding to the P2Y12 receptor at a non-ADP site in a non-competitive, reservable manner. Unlike the thienopyridine antiplatelets, ticagrelor does not require metabolic activation and is orally active. It renders a faster onset within 30 mins with peak effects in 2 hours and stronger platelet inhibition than clopidogrel.[22,27] It still undergoes hepatic metabolism by CYP3A4/5 to an active metabolite, but due its "reversible" antagonism on ADP, platelets can recover their full function depending on the serum concentration of the active metabolite. Ticagrelor's elimination half-life is around 9 hours, and it is mostly excreted through feces.[27] There is no dosing adjustment necessary for patients with renal and mild hepatic impairment; however, it should be avoided in those with severe hepatic impairment.[28] Other than the risk of fatal intracranial bleeding, ticagrelor has distinct adverse effects of bradycardia and self-limiting dyspnea.[27] Overall, ticagrelor is more consistent, potent, and rapid in preventing platelet aggregating compared to thienopyridines class.

SINGLE, DOUBLE, TRIPLE ANTIPLATELET THERAPY (SAPT), (DAPT), (TAPT)

A wide range of antiplatelets have become available for management of thromboembolic events associated with cardiovascular, cerebrovascular and peripheral vascular systems. Single antiplatelet therapy (SAPT) and dual antiplatelet therapy (DAPT) consisting of ASA and a P2Y12 inhibitor have been recommended to reduce the risk of recurrent ischemic events during the first year following acute coronary syndrome (ACS).[29] The combined use of aspirin and clopidogrel as (DAPT) has been a mainstay for management of coronary artery disease. In general, DAPT is recommended in patients with a history of ACS either undergo medical treatment alone or percutaneous intervention (PCI) with or without stent placement, symptomatic peripheral vascular disease undergoing percutaneous lower extremity revascularization, as well as stroke prevention.[29–31] However, newer P2Y12 inhibitors such as prasugrel and ticagrelor have gradually replaced the use of clopidogrel in preventing thrombosis events due to their more favorable pharmacokinetics.[30] Indications on DAPT use are outlined by the 2016 American College of Cardiology (ACC) and the American Heart Association (AHA) as summarized in **Table 3**.[31] In those who developed restenosis, recurrent myocardial infarction, and stent thrombosis after DAPT, a cilostazol-based triple antiplatelet therapy (TAPT) has been introduced to improve the outcome of coronary intervention.[32]

ASSESSMENT OF BLEEDING RISK

It is not uncommon to encounter patients who chronically receive antithrombotic therapy. Some may be on DAPT, TAPT or a triple antithrombotic therapy (DAPT plus one DOAC). Prior to dental treatment, it is imperative to evaluate if temporary discontinuation of the antithrombotic therapy is justified and will not cause a life-threatening

Table 3
Indications on DAPT use in coronary artery disease

Types of Coronary Artery Disease	Types of Intervention (Medical/PCI)	P2Y12 Inhibitor & Aspirin (DAPT)
Acute Coronary Syndrome (ACS)	Medical Therapy Only (STEMI & NSTEMI)	Clopidogrel or Ticagrelor at least 12 mo
Stable Ischemic Heart Disease (SIHD)	Bare Metal Stent (BMS)	Clopidogrel at least 1 mo
Stable Ischemic Heart Disease (SIHD)	Drug Eluted Stent (DES)	Clopidogrel at least 6 mo
Acute Coronary Syndrome (ACS)	Bare Metal Stent (BMS) Drug Eluted Stent (DES)	Prasugrel or Ticagrelor at least 6 mo

Abbreviations: ACS = Acute coronary syndrome including both ST-Elevation myocardial infarction (STEMI) and Non-ST-Elevation myocardial infarction (NSTEMI). PCI = Percutaneous Intervention, SIHD = Stable ischemic heart disease. BMS = Bare metal stent. DES = Drug-eluting stent.
Adapted from ACC/AHA.[30,31]

thromboembolic event. Therefore, it is crucial to predict the bleeding risk associated with the procedure being performed to help assess the necessity for interruption.

The International Society on Thrombosis and Haemostasis (ISTH) proposed three perioperative bleeding risk stratifications (minimal, low, and high) shown in **Table 4** with some common dental procedures being considered as the minimal bleeding risk category.[33] In 2021, The European Heart Rhythm Association (EHRA) published a classification of elective surgical interventions according to bleeding risk, classifying interventions as minor, low-risk, or high-risk. Examples of some dental procedures classified as minor risks and more complex procedures are in low-risk category shown in **Table 5**.[34]

When distinguishing different bleeding risks within dental procedures, there are currently no universal standards. The most recent guidelines published by Scottish Dental Clinical Effectiveness Program (SDCEP) in 2022 compartmentalized dental procedures into 3 categories: unlikely to cause bleeding, low bleeding, and high bleeding shown in **Table 6**.[35] Moreover, an alternative set of review articles collaboratively proposed a list of dental procedures and categorized them into four bleeding risks groups (low, intermediate, moderate, high), as illustrated in **Table 7**.[36,37]

Due to the wide variation in invasiveness in dental procedures, there is no existing consensus when categorizing each dental procedure into one specific bleeding risk. However, some agree that procedures including simple extractions of up to three teeth, incision and drainage of intraoral swelling, endodontic treatment, and supragingival cleaning are considered as low bleeding risk. Major maxillofacial surgical procedures such as fracture repair and orthognathic surgery belong to the high bleeding risk group.[38,39]

A meta-analysis assessing post-operative bleeding risks for dental patients receiving oral anticoagulants suggested that the incidence of bleeding for patients

Table 4
Perioperative bleeding risk stratifications by International Society on Thrombosis and Haemostasis (ISTS).[33]

Minimal	Low	High
Minor dermatologic procedures	Arthroscopy	Major surgery with extensive tissue injury
Cataract procedures	Cutaneous/lymph node biopsies	Major orthopedic surgery
Minor dental procedures (dental cleanings, extractions, restorations, prosthetics, endodontics)	Coronary angiography	Reconstructive plastic surgery
	Shoulder/foot/hand surgery	Tumor resection or ablation
	Abdominal hysterectomy	Bowel resection
	Laparoscopic cholecystectomy	Surgery involving highly vascularized organs (kidneys, liver, spleen)
	Abdominal hernia repair	Cardiac, intracranial, or spinal surgery
	Hemorrhoidal surgery	Urologic or gastrointestinal surgery
	Bronchoscopy	Any major operation > 45 min

Table 5 Classification of elective surgical interventions according to bleeding risk by European Heart Rhythm Association (EHRA)	
Minor Risk	**Low-Risk**
Dental extractions (1–3 teeth), periodontal surgery, implant positioning, subgingival scaling/cleaning	Complex Dental Procedures

Adapted from Steffel and modified to reflect listed dental procedures.[34]

taking oral anticoagulants is low.[40] Although the bleeding rate in anticoagulated patients is higher (4.3%) than non-anticoagulated patients (1.1%), local hemostatic measures are sufficient to prevent adverse bleeding events. Only less than 0.1% of patients who did not discontinue their anticoagulant regimen required hospitalization for further bleeding control.[40] Topical hemostatic agents used in oral and maxillofacial surgery and their properties are summarized in **Table 8**.

PERIOPERATIVE MANAGEMENT FOR ANTITHROMBOTIC THERAPY

Perioperative management of patients taking antithrombotic medications can be challenging due to the risk of thromboembolism during interruption. However, invasive procedures also pose a threat of prolonged bleeding. A balance between managing bleeding risk and prevention of thromboembolism must be achieved.[29–32]

PERIOPERATIVE MANAGEMENT FOR ANTIPLATELETS

When proceeding to procedures with a low and moderate bleeding risk, antiplatelet therapy should not be discontinued even when the patient is on DAPT, as the risks

Table 6 Adapted from The Scottish Dental Clinical Effectiveness Programme (SDCEP) based dental procedures into those that are unlikely to cause bleeding, low, and high bleeding risk.[35]		
Dental Procedures that are Unlikely to Cause Bleeding	**Low Bleeding Risk Procedures**	**High Bleeding Risk Procedures**
Local anesthesia by local infiltration or other regional nerve blocks	Simple extractions of 1–3 teeth with limited wound size	Extractions of more than 3 teeth or complex extractions with large surgical wound
Basic periodontal examination	Incision and drainage of intraoral swellings	Flap raising procedures including dental implants, periodontal surgery, surgical extractions, crown lengthening, and pre-prosthetic procedures
Supragingival dental cleaning	Six-point full periodontal examination	Gingival recontouring
Supragingival restorations	Scaling and Root Planning	Biopsies
Root Canal Therapy	Subgingival restorations	
Prosthetic Procedures including dental impression		
Fitting and adjustment of orthodontic appliances		

Table 7
Bleeding risk stratifications in oral surgery procedures

Low Bleeding Risk Procedures	Intermittent Bleeding Risk Procedures	Moderate Bleeding Risk Procedures	High Bleeding Risk Procedures
Simple extractions of <5 teeth, soft tissue biopsy less than 1 cm in size	Simple extractions of 5–10 teeth, soft tissue biopsy 1.0–2.5 cm in size, simple implant placement	Extraction of impacted wisdom teeth, simple extractions of more than 10 teeth, tori removal, multiple implant placement, osseous biopsy, alveoloplasty	Repair of facial fractures, facial osteotomies, bone grafts

Adapted from Doonquah & Mitchell, Ward & Smith.[36,37]

of post-op bleeding events are minimal (**Table 9**). This is supported by a systematic review demonstrating no clinically significant bleeding risk for patients who are on SAPT or DAPT from invasive dental procedures such as multiple odontotomies, alveoloplasty, apicoectomy, tori removal, deep scaling and root planning, and excisional biopsies.[38] In a prospective comparative study assessing post extraction bleeding risk in patients receiving SAPT, approximately one-third experienced postoperative bleeding episodes, but resolved within 3 days using gauze pads.[41] In 548 cases (489 simple and 59 complicated dental extractions), postoperative bleeding was evident in 1.1%, 3.1% and 4.2% of the patients' prescribed aspirin, clopidogrel and DAPT (combination of aspirin and clopidogrel), respectively.[42] All bleeding episodes were eventually controlled by local hemostatic measures, further suggesting that it is not necessary to discontinue SAPT or DAPT prior to dental procedures with low to moderate bleeding risk.

Table 8
Local hemostatic measures used in oral surgery procedures

Name	Properties
Gelatin Foam (*Gelfoam*)	Provides a clotting framework that inhibits small-vessel bleeding
Cellulous (*Surgicel*)	Provides an absorbable physical matrix for clotting; lowers pH of surrounding tissue
Microfibrillar Collagen (*Avitene*)	Attracts platelets to its fibrils and initiates platelets aggregation
Tranexamic acid 4.8% oral rinse	Antifibrinolytic agent that stabilizes clots by competitively inhibiting plasminogen
Fibrin Glue	Consists of fibrinogen and thrombin to make a fibrin clot
Ostene	Water-soluble bone hemostatic agent that is eliminated by the body within 48 h
HemCon Dental Dressing	A hemostatic, bacteriostatic sponge made from chitosan
Tannic Acid	A commercial compound that prevents mucosa bleeding via vasoconstriction
Sutures	Allows for physical compression of wound edges

Adapted from Doonquah & Mitchell.[36]

Table 9
Perioperative management of antiplatelet regiment for patients with low, moderate, and high thrombosis risks

Intraoperative Bleeding Risk	Thrombosis Risk	
	Low and Moderate	High
Low	Do not interrupt SAPT, DAPT, or TAPT	
Moderate	Do not interrupt SAPT, DAPT, or TAPT	
High	Consider staging treatment in separate appointments converting the bleeding risk to low and moderate level Seek cardiology consult before with holding a P2Y12 inhibitor (5 d for clopidogrel and 7 d for prasugrel) prior to the procedure, while maintaining ASA Resume the P2Y 12 post-op (24–72 h)	Postpone all elective procedures until the completion of recommended regimen Consider staging the treatment in separate appointments converting the bleeding risk to low and moderate level In urgent cases, seek cardiology consult before withholding a P2Y 12 inhibitor (5 d for clopidogrel and 7 d for prasugrel) prior to the procedure, while maintaining ASA Resume the P2Y12 post-op (24–72 h)

Abbreviations: DAPT, dual antiplatelet therapy; SAPT, single antiplatelet therapy; TAPT, triple antiplatelet therapy.
Data from Refs.[35,39,42,43]

Similarly, bleeding episodes after dental procedures with TAPT have not been reported to be associated with the need for hospitalization or transfusion. In a study performed on patients on DAPT (59%) and TAPT (41%) with drug eluded stents (DES) that underwent dental extractions of one to six teeth, 0.2% were reported to experience postoperative bleeding for 4 to 5 hours, which were eventually controlled by local measures. Patients enrolled within this study had dental extractions after DES placement with the earliest reported on post-op day 9.[43] These results suggested that it is safe to proceed with dental procedures of low to moderate bleeding risks without interrupting DAPT or TAPT after successful PCI.

When the surgical bleeding risk is deemed high, but the patient has a low to moderate risk of thrombosis, a P2Y12 inhibitor such as clopidogrel should be discontinued 5 days prior to the scheduled procedure if permitted from the treating cardiologist, while ASA treatment should not be interrupted. The discontinued antiplatelet is usually resumed within 24 to 72 hours postoperatively.

When both intraoperative bleeding risk and thromboembolic risk are high, elective procedures should be delayed until the end of the antiplatelet regimen (see **Table 3**). In emergency cases, a cardiologist consultation is warranted, and, if allowed, clopidogrel and other P2Y12 inhibitors should be withdrawn 5 days before the procedure, while prasugrel, in specific, should be withheld for 7 days. Ideally, these combined high-risk cases are best performed in a hospital setting where an interventional radiologist is available in the event of thrombosis.[39] A similar review in the UK recommended the duration of clopidogrel interruption to be 7 days instead of 5 for high bleeding risk procedures. Furthermore, the same reviewer recommended to delay elective surgery for both moderate and high thrombosis groups. This is not in line with Wójcik's recommendation such that only those with high risk of thrombosis need to have their surgeries postponed.[44] Alternatively, the 2022 SDCEP guidelines suggest instead of discontinuing P2Y12 inhibitors before high bleeding risk procedure, practitioners should consider sequencing these treatments in separate appointments by down-grading the bleeding risk and perform them without drug interruption.[35]

PERIOPERATIVE MANAGEMENT FOR VITAMIN K ANTAGONIST

In patients who are on a continuous prescription of vitamin K antagonist, therapy should not be discontinued for procedures which entail a low to moderate risk of bleeding. The INR value should always be tested 24 hours prior to the procedure and should be under 3. If the value is above 3, treatment should be postponed until the value is within the targeted range. When the treatment is deemed to have a high risk of bleeding, the physician should be consulted prior to treatment. This strategy usually requires adjusting the INR level to 2.0 - 2.5 under the direction of the special-ists. For patients who have a high risk of thromboembolism, physicians may propose bridging anticoagulation therapy in the period preceding a high-risk procedure, re-flected in **Table 10**. If necessary, physicians may also consider vitamin K therapy to optimize patients perioperatively, outlined in **Table 11**.[45–47]

Some prescribing physicians may recommend bridging longer acting anticoagulant agents, such as warfarin, typically with the administration of a short-acting anticoag-ulant such as a low molecular weight heparin (LMWH). There is increasing evidence that in many patients, bridging does not reduce the risk of thromboembolism, and in fact may increase the risk of bleeding. When bridging is indicated, it is typically initi-ated 3 days prior to the procedure, and 2 days after the interruption of warfarin. Sub-cutaneous LMWH is then discontinued 24 hours prior to the procedure, based on its biological half-life of three to 5 hours. There is no increased incidence of bleeding from patients who pause LMWH 12 or 24 hours prior to their procedure. However, in studies assessing a marker for bleeding (factor Xa) when LMWH was discontinued 12 hours, 90% of patients had a detectable level of anticoagulant and 34% were still at a ther-apeutic range.[49] The most recent guidelines by the American College of Surgeons and the American Society of Regional Anesthesia recommend to withhold LMWH 24 hours prior to surgery.[50]

PERIOPERATIVE MANAGEMENT FOR DIRECT ORAL ANTICOAGULANTS
Direct Oral Anticoagulants with Alteration/Interruption/Continuance Strategy

The 2021 European Heart Rhythm Association (EHRA) practical guide states that pa-tients receiving DOAC *generally* do not require any perioperative bridging with low mo-lecular weight heparins (LMWH) or unfractionated heparin (UFH) (**Table 12**). However, the current EHRA's position does advise either altering, with or without interrupting

Table 10	
INR values and bleeding risk	
INR	**Bleeding Risk**
< 2	Low
2–3	Moderate
> 4.5	High

Abbreviation: INR, International Normalized Ratio.
   Data from Ref.[48]

Table 11
Perioperative management of patients taking vitamin K antagonist (VKA) using vitamin K therapy

Indications for Vitamin K Administration	Timing of Vitamin K/PCC's Administration	INR Monitoring
Urgent surgery or bleeding in patients with elevated INR	KCENTRA™ (4 Factor unactivated PCC)	Monitor INR at baseline and 30 min post dose
Elective surgery in patients on warfarin with elevated INR	Vitamin K 3 mg IV or 1 mg PO Day before surgery	Monitor INR; repeat vitamin K dosing as needed based on INR

Abbreviations: INR, international normalized ratio; IV, intravenous; PCC, prothrombin complex concentrates; PO, oral.
  Data from Refs.[45–47].

anticoagulant intake under certain circumstances. This is depending on upon the drug's plasma concentration and renal function, dosage scheduling, and anticipated bleeding risk.[34]

For minor bleeding risk procedures (eg,; up to 3 simple tooth extractions), it is recommended to perform the procedure at the drug's trough level (12 - 24 hours after the last dose) and resume 6 hours later (alteration strategy) or skip a dose and resume the next one at the regular schedule (interruption strategy). For example, BID regimen may consider a pause of the medication in the morning of surgery and patient can resume the evening dose after hemostasis is achieved (interruption strategy). As stated above, the consideration of withholding a preoperative dose is dependent on (eg,; drug's plasma concentration and renal clearance and other drug-drug interactions affecting DOAC's elimination, and so forth). As for QD regimen taken in the morning time, this dose can be withheld in the morning of surgery and resume 6 hours after procedure (alteration strategy). Lastly, if the QD dose is taken in the evening, surgery can be performed in the following morning with the next dose intake during evening time (continuance strategy).[34]

Table 12
Management of timing of last DOAC intake prior to elective procedure, depending on renal function and bleeding risk

	Dabigatran		Rivaroxaban, Apixaban, Edoxaban	
Minor risk bleeding procedures: • Perform procedure at DOAC's trough level (eg,; ≥ 12–24 h after last dose) • Resume ≥ 6 h after surgery				
Renal Function (C_RC_L ml/min)	*Low risk*	*High risk*	*Low risk*	*High risk*
80 mL/min (Normal)	≥ 24 h	≥ 48 h	≥ 24 h	≥ 48 h
50–79 mL/min (Mild)	≥ 36 h	≥ 72 h	≥ 24 h	≥ 48 h
30–49 mL/min (Moderate)	≥ 48 h	≥ 96 h	≥ 24 h	≥ 48 h
15–29 mL/min (Severe)	Contraindicated		≥ 36 h	≥ 48 h
<15 mL/min (Failure)	Contraindicated			

Abbreviations: CrCl, Creatinine Clearance; LMWH, low molecular weight heparin; UFH, unfractionated heparin.
  Adapted from 2021 European Heart Rhythm Association Practical Guide on the Use of Non-Vitamin K Antagonist Oral Anticoagulants in Patients with Atrial Fibrillation. hr = hours[34]

For dental procedures entailing more complexity than 3 extractions, defined as low risk, dabigatran patients with normal renal function (CrCl > 80 mL/min) must pause 24 hours prior. Patients with mild renal impairment (CrCl 50 - 79 mL/min) must pause 36 hours prior. For moderate renal impairment (CrCl 30 - 49 mL/min), patients must pause 48 hours prior while Dabigatran is not indicated for severe or renal failure group. All high bleeding risk should pause according to their renal function (48–96 hr).[34]

For dental procedures entailing more complexity than 3 extractions, defined as low risk, dabigatran patients with normal renal function (CrCl > 80 mL/min) must pause 24 hours prior and 48 hours prior for high-risk bleeding procedures. Patients with mild renal impairment (CrCl 50 - 79 mL/min) must pause 36 hours prior for low-risk procedures, and 72 hours prior for high-risk bleeding procedures. For moderate renal impairment (CrCl 30 - 49 mL/min) patients must interrupt 48 hours prior for low-risk bleeding procedures, and 96 hours prior for high-risk bleeding procedures. Dabigatran is not indicated for severe or renal failure group.[34]

Patients undergoing factor Xa inhibitors for low bleeding risk will pause medication 24 hours prior for normal, mild, and moderate renal impairment group (CrCl 30 - 80+ ml/min). As for severe renal impairment, a 36-h pause is recommended. All high-risk bleeding procedures will need to pause for at least 48 hours.[34]

Again, minor risk bleeding group should resume medication ≥ 6 hours after surgery while low risk and high bleeding risk groups should resume within 24 hours and 48 to 72 hours respectively.[34]

DIRECT ORAL ANTICOAGULANTS WITHOUT INTERRUPTION STRATEGY

There are many who support the continuance of DOACs for low-risk bleeding procedures when proper local measures and post-op instructions can be employed[51–58] and uncomplicated extractions up to 3 teeth.[54,56,59] Furthermore, Clemm and colleagues's prospective study demonstrated multiple implant placement with concurrent autogenous sinus augmentation is possible without interruption when compared to all antithrombotic therapy studied (Antiplatelet, vitamin K antagonist, LMWH ± bridging, and DOACs).[60] The American Dental Association also supports, albeit limited data, without pausing DOAC's for non-high risk bleeding procedures based on couple of systemic reviews.[61,62]

POST-OP BLEEDING OUTCOME ASSESSMENT (DIRECT ORAL ANTICOAGULANTS VS WARFARIN)

Prospective studies on DOACs versus warfarin had good outcome and low propensity for post-op bleeding for both groups when dental extractions were performed. No difference in bleeding was noted between the DOACs and vitamin K antagonist group.[52] In another study on single tooth extraction, one post-op bleed was reported from the DOAC group and two from the vitamin K antagonist group with both groups managed by local measures.[55] Equally, teeth extraction (up to 5 teeth) demonstrated four bleeding events by the DOAC group. All four were managed by local measures with two patients requiring to skip the next dose due to prolonged bleeding.[54]

POST-OP BLEEDING OUTCOME ASSESSMENT (DIRECT ORAL ANTICOAGULANTS VS VITAMIN K ANTAGONIST VS ANTIPLATELETS VS LOW MOLECULAR WEIGHT HEPARIN VS NO MEDICATIONS)

Additionally, a recent prospective study support to maintain daily intake of DOACs, antiplatelets, and vitamin K antagonists for both low and high risks procedures, from simple tooth extraction to multiple teeth (extraction >3 per quadrant) and greater than 1 implant placement per arch.[41] Even though this prospective study noted most bleeding was in this descending order antiplatelets (n = 16/51) > DOAC (n = 8/27) > warfarin (n = 1/16), it was mild and managed with local measures and persistent pressure with gauze pads.[41] Conversely, a prospective study compared users of antiplatelet, vitamin K antagonist, DOACs, and LMWH against control group and found most bleeding came from the vitamin K antagonist group (with statistical difference). Although four patients required hospitalizations, all bleeders were also controlled with local measures. Additionally, the type of surgical procedure (Number of teeth extracted or tooth osteotomies) did not influence the degree of bleeding.[63]

In reference to post-op bleeding for dentoalveolar surgeries, a meta-analysis concluded there were no difference between the anticoagulated and the control group for high-risk bleeding events. The DOACs had less post-op bleeding than vitamin K antagonist group when implant procedures were compared, and overall increased bleeding was noted in the anticoagulated group than control group. Nevertheless, all bleeding events were controlled effectively with local hemostasis.[40] The author also cautioned that International Normalized Ratio (INR) was not controlled in their analysis and future controlled studies are needed. Another systematic review in 2021 also found DOACs had less postoperative bleeding than patients on vitamin K antagonists, however they claimed the quality of evidence is low due to the sheer lack of larger scale studies. Additionally, they believed the shorter half-life of DOACs and better safety profile are contributing factors to the decreased incidence of postoperative hemorrhage.[64]

With much controversy swirling around the preoperative management decisions, published findings have discussed the frequency of postoperative bleeding. One anticoagulant study found approximately 1.7% of all analyzed dental patient appointments to have postoperative bleeding, with the highest risk being warfarin at 3.9% of incidents. Clopidogrel interestingly carried almost 0% risk of bleeding.[58] Another study compared 2102 patients taking oral anticoagulants (vitamin K inhibitors/antagonists, rivaroxaban, dabigatran) to 2271 control patients (no medication) and they found a bleeding risk of 4.33% and 1.1% respectively.[40] Yet another study compared DOAC patients to those on warfarin and found a postoperative bleeding rate of 1.65% for dabigatran and 3.63% for warfarin. And for the medication naïve, the bleeding rate was reported at 0.39%.[65]

Although most postoperative bleeding is resolved with local measures, it is possible for more serious bleeding events to occur. One case report in 2019 described a serious bleeding event where a 74-year-old patient with multiple comorbidities required hospitalization due to severe oral bleeding after the extraction of 5 teeth. The authors noted this patient was prescribed apixaban and was bridged with heparin. Despite the severity of bleeding and patient's medical history, the authors noted the oral bleed was managed by removal of the unorganized clot, resutured the site and placement of tranexamic acid-soaked gauze. The authors also emphasized the unnecessary bridging for this situation given the patient's decreased renal function. It would have been more prudent to allow the medication to be metabolized and eliminated without supplementation based upon this patient's GFR status.[66]

DISCUSSION

The degree of anticipated postoperative bleeding should be weighed against the risk of stroke and/or adverse thromboembolic events from withholding these antithrombotic(s) during the perioperative phase for each patient. There is 0.8% risk and

0.2% fatality when there is an interruption or bridging for vitamin K antagonist medications.[67] Additionally, DOAC patients encountered perioperative thrombosis at 2.6% percent when interrupted.[68] Although low quality studies were analyzed in the latest systematic review and meta-analysis, bleeding from extractions postoperatively were lower in DOACs than in the vitamin K antagonist group.[64]

While the older regiment (ASA, clopidogrel, and warfarin) has been well studied, the newer drugs notably the DOACs have limited prospective studies supporting the continuance of their medications. Recently, Scottish Dentists were surveyed and only 38% were compliant with their national guideline for low-risk bleeding procedures.[69] Furthermore, a multicentric study survey concluded 73.8% would follow the same protocol.[70] Both surveys revealed their practitioners were more comfortable treating patients on vitamin K antagonist than DOACs. Perhaps having a tangible preoperative blood test (INR) provides a sense of security.

There appears to be an increasing number of studies showing continuance of DOACs while performing low-risk procedures do carry a good outcome[51-56,58] and other practitioners had equally good outcome in complex high-risk cases.[60,63]

The perioperative decision to either pause, alter or continue DOAC dosage should be tailored to the individual based on the following factors: 1) bleeding risk, 2) type of procedure, 3) clearance of the drug based on elimination half-life and the functionality of the organ involved, 4) other systemic diseases impacting coagulopathy. The European Heart Rhythm Association (EHRA) recommends these medications to be at its nadir for the minor bleeding risks surgeries and pausing from 24 to 96 hours (pending on drug and renal clearance) for low to high-risk bleeding procedures. And when post-op bleeding is encountered, the vast majority are managed by local measures without any case of reported fatalities.[34,71]

When faced with multiple dental extractions to be performed, it may be prudent to downgrade the number of teeth and convert them into multiple appointments to circumvent skipping a dose.[56] And while several prospective studies demonstrated by using this strategy is safe and effective, some practitioners have documented postoperative bleeding requiring hospitalizations just from simple teeth extractions.[63,66]

Although DAPT and TAPT have been shown to increase the post operative bleeding compared to SAPT, most of the bleeding episodes can be controlled by local measures.[43,72] The consensus is that it is not necessary to interrupt DAPT and TAPT before procedures with low to moderate bleeding risks. However, in the setting of high bleeding risk, the P2Y12 inhibitor should be held for 5 to 7 days when the thrombosis risk is low, and elective procedures should be postponed until the completion of the antiplatelet regimen for those with a high thrombosis risk. This antiplatelet regimen is generally prescribed for 1, 6, or 12 months depending on the cardiac situation and the type of stent used. A cardiology consultation is always warranted prior to discontinuing any P2Y12 inhibitor(s).

Because the newer generation of antiplatelets such as prasugrel and ticagrelor only debuted in the late 2000s, there is not enough evidence to suggest the perioperative management of these medications.[73] With a faster onset and more potent antiplatelet effects, prasugrel and ticagrelor are associated with a higher incidence of bleeding compared to clopidogrel. However, the bleeding risk for patients who are taking either prasugrel or ticagrelor as part of their DAPT is found not to be remarkably different than those taking ASA and clopidogrel, suggesting that it is not necessary to interrupt these new generations of DAPT.[73,74] It is noteworthy that the number of patients taking prasugrel or ticagrelor as part of DAPT regimen is still far lower than the current combination of ASA and clopidogrel, making the existing evidence of the newer generations very limited for perioperative management.[73]

To further mention, the risk stratification of surgery is highly variable so making a direct comparison is difficult. There are those who classify biopsy as low risk[56] and others as high (2022 SDCEP's guideline). To further mention, the risk stratification of surgery is highly variable so making a direct comparison is difficult. There are those who classify biopsy as low risk[56] and others as low/high risk (2022 SDSEP's guideline). Despite these disparities, there are some common dominators when low risk surgeries are categorized (eg,: simple tooth extraction 1–3 teeth)[14,34,35,51,56,57,59] to high risks (eg,: maxillofacial procedures requiring plating). However, a large majority of the procedures are still in a "gray area" and perhaps standardizing this specifically for dentistry would be helpful for future direction.

Although post-op bleeding associated with antithrombotic medication(s) can be managed by proper local measures, the need for the practitioner to provide alternative venues, especially after office hours, when patients are experiencing uncontrollable bleed despite their best attempt at home. Available and direct contact with the surgeon or, if critical, access to the local emergency room should be outlined. Again, a vast majority of these bleeds are controlled successfully with local measures. Reversal agents are available at the emergency physician or specialist's discretion and are usually reserved for life threatening situations. A close collaboration among all parties involved, including educating patients can mitigate sometimes even foreseen circumstances.

SUMMARY

SAPT, DAPT, and TAPT should not be interrupted for procedures of low and moderate bleeding risks. For procedures of high bleeding risk, P2Y12 inhibitors should be held for 5 to 7 days, and elective procedures should be postponed until the completion of the antiplatelet regimen. It would be prudent to seek physician's consultation for all high-risk for thrombosis and bleeding procedures. Given limited data thus far on DOACs, it is not necessary to interrupt the medication for simple tooth extractions of up to 3 teeth and the most optimal circumstance is to have the procedure done at the drug's trough level of 12 to 24 hours of last intake. A decision to alter or skip a dose will be based on the bleeding risk, type of procedure, GFR and other factors affecting drug clearance. As for high-risk bleeding procedures for patients with decreased renal function, a hold on DOAC may be indicated for up to 48 - 96 hours, typically without the need for bridging. Local measures along with patient maintaining biting direct pressure with gauze pad should manage most post-op bleeds. A larger prospective controlled study would certainly provide more sound empirical data. Additionally, standardizing the procedure's risk stratification reflecting bleeding risks can also be helpful for direct comparison.

CLINICS CARE POINTS

- It is not necessary to stop SAPT, DAPT or TAPT when performing low to moderate risk bleeding dental procedures.
- The decision to pause, alter, or continue DOAC dosage during the perioperative period should be based on bleeding risk, type of procedure, drug clearance, organ functionality, and other systemic diseases affecting coagulopathy.
- Limited data demonstrating low-risk bleeding procedures have good clinical outcome without pausing DOAC medication
- Local hemostatic measures, good post-op instructions and an outlined emergency plan for patient to following in the event of a true "bleeding" emergency.

- Downgrading the number of teeth and scheduling multiple appointments for dental extractions may be advisable to prevent the need to skip or alter a dose.

- No mortalities were documented for those who continued their antithrombotic. However, there is a 0.8% risk and 0.2% fatality with an interruption or bridging for vitamin K antagonist medications. Also, 2.6% of perioperative thrombosis occurred when DOAC was withheld.

DISCLOSURE

The authors listed above have nothing to disclose.

REFERENCES

1. ClinCalc. ClinCalc DrugStats Database; Available at: https://clincalc.com/DrugStats/. Accessed March 18, 2023.
2. Chaudhry R, U.S., Babiker HM. Physiology, Coagulation Pathways. 2022 ; Available at: https://www.ncbi.nlm.nih.gov/books/NBK482253/. Accessed March 8, 2023
3. Lee CA, Kessler CM, Varon D, et al. Newer concepts of blood coagulation. Haemophilia 1998;4(4):331–4.
4. Kessler CM. Urgent reversal of warfarin with prothrombin complex concentrate: where are the evidence-based data? J Thromb Haemost 2006;4(5):963–6.
5. UpToDate. Warfarin: Drug Information. 2023. Available at: https://www.uptodate.com/contents/warfarin-drug-information. Accessed March 2, 2023.
6. Boehringer Ingelheim Pharmaceuticals, I. Pradaxa (prescribing information). 2023 March 4, 2023.
7. Janssen Pharmaceuticals, I. Xarelto (Prescribing Information). 2023. Available at: https://www.janssenlabels.com/package-insert/product-monograph/prescribing-information/XARELTO-pi.pdf. Accessed March 4, 2023
8. Squibb, B.-M. Eliquis: Prescribing Information. 2023; Available at: https://packageinserts.bms.com/pi/pi_eliquis.pdf. Accessed March 4, 2023.
9. Powell JR. Are new oral anticoagulant dosing recommendations optimal for all patients? JAMA 2015;313(10):1013–4.
10. Daiichi Sankyo, I. Savaysa: Prescribing Informatiton. 2015 March 4, 2023; Available at: https://www.accessdata.fda.gov/drugsatfda_docs/label/2015/206316lbl.pdf.
11. Lu G, Conley PB, Leeds JM, et al. A phase 2 PK/PD study of andexanet alfa for reversal of rivaroxaban and edoxaban anticoagulation in healthy volunteers. Blood Adv 2020;4(4):728–39.
12. Aldhaeefi M, Badreldin HA, Alsuwayyid F, et al. Practical Guide for Anticoagulant and Antiplatelet Reversal in Clinical Practice. Pharmacy (Basel) 2023;11(1).
13. Tripodi A, Ageno W, Ciaccio M, et al. Position Paper on laboratory testing for patients on direct oral anticoagulants. A Consensus Document from the SISET, FCSA, SIBioC and SIPMeL. Blood Transfus 2018;16(5):462–70.
14. Lupi SM, Rodriguez YBA. Patients Taking Direct Oral Anticoagulants (DOAC) Undergoing Oral Surgery: A Review of the Literature and a Proposal of a Peri-Operative Management Protocol. Healthcare (Basel) 2020;8(3):281.
15. Patel S, Singh R, Preuss CV, et al. Warfarin. [1-10] StatPearls, 2022, StatPearls Publishing Copyright © 2022. Treasure Island, FL: StatPearls Publishing LLC; 2022.
16. UpToDate. Dabigatran: Drug Information. 2023 March 4, 2023; Available at: https://www.uptodate.com/contents/dabigatran-drug-information.

17. Broos K, Feys HB, De Meyer SF, et al. Platelets at work in primary hemostasis. Blood Rev 2011;25(4):155–67.
18. Woulfe D, Yang J, Brass L. ADP and platelets: the end of the beginning. J Clin Invest 2001;107(12):1503–5.
19. Le TBV, Sochat M. First aid for the USMLE step 1 2021. New York: McGraw-Hill Education; 2021.
20. Warner TD, Nylander S, Whatling C. Anti-platelet therapy: cyclo-oxygenase inhibition and the use of aspirin with particular regard to dual anti-platelet therapy. Br J Clin Pharmacol 2011;72(4):619–33.
21. Bayer. Aspirin Product Monograph. 2022; Available at: https://www.bayer.com/sites/default/files/2020-11/aspirin-pm-en.pdf. Accessed March 30, 2023.
22. Damman P, Woudstra P, Kuijt WJ, et al. P2Y12 platelet inhibition in clinical practice. J Thromb Thrombolysis 2012;33(2):143–53.
23. Genpharm. Ticlopidine Prescriber Information. 1998; Available at: https://www.accessdata.fda.gov/drugsatfda_docs/anda/99/75161_Ticlopidine%20Hydrochloride_Prntlbl.pdf. Accessed March 24, 2023.
24. Iqbal AM, Lopez RA, Hai O. Antiplatelet Medications. In: StatPearls. Treasure Island (FL): [1-7] StatPearls Publishing Copyright © 2023, StatPearls Publishing LLC; 2023.
25. Squibb/Sanofi, B.-M. Plavix Prescribing Information. 2009; Available at: https://www.accessdata.fda.gov/drugsatfda_docs/label/2009/020839s044lbl.pdf. Accessed April 1, 2023.
26. Lilly, D.S.E. Effient Prescriber Information. 2009; Available at: https://www.accessdata.fda.gov/drugsatfda_docs/label/2012/022307s007lbl.pdf. Accessed March 24, 2023.
27. Dobesh PP, Oestreich JH. Ticagrelor: pharmacokinetics, pharmacodynamics, clinical efficacy, and safety. Pharmacotherapy 2014;34(10):1077–90.
28. AstraZeneca. Brilinta Prescriber Information. 2011. Available at: https://www.accessdata.fda.gov/drugsatfda_docs/label/2020/022433s029lbl.pdf. Accessed March 24, 2023.
29. Dézsi CA, Dézsi BB, Dézsi AD. Management of dental patients receiving antiplatelet therapy or chronic oral anticoagulation: A review of the latest evidence. Eur J Gen Pract 2017;23(1):196–201.
30. Stawiarski K, Kataria R, Bravo CA, et al. Dual-antiplatelet Therapy Guidelines and Implications for Perioperative Management. J Cardiothorac Vasc Anesth 2018; 32(2):1072–80.
31. Levine G.N., Bates E.R., Bittl J.A., et al., 2016 ACC/AHA Guideline Focused Update on Duration of Dual Antiplatelet Therapy in Patients With Coronary Artery Disease: A Report of the American College of Cardiology/American Heart Association Task Force on Clinical Practice Guidelines: An Update of the 2011 ACCF/AHA/SCAI Guideline for Percutaneous Coronary Intervention, 2011 ACCF/AHA Guideline for Coronary Artery Bypass Graft Surgery, 2012 ACC/AHA/ACP/AATS/PCNA/SCAI/STS Guideline for the Diagnosis and Management of Patients With Stable Ischemic Heart Disease, 2013 ACCF/AHA Guideline for the Management of ST-Elevation Myocardial Infarction, 2014 AHA/ACC Guideline for the Management of Patients With Non-ST-Elevation Acute Coronary Syndromes, and 2014 ACC/AHA Guideline on Perioperative Cardiovascular Evaluation and Management of Patients Undergoing Noncardiac Surgery. Circulation. 2016;134(10):e123-1255.
32. Zhao S, Zhong Z, Qi G, et al. Effects of Cilostazol-Based Triple Antiplatelet Therapy Versus Dual Antiplatelet Therapy After Coronary Drug-Eluting Stent

Implantation: An Updated Meta-Analysis of the Randomized Controlled Trials. Clin Drug Investig 2019;39(1):1–13.

33. Spyropoulos AC, Al-Badri A, Sherwood MW, Douketis JD. Periprocedural management of patients receiving a vitamin K antagonist or a direct oral anticoagulant requiring an elective procedure or surgery. J Thromb Haemost 2016;14(5):875–85.

34. Steffel J., Collins R., Antz M., et al., 2021 European Heart Rhythm Association Practical Guide on the Use of Non-Vitamin K Antagonist Oral Anticoagulants in Patients with Atrial Fibrillation. Europace. 2021;23(10):1612-1676.

35. Woolcombe SA, Ball RE, Patel JP. Managing direct oral anticoagulants in accordance with the Scottish Dental Clinical Effectiveness Programme guidance for patients undergoing dentoalveolar surgery. Br Dent J 2022;232(8):547–54.

36. Doonquah L, Mitchell AD. Oral surgery for patients on anticoagulant therapy: current thoughts on patient management. Dent Clin North Am 2012;56(1):25–41, vii.

37. Ward BB, Smith MH. Dentoalveolar procedures for the anticoagulated patient: literature recommendations versus current practice. J Oral Maxillofac Surg 2007;65(8):1454–60.

38. Napeñas JJ, Oost FC, DeGroot A, et al. Review of postoperative bleeding risk in dental patients on antiplatelet therapy. Oral Surg Oral Med Oral Pathol Oral Radiol 2013;115(4):491–9.

39. Wójcik S, Mocny-Pachońska K, Bisch-Wójcik S, et al. Perioperative Management of Dental Surgery Patients Chronically Taking Antithrombotic Medications. Int J Environ Res Public Health 2022;19(23).

40. Shi Q, Xu J, Zhang T, et al. Post-operative Bleeding Risk in Dental Surgery for Patients on Oral Anticoagulant Therapy: A Meta-analysis of Observational Studies. *Front Pharmacol* 2017;8:58.

41. Buchbender M, Schlee N, Kesting MR, et al. A prospective comparative study to assess the risk of postoperative bleeding after dental surgery while on medication with direct oral anticoagulants, antiplatelet agents, or vitamin K antagonists. BMC Oral. Health 2021;21(1):504.

42. Lu SY, Lin LH, Hsue SS. Management of dental extractions in patients on warfarin and antiplatelet therapy. J Formos Med Assoc 2018;117(11):979–86.

43. Park MW, Her SH, Kwon JB, et al. Safety of dental extractions in coronary drug-eluting stenting patients without stopping multiple antiplatelet agents. Clin Cardiol 2012;35(4):225–30.

44. Mahmood H, Siddique I, McKechnie A. Antiplatelet drugs: a review of pharmacology and the perioperative management of patients in oral and maxillofacial surgery. Ann R Coll Surg Engl 2020;102(1):9–13.

45. Burbury KL, Milner A, Snooks B, et al. Short-term warfarin reversal for elective surgery–using low-dose intravenous vitamin K: safe, reliable and convenient*. Br J Haematol 2011;154(5):626–34.

46. Woods K, Douketis JD, Kathirgamanathan K, et al. Low-dose oral vitamin K to normalize the international normalized ratio prior to surgery in patients who require temporary interruption of warfarin. J Thromb Thrombolysis 2007;24(2):93–7.

47. Medicine J.H. John Hopkins Anticoagulation Reversal Guide for Physicians. 2023; Available at: https://www.hopkinsmedicine.org/suburban_hospital/for_physicians/_docs/anticoagulation_reversal_guide.pdf. Accessed June 10, 2023.

48. Pagano MB, Chandler WL. Bleeding risks and response to therapy in patients with INR higher than 9. Am J Clin Pathol 2012;138(4):546–50.

49. Douketis J.D., Spyropoulos A.C., Spencer F.A., et al., Perioperative management of antithrombotic therapy: Antithrombotic Therapy and Prevention of Thrombosis, 9th ed: American College of Chest Physicians Evidence-Based Clinical Practice Guidelines. Chest. 2012;141(2 Suppl):e326S-e350S.

50. Polania Gutierrez JJ, Rocuts KR. Perioperative Anticoagulation Management. In: StatPearls [1-19]. Treasure Island (FL): StatPearls Publishing Copyright © 2023, StatPearls Publishing LLC; 2023.

51. Breik O., Cheng A., Sambrook P., Goss A., Protocol in managing oral surgical patients taking dabigatran. Aust Dent J. 2014;59(3):296-301; quiz 401.

52. Mauprivez C, Khonsari RH, Razouk O, et al. Management of dental extraction in patients undergoing anticoagulant oral direct treatment: a pilot study. Oral Surg Oral Med Oral Pathol Oral Radiol 2016;122(5):e146–55.

53. Patel JP, Woolcombe SA, Patel RK. Managing direct oral anticoagulants in patients undergoing dentoalveolar surgery. Br Dent J 2017;222(4):245–9.

54. Yoshikawa H, Yoshida M, Yasaka M, et al. Safety of tooth extraction in patients receiving direct oral anticoagulant treatment versus warfarin: a prospective observation study. Int J Oral Maxillofac Surg 2019;48(8):1102–8.

55. Berton F, Costantinides F, Rizzo R, et al. Should we fear direct oral anticoagulants more than vitamin K antagonists in simple single tooth extraction? A prospective comparative study. Clin Oral Investig 2019;23(8):3183–92.

56. Felix J, Chaban P, Ouanounou A. Dental Management of Patients Undergoing Antithrombotic Therapy. J Can Dent Assoc 2020;86:k17.

57. Brennan Y., Gu Y., Schifter M., et al., Dental extractions on direct oral anticoagulants vs. warfarin: The DENTST study, *Res Pract Thromb Haemost*, 4 (2), 2020, 278–284.

58. AlSheef M, Gray J, AlShammari A. Risk of postoperative bleeding following dental extractions in patients on antithrombotic treatment. The Saudi Dental Journal 2021;33(7):511–7.

59. Syyed N, Ansell M, Sood V. Dabigatran (Pradaxa(®)): surgeon's friend or foe? Br Dent J 2014;217(11):623–6.

60. Clemm R, Neukam FW, Rusche B, et al. Management of anticoagulated patients in implant therapy: a clinical comparative study. Clin Oral Implants Res 2016; 27(10):1274–82.

61. Manfredi M, Dave B, Percudani D, et al. World workshop on oral medicine VII: Direct anticoagulant agents management for invasive oral procedures: A systematic review and meta-analysis. Oral Dis 2019;25(Suppl 1):157–73.

62. Lusk KA, Snoga JL, Benitez RM, Sarbacker GB. Management of Direct-Acting Oral Anticoagulants Surrounding Dental Procedures With Low-to-Moderate Risk of Bleeding. J Pharm Pract 2018;31(2):202–7.

63. Schmitt CM, Rusche B, Clemm R, et al. Management of anticoagulated patients in dentoalveolar surgery: a clinical comparative study. Clin Oral Investig 2020; 24(8):2653–62.

64. Hua W, Huang Z, Huang Z. Bleeding Outcomes After Dental Extraction in Patients Under Direct-Acting Oral Anticoagulants vs. Vitamin K Antagonists: A Systematic Review and Meta-Analysis. Front Pharmacol 2021;12:702057.

65. Hiroshi I, Natsuko SY, Yutaka I, et al. Frequency of hemorrhage after tooth extraction in patients treated with a direct oral anticoagulant: A multicenter cross-sectional study. PLoS One 2022;17(4):e0266011.

66. Ehrhard S, Burkhard JP, Exadaktylos AK, Sauter TC. Severe Enoral Bleeding with a Direct Oral Anticoagulant after Tooth Extraction and Heparin Bridging Treatment. Case Rep Emerg Med 2019;2019:6208604.

67. Wahl MJ, Pinto A, Kilham J, Lalla RV. Dental surgery in anticoagulated patients–stop the interruption. Oral Surg Oral Med Oral Pathol Oral Radiol 2015;119(2): 136–57.
68. Vanga SR, Satti SR, Williams J, et al. Discontinuation of oral anticoagulation preceding acute ischemic stroke–prevalence and outcomes: Comprehensive chart review. Postgrad Med 2015;127(8):791–5.
69. Kelly N, Beaton L, Knights J, et al. The practices and beliefs of dental professionals regarding the management of patients taking anticoagulant and antiplatelet drugs. BDJ Open 2023;9(1):1.
70. Precht C, Demirel Y, Assaf AT, et al. Perioperative Management in Patients With Undergoing Direct Oral Anticoagulant Therapy in Oral Surgery - A Multicentric Questionnaire Survey. In. Vivo 2019;33(3):855–62.
71. Heidbuchel H, Verhamme P, Alings M, et al. Updated European Heart Rhythm Association Practical Guide on the use of non-vitamin K antagonist anticoagulants in patients with non-valvular atrial fibrillation. Europace 2015;17(10):1467–507.
72. Ockerman A, Bornstein MM, Leung YY, et al. Incidence of bleeding after minor oral surgery in patients on dual antiplatelet therapy: a systematic review and meta-analysis. Int J Oral Maxillofac Surg 2020;49(1):90–8.
73. Johnston S. An evidence summary of the management of the care of patients taking novel oral antiplatelet drugs undergoing dental surgery. J Am Dent Assoc 2016;147(4):271–7.
74. Olmos-Carrasco O, Pastor-Ramos V, Espinilla-Blanco R, et al. Hemorrhagic complications of dental extractions in 181 patients undergoing double antiplatelet therapy. J Oral Maxillofac Surg 2015;73(2):203–10.

Short Implants
Their Role in Implant Reconstruction

Raza A. Hussain, BDS, DMD[a,b,c,*], Jennifer B. Cohen, DDS[a,b],
Benjamin Palla, DMD, MD[b,c,1]

KEYWORDS

• Dental implants • Short implants • Complications • Reconstruction

KEY POINTS

- Minimally invasive surgical techniques are being advocated for in all specialties.
- The prevalence of short dental implants is increasing in various clinical scenarios.
- Short implants have many advantages over standard length implants.
- Various factors (surgical, biomechanical, and restorative) lead to improved success rates of short implants.
- While more long-term studies are needed, the literature indicates success rates of short implants are comparable to those of longer length implants.

INTRODUCTION

Since Branemark's discovery of titanium dental implants in the 1960s, the process of replacing missing dentition has evolved significantly due to improvements in implant design, as well as surgical and restorative techniques. Modern day dental implants come in a variety of lengths which, among other factors, can influence the long-term success rate. The discussion of short versus conventional length implants has created controversy in the sense that there are conflicting opinions on where to draw the line between these 2 categories. The definition of a short implant in particular is variable, but generally considered to be less than 10 mm. Many of the earlier cases of endosseous implant placement in edentulous mandibles involved 13-16 mm transmandibular implants,[1] which were placed in a bicortical fashion (**Fig. 1**). As time went on, the use of shorter implants became more common. In some of Brånemarks original studies, the length of dental implants used was 10 mm.[2] In 2006, the State of the in Implant Dentistry (SSID) Conference defined short implants as those with 8 mm or less of Designed

---

[a] Jesse Brown VA Medical Center, 820 South Damen Avenue, Chicago, IL 60612, USA; [b] Dental/OMS Service, 4th Floor Damen; [c] Department of Oral & Maxillofacial Surgery, University of Illinois Chicago, Chicago, IL, USA
[1] Present address: 820 South Damen Avenue, Chicago, IL 60612.
* Corresponding author. Jesse Brown VA Medical Center, 820 South Damen Avenue, 4th Floor Damen, Chicago, IL 60612.
E-mail address: raza.hussain@va.gov

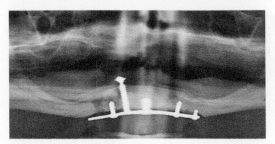

Fig. 1. Transmandibular implant (Infected).

Intrabony length (DIL).[3] Renouard also defined a short implant as one being less than 8 mm, and an ultrashort implant being < 5 mm.[4,5] Benefits of short implants specifically revolve around the ability to avoid bone augmentation and overcome anatomic limitations. Therefore, short implants can be considered less invasive, less complex, and both time and cost-saving.[6] For the purposes of our discussion we will consider short implants as any implant with a length of less than 10 mm.

WHAT IS A SHORT IMPLANT?

As previously stated, short dental implants are 2-piece implants of standard width and less than 10 mm in length. They are placed via osteotomy preparation and have various integration times based on anatomic location. Short dental implants were developed with the purpose of acting as "permanent" replacements for missing dentition, not to be confused with mini dental implants which have a narrow diameter and are designed to temporarily retain a preliminary prosthesis. Short implants less than 5-6 mm are commonly referred to as ultrashort. An implant less than 4 mm begins to encroach on the internal implant components that allow attachment to the clinical crown.

ADVANTAGES OF SHORT IMPLANTS

1. *Overcome anatomic limitations:* Such anatomic structures include the maxillary sinus, nasopalatine canal, and inferior alveolar canal (**Fig. 2**).
2. *Avoid complex surgery:* Prior to the development of short implants many patients underwent extensive grafting or reconstructive procedures in preparation for dental implant placement. These procedures could be as extensive as major autogenous bone graft procurement from sites such as the anterior iliac crest. LeFort I osteotomies with interpositional bone grafting were also at times utilized in order to

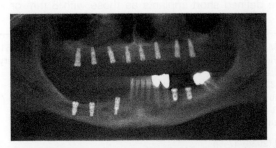

Fig. 2. Right side with nerve lateralization and standard length implants, left side with short implants.

provide sufficient bone for maxillary implant placement (**Fig. 3**). Additionally, nerve lateralization procedures have been proposed for the posterior mandible when minimal vertical bone stock exists. These procedures are technique sensitive and risk transient nerve injury (**Fig. 4**).

3. *Shorter treatment time*: In the case of an atrophic mandible, for example, the elimination of ridge augmentation via short implant placement leads to faster loading and restoration.
4. *Fewer post-op complications*: Naturally with fewer surgical steps, post-op complications are less likely to arise
5. *More cost-effective*: For both the clinician and patient

In a study by Stellingsma in 2003, the authors compared 3 different implant treatment methods for implant overdentures in the severely resorbed mandible.[7] The first group received transmandibular implants, the second received bony augmentation and axial implants, and the third group received short implants without augmentation. The authors found all 3 methods improved the patient's quality of life, but the treatment time and morbidity from autologous grafting was the least favorable option by the subjects.[7]

In the 4th European Association of Osseointegration (EAO) Conference in 2015, three systematic reviews evaluated the role of short implants in immediate extraction sites, as well as the posterior maxilla and mandible with or without bone augmentation.[8] The Conference concluded both options were viable, but that the placement of short implants had fewer complications.[8]

A systematic review in 2016 analyzed 14 RCTs comparing implant restoration in the posterior mandible with either short implants, or long implants following vertical bony augmentation.[9] The study found no differences in implant failure or prosthetic failure, however, complications were higher with vertical bony augmentation (OR 8.3).[9]

FACTORS FOR SUCCESS

There are numerous factors which contribute to a successful outcome of an implant. For a short implant to have comparable success rates to standard length implants, biomechanics must be optimized and a thoughtful restorative plan must be incorporated. With the use of standard-length dental implants, excessive forces can often be countered via increased implant length and engaging buttress bone for additional stability. Short implants, on the other hand, do not have this advantage and therefore the clinician must utilize different techniques to offset occlusal forces.

1. *Implant surface design*: Increased surface area is more optimal, especially for implants lacking length. This can be accomplished by increasing the number of

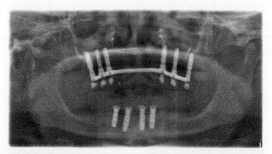

Fig. 3. Maxillary reconstruction with LeFort I osteotomy and Interpositional Ilium graft (Raza A. Hussain, BDS, DMD, FACS).

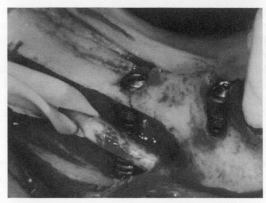

Fig. 4. Nerve lateralization procedure prior to implant placement.

threads, increasing the depth, and using a square thread design as opposed to v-shaped.

2. *Bone quality:* In general, all implants will be more stable and have greater long-term success if placed in Type I or Type II bone. If a short implant needs to be placed in an area of lower quality bone (for example, in the posterior maxilla to avoid sinus lift), there are certain biomechanical factors, as discussed later in discussion, that can compensate and enhance success.

   Lekhom and Zarb Classification of Bone Quality[10]:

   Type I- Homogenous Cortical Bone.

   Type II- Thick cortical bone with marrow cavity.

   Type III- Thin cortical bone with dense trabecular bone of good strength.

   Type IV- Very thin cortical bone with low-density trabecular bone of poor strength.

3. *Increased number of implants*: Increasing the number of implants provides additional implant-to-bone contact, leading to improved stability. This is especially important in areas where standard length implants are not ideal (**Fig. 5**).

4. *Implant Diameter:* Studies have shown that occlusal forces are localized and primarily impact the coronal 3-5 mm of a dental implant.[11] Increasing the diameter allows for improved distribution of forces at the bone-implant interface. Therefore, utilizing a wider implant is another means of providing additional stability to a shorter length implant.

5. *Splinting:* While controversial among providers, splinting can be a useful technique when restoring short implants in that it distributes excess forces across multiple interfaces (**Figs. 6** and **7**).

6. *Crown-to-Implant Ratio:* It was previously assumed that a greater crown-to-implant ratio could result in bone loss and potential failure. More recent studies have shown that even short implants with a higher crown-to-implant ratio are not associated with higher failure rates.[2,12]

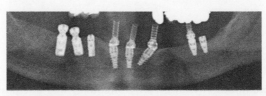

Fig. 5. Multiple splinted implants with lower left short implants for full arch reconstruction.

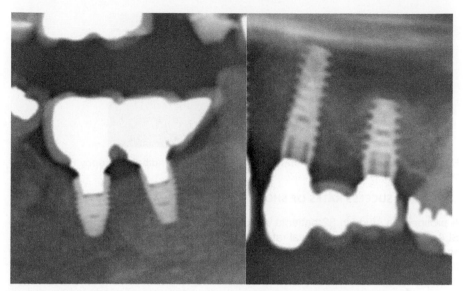

Fig. 6. Splinted short implants. (*Courtesy* Raza A. Hussain, BDS, DMD, FACS.)

PATIENT SELECTION

When considering whether a patient is a good candidate for implant surgery, the same criteria applies to implants of all length. In patients with complex medical issues, such as uncontrolled diabetes, heart disease, and immunosuppressive disorders, implant placement may not be the most ideal treatment plan.[13] Implants are typically not ideal in patients who have undergone head and neck radiation, or have a history of antiresorptive therapy. In addition, smoking can have negative effects on the long-term outcome of an implant. An advantage of short implants, as opposed to longer standard length implants, is that they allow for patients with medical issues a less invasive, safer approach to restoring their dentition (**Fig. 8**).

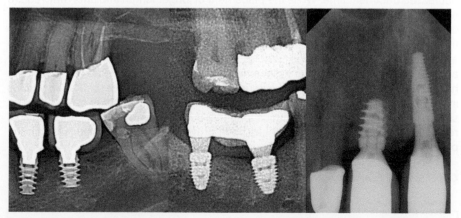

Fig. 7. Multiple short implants in function for between 5 and 10 years. (*Courtesy* Raza A. Hussain, BDS, DMD, FACS.)

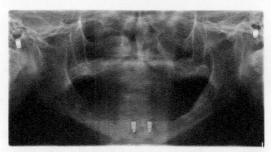

Fig. 8. Short implants placed in an elderly patient with mandibular atrophy (Raza A. Hussain, BDS, DMD, FACS).

LONG-TERM SUCCESS RATES OF SHORT VERSUS LONG IMPLANTS

A prospective study in 32 patients evaluated ultra-short implants (4 mm Straumann SLActive) and found the survival rate to be 95.7% at 2 years.[14] In a subsequent publication of this same group, Slotte found the 5 year survival rate was 92.2%.[15] These findings were consistent with 4-mm implants placed in the posterior jaws to support fixed partial dentures which had a 97.5% survival rate at 1 year.[16] Other systematic reviews have found that long implants (>6 mm) had higher complication rates when compared to short implants (≤6 mm), 32.8% versus just 6.8% respectively.[16] A systematic review in 2018 by the International Team for Implantology (ITI) included 10 RCTs, and over 1,200 implants.[16] Short implants (≤6 mm) performed similar to long implants (>6 mm), with a survival rate at 1-5 years of 96% versus 98% respectively.[16] The authors speculated this was related to the need for simultaneous bone augmentation with longer implants. Felice and colleagues[17] compared short (5 mm) implants with the bony augmentation and placement of 10 mm implants in the posterior mandible in a split mouth study. Results showed similar implant survival, and patients had no preference for one treatment option versus the other.

SUMMARY

The prevalence of short dental implants is increasing across various dental specialties. They provide an option to patients that involve less surgical trauma, lower cost, and decreased treatment time. While the placement of longer length implants may require additional surgical procedures such as ridge augmentation or maxillary sinus lift, the use of short implants can avoid these procedures altogether, benefitting both the patient and clinician. Strict adherence to reliable surgical and restorative principles is essential for an ideal outcome, among other factors such as patient compliance and medical history. As implant placement in general has evolved over time, there has been a considerable amount of literature comparing the success rates of various implant lengths. Compared to early literature, more recent studies have shown a similar rate of success in short versus long implants. While the use of short implants remains somewhat controversial, it has been proven that they can offer a long term, predictable outcome for almost any clinical scenario.

CLINICS CARE POINTS

- The use of short dental implants for many different clinical scenarios in dentistry is rapidly increasing.

- With many of the non-surgical based specialties in dentistry now offering dental implant placement the thought of decreasing potential significant complications is very appealing.
- Short dental implants can be complete with less surgical trauma and often in less time.
- The clinician must take into consideration each particular scenario and ensure that short dental implant placement is in the patient's best interest.
- Strict adherence to tried and true surgical and prosthodontic principles is key for an ideal outcome.
- Short dental implants can offer a long term, predictable outcome for almost any clinical scenario.

DISCLOSURE

All authors have no financial conflicts of interest to disclose.

REFERENCES

1. Bosker H, van Dijk L. The transmandibular implant: a 12-year follow-up study. J Oral Maxillofac Surg 1989;47(5):442–50.
2. Brånemark PI. Osseointegration and its experimental background. J Prosthet Dent 1983;50(3):399–410.
3. State of the science on implant dentistry. Consensus conference proceedings, August 3-6, 2006. Int J Oral Maxillofac Implants 2007;22(Suppl):7–226.
4. Nisand D, Renouard F. Short implant in limited bone volume. Periodontal 2000 2014;66(1):72–96.
5. Renouard F, Nisand D. Impact of implant length and diameter on survival rates. Clin Oral Implants Res 2006;17(Suppl 2):35–51.
6. Pistilli R, Felice P, Cannizzaro G, et al. Posterior atrophic jaws rehabilitated with prostheses supported by 6 mm long 4 mm wide implants or by longer implants in augmented bone. One-year post-loading results from a pilot randomized controlled trial. Eur J Oral Implantol 2013;6(4):359–72.
7. Stellingsma K, Bouma J, Stegenga B, et al. Satisfaction and psychosocial aspects of patients with an extremely resorbed mandible treated with implant-retained overdentures. A prospective, comparative study. Clin Oral Implants Res 2003;14(2):166–72.
8. Sanz M, Donos N, Alcoforado G, et al. Therapeutic concepts and methods for improving dental implant outcomes. Summary and consensus statements. The 4th EAO Consensus Conference 2015. Clin Oral Implants Res 2015;26(Suppl 11):202–6.
9. Camps-Font O, Burgueño-Barris G, Figueiredo R, et al. Interventions for dental implant placement in atrophic edentulous mandibles: vertical bone augmentation and alternative treatments. A meta-analysis of randomized clinical trials. J Periodontol 2016;87(12):1444–57.
10. Lekholm U, Zarb GA. Patient selection and preparation. In: Branemark PI, Zarb GA, Albrektsson T, editors. Tissue integrated prosthesis: osseointegration in clinical dentistry. Chicago, IL: Quintessence Publishing; 1985. p. 199–209.
11. Bedrossian E. Compendium July/August 2020 Volume 41. Issue 7.
12. Tawil G, Aboujaoude N, Younan R. Influence of prosthetic parameters on the survival and complication rates of short implants. Int J Oral Maxillofac Implants 2006; 21(2):275–82.

13. Shokouhi B, Cerajewska T. Radiotherapy and the survival of dental implants: a systematic review. Br J Oral Maxillofac Surg 2022;60(4):422–9.
14. Slotte C, Grønningsaeter A, Halmøy AM, et al. Four-millimeter implants supporting fixed partial dental prostheses in the severely resorbed posterior mandible: two-year results. Clin Implant Dent Relat Res 2012;14(Suppl 1):e46–58.
15. Slotte C, Grønningsaeter A, Halmøy AM, et al. Four-millimeter-long posterior-mandible implants: 5-year outcomes of a prospective multicenter study. Clin Implant Dent Relat Res 2015;17(Suppl 2):e385–95.
16. Jung RE, Al-Nawas B, Araujo M, et al. Group 1 ITI consensus report: the influence of implant length and design and medications on clinical and patient-reported outcomes. Clin Oral Implants Res 2018;29(Suppl 16):69–77.
17. Felice P, Checchi V, Pistilli R, et al. Bone augmentation versus 5-mm dental implants in posterior atrophic jaws. Four-month post-loading results from a randomised controlled clinical trial. Eur J Oral Implantol 2009;2(4):267–81.

Applications of Cone Beam Computed Tomography Scans in Dental Medicine and Potential Medicolegal Issues

Zachary A. Heller, DO, DMD[a],*, Maritzabel Hogge, MS, DDS[b],
Michael R. Ragan, DMD, JD, LLM[a],
Jason E. Portnof, DMD, MD, FACD, FICD[a,c]

KEYWORDS

- CBCT • Cone beam • Panoramic • Plan film • Maxillofacial • FOV • Radiography

KEY POINTS

- A cone beam computed tomography (CBCT) scan produces images in orthogonal and non-orthogonal with great spatial resolution.
- When a dental health care practitioner (DHP) orders a CBCT scan, they should consider if it is truly indicated, as CBCT scans carry up to four times the dosage of radiation compared to panoramic radiographs.
- Any diagnostic imaging obtained of a patient should include a formal interpretive report commenting on the findings within the imaging.
- Ordering of limited field of view (FOV) CBCT scans and failing to report on abnormal findings present outside of the region of interest (ROI) is a potential medicolegal issue.

BACKGROUND

Cone beam computed tomographic (CBCT) imaging was initially developed for medical applications in angiography in the early 1980's. The first CBCT machines were introduced in Europe in 1996 and made their way to the United States in 2001.[1] There are three main components to CBCT imaging: image production, visualization, and interpretation. A CBCT scan is performed using a rotating platform carrying an x-ray source and detector. The collimator in the x-ray tube helps to generate a cone-

[a] Department of Oral and Maxillofacial Surgery, Nova Southeastern University College of Dental Medicine, 3050 South University Drive, Davie, FL 33314, USA; [b] Department of Maxillofacial Medicine, Nova Southeastern University College of Dental Medicine, 3050 South University Drive, Davie, FL 33314, USA; [c] Private Practice, 9980 North Central Park Boulevard, Suite 113, Boca Raton, FL 33428, USA
* Corresponding author. 9980 North Central Park Boulevard, Suite 113, Boca Raton, FL 33428
E-mail address: heller.zach@gmail.com

Dent Clin N Am 68 (2024) 55–65
https://doi.org/10.1016/j.cden.2023.07.009
0011-8532/24/© 2023 Elsevier Inc. All rights reserved.

shaped beam. The source of radiation is directed through the region of interest (ROI), and the residual attenuated radiation beam is projected onto an area x-ray detector on the opposite side.[2] During the rotation, multiple planar projection images (ranging from 150 to 599 unique radiographic views) are captured sequentially. The complete series of these images is referred to as the projection data.[1]

Using sophisticated algorithms, imaging software reconstructs the projection data, producing a digital volume of anatomic data that can be visualized three dimensionally in voxel resolution. A voxel is the smallest subunit of a digital volume. CBCT voxels are generally isotropic (the X, Y, and Z dimensions are all equal) and range in size from approximately 0.07 mm to 0.40 mm per side.[1,3] The projection data in these three orthogonal planes is limited by the dimensions of the scan volume, also known as the field of view (FOV). CBCT units are classified according to the maximum FOV incorporated from the scan. Large FOV scans provide images of the entire craniofacial skeleton. A medium FOV scan provides images of the maxilla or mandible. A focused or limited FOV scan provides high-resolution images of limited regions.[4]

Cone-beam imaging has numerous features compared to multidetector computed tomography (MDCT) that makes it suitable for dental applications. These include: size & cost, speed of image acquisition, image resolution, and radiation dose. A CBCT machine has a smaller physical footprint and costs approximately one-fourth to one-fifth as much as an MDCT machine.[5] Additionally, with more recent advances in solid-state detector achievable frame rates and computer processing speeds, most CBCT scanning can be performed in less than 30 seconds.[4,6] According to the 2007 recommendations from the International Commission on Radiological Protection, the effective dose for various CBCT machines ranges from 25 to 1025 uSv. These values are roughly equivalent to 1 to 42 digital panoramic radiographs (approximately 24 uSv) or 3 to 123 days' equivalent per capita natural background radiation (approximately 3000 uSv in the United States) (**Table 1**).[7]

CONE BEAM CENTRAL TOMOGRAPHY AND DENTAL IMPLANT PLANNING

Today, roughly every fourth article published on CBCT is related to the use of CBCT scans in implant dentistry, with two out of three on the presurgical use of CBCT scans, primarily for presurgical planning and transfer to implant placement.[8] Radiographic assessment of the 3D implant position, angulation, and restorative space is essential

Table 1
Range of radiation doses

	Range of Dose of Radiation
CBCT	11–674 μSv (median value 61 μSv) for small and medium FOV scans (volumes <10 cm) 30–1073 μSv (median value 87 μSv) for large FOV scans (volumes > 10 cm)
Panoramic Radiograph	9–26 μSv
Intraoral full mouth radiographic series	34.9 μSv (PSP plates/F-speed film, rectangular collimation) 170.7 μSv (PSP plates/F-speed film, round collimation) 388 μSv (D-speed film, round collimation)
MDCT	290–1410 μSv
Average Background Radiation in USA	8 μSv per day

Adapted from Tamimi D, Hatcher D. Specialty Imaging Temporomandibular Joint 1st Edition. Elsevier 2016, Philadelphia, PA.

during presurgical diagnostics and treatment planning of implant sites within the residual alveolar bone.[9] CBCT scans provide cross-sectional images of the alveolar bone height, width, and angulation and accurately depict vital structures, such as the inferior alveolar dental nerve canal or the maxillary sinus (**Figure 1**).[10]

When a CBCT scan is performed on patients with preexisting metallic dental materials (ie, amalgam restorations, porcelain fused to metal (PFM) crowns, dental implants), these materials can create artifacts in the scan due to the beam hardening phenomena. This phenomenon occurs when an x-ray beam composed of polychromatic energies passes through an object, leaving only high energy photons to contribute to the beam and thus the mean beam energy is increased or "hardened."[11] This can result in a streaking artifact, which manifests as multiple dark streaking bands positioned between two dense objects. The presence of these artifacts decreases the overall image quality and if severe enough can render the scan useless.[12]

Implant planning software, utilizing CBCT imaging, allows greater sophistication in analysis and planning, providing interactive methods of translating prosthetic planning to the surgical site. In implant planning, software can be used to select and direct the placement of implant bodies either directly by the use of CBCT image-guided navigation or indirectly via the construction of 3-D printed surgical guides fabricated to the patient's specific measurements obtained on CBCT imaging.[13] Currently, there is no literature to support placing implants via computer-guided surgery being superior to conventional methods. Implants placed utilizing computer-guided surgery with a follow-up period of at least 12 months demonstrate a mean survival rate of 97.3% (n = 1941), which is comparable to implants placed following conventional procedures.[14]

When planning dental implants in an edentulous patient, CBCT scans can assist with virtual implant placement and fabrication of surgical guides. In the edentulous patient, a new denture can be fabricated and used as a radiographic stent. The patient then has a CBCT scan performed with the radiographic stent in place. When obtaining this scan, it is paramount that the intaglio surface of this denture fits perfectly to the mucosa with no "air" pockets. If cross-sections of the CBCT scan show space

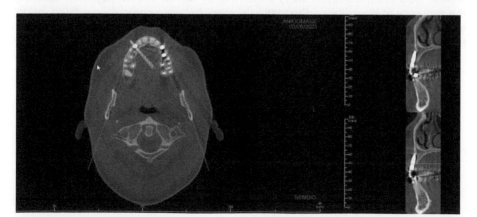

Fig. 1. The left image is a CBCT axial cut of the maxilla, the green lines indicate the location of the axial view in relation to the sagittal view. The images in the right-hand column are the sagittal views in the locations of the green lines from the right-hand image. In this view, the relationship to vital structures, such as the nasal floor, and the apex of the implant can be appreciated. As well as the angle of the implant's inclination.

between the mucosa and the stent, then the surgical guide stent fabricated using this scan will not fit, and the implant placement will be inaccurate.[15,16]

Proponents for the use of CBCT scans in dental implantology argue that the benefits of planning implants for the edentulous patient assisted by CBCT scan and static surgical guide include: complete knowledge of the bone morphology before surgery, use of a flapless surgical technique which shortens the surgical time and reduces postoperative pain and swelling, and laboratory preparation of the denture based on the transfer of the CBCT plan to a working model.[15,16,17] However, this all falls under the pretense that the CBCT scan was obtained accurately and that the provider ordering the scan is capable of interpreting any errors before moving forward with any stent fabrication.

CONE BEAM CENTRAL TOMOGRAPHY AND VIRTUAL SURGICAL PLANNING

Today the use of CBCT imaging for presurgical orthognathic treatment has begun to overtake conventional model surgery in popularity amongst providers performing these procedures. From a presurgical imaging standpoint, the increased adoption of CBCT can partly be attributed to a CBCT machine's ability to obtain high-resolution images in under 30 seconds, allowing for a two-dimensional (2D) cephalometric analysis to be visualized in the three-dimensional (3D) realm.[4,18] As computer software technology has continued to advance, the software environments which allow virtual surgical planning (VSP) have been shown to be less time-consuming and in some ways more accurate than conventional model surgery.[17,19] The key feature that makes systems interoperable is the use of image files that are conformant with the Digital Imaging and Communications in Medicine (DICOM) standard file format.[19] When using VSP for orthognathic surgery, DICOM data from CBCT scans can be used to construct physical stereolithographic models or to generate virtual 3-D models (**Figure 3**).[20] These reconstructions can then be used as aids intraoperatively to adapt custom cutting guides and analyze the spatial relationship of neighboring structures[21] (**Figure 2**).

A reason VSP and subsequently CBCT has become so widely adopted, is its high level of recorded accuracy. A study performed by De Riu and colleagues, measuring the accuracy of bimaxillary orthognathic surgery between computer-assisted model surgery and conventional model surgery at the immediate postoperative time point, found angular measurements were more accurate with computer-assisted surgery

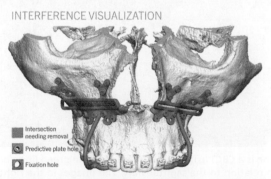

INTERFERENCE VISUALIZATION

Intersection needing removal
Predictive plate hole
Fixation hole

Fig. 2. 3-D rendering created from a preoperative CBCT scan highlighting anticipated bony interferences and placement of custom cutting guides for a planned LeFort 1 osteotomy advancement.

than with conventional presurgical planning with 1.19° difference between planned and actual movements.[22]

Despite the recorded increase in accuracy of virtual surgical planning over conventional model surgery, there are still areas in which error can be introduced. One crucial step in virtual surgical planning that can introduce significant error is the acquisition of the CBCT scan. In maxilla-first virtual surgical planning, the CBCT scan, is in essence, the facebow transfer for the model surgery. Therefore, the CBCT scan must be obtained in centric relation for maxilla-first virtual surgical planning. If the patient is not in centric relation with their condyle in the fossa, then the intermediate splint will be inaccurate and place the maxilla off from the pre-planned position.[23]

Another major limitation to the use of CBCT when performing VSP is CBCT technology currently lacks the ability to capture the teeth and their occlusal surfaces with high accuracy. In order to produce accurate CAD/CAM splints for intraoperative use, it is necessary to replace inaccurate occlusal surfaces from CBCT scans with high-resolution scans of the maxillary and mandibular arches utilizing digital intraoral scanners.[24]

CONE BEAM CENTRAL TOMOGRAPHY AND ENDODONTICS

Success in endodontics is assessed in healing of the periapical bone adjacent to obturated canals. Goldman and colleagues showed that in evaluating healing of periapical lesions using 2-D periapical radiographs there was only 47% agreement between six examiners.[25,26] Goldman and colleagues also reported that when those same examiners evaluated the same films at two different times, they only had 19%–80% agreement between the two evaluations.[27] The limitations associated with traditional 2-D intraoral radiography, has led to a greater adoption of CBCT imaging in endodontics.

Bernardes and colleagues retrospectively compared conventional periapical radiographs and CBCT images for 20 patients with suspected root fractures. They found that CBCT was able to detect fractures in 18 (90%) of patients whereas conventional periapicals could only detect fractures 6 to 8 of the cases (30% to 40%) and indicated that CBCT was an excellent supplement to conventional radiography in the diagnosis of root fractures[28] (see **Figure 3**). Stavropoulos and Wenzel compared CBCT to digital- and film-based intraoral periapical radiography for the detection of periapical bone defects on 10 frozen pig mandibles by four calibrated examiners. They reported

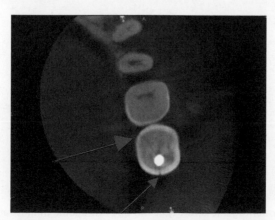

Fig. 3. Axial cut of a CBCT scan highlighting a vertical crown root fracture of a mandibular second molar.

that CBCT provides greater diagnostic accuracy (61%) compared with digital (39%) and (44%) conventional radiographs.[29]

Despite the advantages of CBCT imaging in endodontics, conventional intraoral radiography provides clinicians with an accessible, cost effective, high-resolution imaging modality that continues to be of value in endodontic therapy. There are, however, specific situations, both pre- and postoperatively, where the understanding of spatial relationships afforded by CBCT imaging facilitates diagnosis and influences treatment. CBCT imaging is a useful task-specific imaging modality and should be limited to the assessment and treatment of complex endodontic conditions.[25]

CONE BEAM CENTRAL TOMOGRAPHY AND PATHOLOGY

CBCT can be used as a noninvasive diagnostic technique in maxillofacial pathosis (see **Fig. 3**). Simon and colleagues compared the diagnosis of large periapical lesions (granulomas vs cysts) using CBCT and biopsy. These authors examined 17 lesions with a size equal to or greater than 1 cm × 1 cm, making a preoperative diagnosis based on the density of the lesions measured by CBCT. There was concordance between the preoperative diagnosis based on CBCT and the histologic study in 13 of 17 cases. In four of the 17 lesions, the preoperative diagnosis by CBCT was of a cyst whereas the histologic result was of chronic periapical granuloma.[30] These results suggest that CBCT could be a rapid diagnostic method without invasive surgery and/or prolonged periods of observation to see if a nonsurgical therapy is effective (**Fig. 4**).

The occasional discovery of occult pathologies upon commissioning of maxillofacial imaging is a widespread and well-known occurrence, a study conducted by Bondemark and colleagues in 2006 showed revealed that the panoramic imaging of 8.7% of 496 orthodontic patients displayed radiographic lesions other than those for which the image was commissioned.[31,32] However, CBCT scans with their increased resolution and field of view, have multiplied the range of pathologies that can be incidentally detected. The potential for incidentally encountering an unexpected pathology with a CBCT scan is triple that compared to a panoramic radiograph.[33]

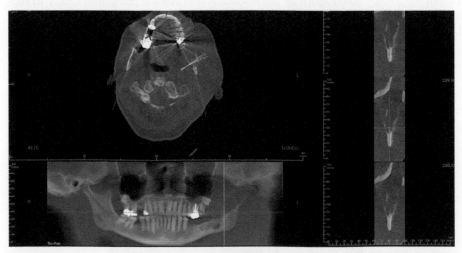

Fig. 4. CBCT of an odontogenic keratocyst. The CBCT is capable of illustrating the extent of lytic bone destruction. Additionally, the coronal views provide the visualization of the buccal and lingual expansion of the mandibular bone.

Interpretation and Reporting of a Cone Beam Central Tomography Image

The essential elements of a cone-beam computed tomographic radiologic report include: patient information, scan information, radiologic findings, and radiologic impression. The most important and often most overlooked components of the radiologic report for a CBCT scan are the radiologic findings and impression. The radiologic findings should include reference to intraoral findings such as: missing teeth, pre-existing restorations, presence of implants, root canal-treated teeth, periapical lesions, alveolar bone status, and edentulous regions. As well as making reference to extraoral findings/structures such as: the temporomandibular joint (TMJ), paranasal sinuses, nasopharyngeal airway, soft tissues of the neck, and intracranial calcifications.[34,35] The radiologic impression component of the report should include a differential diagnosis related to the rationale for the imaging examination or clinically significant incidental findings, a comparison to previous imaging studies (if available), and any recommendations for additional clinical or diagnostic studies to clarify, confirm, or exclude a diagnosis.[36]

DISCUSSION

According to the National Council of Radiation Protection and Measurement, the average annual radiation dose per person in the United States is 6.2 mSv, half of which comes from natural background sources, such as cosmic radiation, naturally occurring radiation in the ground and human body, and the radioactive gasses radon and thoron, which are produced by the radioactive decay of naturally occurring elements such as uranium and thorium.[2,37] Another 48% of the average annual radiation dose a person in the United States is exposed to, comes from medical treatment and diagnostic tests. Of that 48%, half, or 24% of the total dose, comes from CT imaging of one form or another.[37]

Currently, there are multiple different medical device companies manufacturing CBCT machines for medical use. The exposure profile of a CBCT scan varies from machine to machine and is also influenced by the FOV of the scan. A full FOV CBCT scan requires seven times the effective dosage of radiation compared to panoramic imaging.[38] When compared to a medical grade CT scan of the maxilla and mandible, a full FOV CBCT scan of the maxilla and mandible has a fraction of the effective dose of radiation (1800–2100 mSv vs 34–89 mSv respectively).[39,40,41] Which according to the Environmental Protection Agency's Federal Guidance Report, would account for only 2% to 5% of the effective dosage of medical grade CT.[10,42]

The US Food and Drug Administration (FDA) classifies CBCT machines as CT machines.[43] The regulatory standards and practices for CBCT machines vary state to state. In states within the US where a CBCT machine is considered a medical device, a dental technician or assistant may not be qualified to perform a CBCT scan under state law. In these regions, performing a CBCT scan may be restricted to a certified medical radiology technician, radiologist, or a specifically trained individual.[34,44] The importance of a properly trained individual operating a CBCT machine and performing scans is highlighted by the risk of fatal malignancy related to CBCT radiation exposure. In adults, the risk can range from 1 in 100,000. In children, the risk of fatal malignancy related to CBCT radiation exposure can be doubled.[41]

Conventional medical radiology requires an over-read by a medical radiologist and a formal written report. Accredited health care centers are required to use the report as a manifestation of quality and a tool to facilitate peer review of images. Historically, these practices have not been followed by the field of dental medicine, because most dental images are considered diagnostic tools.[38] There is one standard of care for any procedure in dental medicine and the dental health care practitioner (DHP) must meet said standard. Although over-reads are generally not required, the DHP ordering the CBCT study must be capable of reading and interpreting the entire FOV captured by the study, including structures outside the region of interest.[34,45] Dental health care practitioners ordering CBCT scans, should be able to read and interpret any conventional radiograph, including a CBCT scan, and identify and report any identifiable pathology. Whether it is with a conventional panoramic image or CBCT scan, failure to diagnose an identifiable pathology could be a potential medicolegal issue.[46]

As a matter of law, a DHP owes a duty to a patient to use the ordinary skills, means, and methods that are recognized as necessary and which are customarily followed in the particular type of case according to the standard of those who are qualified by training and experience to perform similar services in the community.[47] This standard of care is judged on a local level for generalists or general practitioners, whereas specialists are held to a national standard of care.[48] For one to prevail in a medical malpractice action, a plaintiff must identify the standard of care owed by the DHP, produce evidence that the DHP breached the duty to render medical care in accordance with the requisite standard of care, and establish that the breach proximately caused the injury alleged.[49]

A DHP must perform proper diagnostic imaging for preoperative planning. The issue is whether a DHP can rely solely on periapical and/or panoramic radiographs in their preoperative planning diagnostic imaging, or whether MDCT or CBCT are considered the standard of care.[50] When a DHP does elect to order a CBCT scan, they are responsible for the identification of all pathology within the FOV. Some authors have suggested a solution being the decrease of the FOV to include only those structures within the usual and customary dental view. A potential problem could arise if the FOV is reduced to exclude unfamiliar structures and therefore the ability to diagnose potential conditions. The better course is to include within the FOV all anatomic structures relevant to the treatment planning of the patient. Prudence may dictate that the DHP defer reading of the CBCT to a practitioner with the requisite special knowledge to comprehensively interpret the diagnostic modality. It is the authors' counsel that the DHP strongly consider deferring to an Oral and Maxillofacial Radiologist or to use the services of a CBCT "Over-read" service. These "over-read" services can provide the DHP with a written radiologic analysis and assessment and represent a method of reducing potential exposure for failure to diagnose disease/lesion and/or anatomic abnormalities.

The use of CBCT scans in dental medicine today is becoming an increasingly valuable imaging modality. Today's CBCT scanners are capable of rapidly obtaining high-resolution, three-dimensional imaging of the maxillofacial region. Although CBCT scanners are capable of these measures, because of the increased cost and radiation exposure to the patient, CBCT scans should not be considered the blanket "gold standard" for all maxillofacial imaging in dental medicine. It is the authors' belief that less invasive imaging modalities be performed first in the assessment and diagnosis of patients, reserving CBCT scans as an adjuvant task-specific imaging modality when indicated.

DISCLOSURE

There are no disclosures in relation to this article.

ACKNOWLEDGMENTS

The authors are grateful for the contributions of our authors without whom this work would not have been possible: Avi I. Dumanis, BS, Predoctoral Student, College of Dental Medicine, Nova Southeastern University College of Dental Medicine, Fort

Lauderdale, Florida. Victor P. Celis, DMD, Resident, Department of Oral and Maxillo-facial Surgery, Nova Southeastern University College of Dental Medicine, Fort Lauderdale, Florida.

REFERENCES

1. Hatcher DC. Operational principles for Cone-beam computed tomography. J Am Dent Assoc 2010;141. https://doi.org/10.14219/jada.archive.2010.0359.
2. Scarfe WC. Cone-Beam Computed Tomography: Volume Acquisition. In: Farman AG, editor. Oral radiology principles and interpretation. 7th edition. St.Louis, MO: Elsevier Mosby; 2014. p. 185–98.
3. Pauwels R, Araki K, Siewerdsen JH, et al. Technical aspects of dental CBCT: State of the art. Dentomaxillofacial Radiol 2015;44(1):20140224.
4. Scarfe WC, Li Z, Aboelmaaty W, et al. Maxillofacial Cone Beam Computed Tomography: Essence, elements and steps to interpretation. Aust Dent J 2012; 57:46–60.
5. Angelopoulos C, Scarfe WC, Farman AG. A comparison of maxillofacial CBCT and medical CT. Atlas Oral Maxillofac Surg Clin North Am 2012;1–17, 20.
6. Scarfe WC, Farman AG. What is cone-beam CT and how does it work? Dent Clin 2008;52(4):707–30.
7. The 2007 recommendations of the International Commission on Radiological Protection. IRCP Publication 103. Ann ICRP 2007;37(2–4):9–34.
8. Zhang N, Liu S, Hu Z, et al. Accuracy of virtual surgical planning in two-jaw orthognathic surgery: Comparison of planned and actual results. Oral Surgery, Oral Medicine, Oral Pathology and Oral Radiology 2016;122(2):143–51.
9. Scherer MD. Presurgical implant-site assessment and restoratively driven digital planning. Dent Clin North Am 2014;58(3):561–95.
10. Scarfe WC, Farman AG, Sukovic P. Clinical applications of cone-beam computed tomography in dental practice. J Can Dent Assoc 2006;72(1):75–80. PMID: 16480609.
11. Pessis E, Campagna R, Sverzut JM, et al. Virtual monochromatic spectral imaging with fast kilovoltage switching: reduction of metal artifacts at CT. Radiographics 2013;33(2):573–83.
12. Jaju P. Cone beam computed tomography: Physics and artifacts. Cone Beam Computed Tomography: A Clinician's Guide to 3D Imaging. 2015:4-4. doi:10.5005/jp/books/12484_3.
13. Tyndall DA, Price JB, Tetradis S, et al. Position statement of the American Academy of Oral and Maxillofacial Radiology on selection criteria for the use of radiology in dental implantology with emphasis on cone beam computed tomography. Oral Surg Oral Med Oral Pathol Oral Radiol 2012;113(6):817–26.
14. Bornstein MM, Al-Nawas B, Kuchler U, et al. Consensus statements and recommended clinical procedures regarding contemporary surgical and radiographic techniques in implant dentistry. Int J Oral Maxillofac Implants 2014;29(Suppl): 78–82.
15. Miloro M, Ghali GE, Larsen P, Waite P. In: Peterson's principles of oral and maxillofacial surgeryVol. 2, 3rd edition. Cham: Springer; 2022. p. 311–66.
16. Poeschl PW, Schmidt N, Guevara-Rojas G, et al. Comparison of cone-beam and conventional multislice computed tomography for image-guided dental implant planning. Clin Oral Invest 2013;17(1):317–24.
17. Jayaratne YSN, Zwahlen RA, Lo J, et al. Computer-Aided Maxillofacial Surgery: An Update. Surg Innovat 2010;17(3):217–25.

18. Gateno J, Xia JJ, Teichgraeber JF. New 3-dimensional cephalometric analysis for orthognathic surgery. J Oral Maxillofac Surg 2011;69(3):606–22.
19. Scarfe WC. Cone-beam computed tomography: volume preparation. In: Farman AG, editor. Oral radiology principles and interpretation. 7th edition. St.Louis, MO: Elsevier Mosby; 2014. p. 199–213.
20. Ahmad M, Jenny J, Downie M. Application of cone beam computed tomography in oral and maxillofacial surgery. Aust Dent J 2012;57:82–94.
21. Swennen GR, Mollemans W, Schutyser F. Three-dimensional treatment planning of orthognathic surgery in the era of virtual imaging. J Oral Maxillofac Surg 2009;67(10):2080–92 [published correction appears in J Oral Maxillofac Surg. 2009;67(12):2703].
22. De Riu G, Virdis PI, Meloni SM, et al. Accuracy of computer-assisted orthognathic surgery. J Cranio-Maxillofacial Surg 2018;46(2):293–8.
23. Miloro M, Ghali GE, Larsen PE, et al. Ch 64. Sequencing in Orthognathic Surgery. In: Peterson's principles of oral and maxillofacial surgeryvol 2, 3rd edition. Cham: Springer; 2022. p. 1945–68.
24. Miloro M, Ghali GE, Larsen PE, et al. Ch 61. Model Surgery and Computer-Aided Surgical Simulation for Orthognathic Surgery. In: Peterson's principles of oral and maxillofacial surgeryvol 2, 3rd edition. Cham: Springer; 2022. p. 1825–49.
25. Scarfe WC, Levin MD, Gane D, et al. Use of cone beam computed tomography in endodontics. Int J Dent 2009;2009:634567.
26. Goldman M, Pearson AH, Darzenta N. Endodontic success–who's reading the radiograph? Oral Surg Oral Med Oral Pathol 1972;33(3):432–7.
27. Goldman M, Pearson AH, Darzenta N. Reliability of radiographic interpretations. Oral Surg Oral Med Oral Pathol 1974;38(2):287–93.
28. Bernardes RA, de Moraes IG, Húngaro Duarte MA, et al. Use of cone-beam volumetric tomography in the diagnosis of root fractures. Oral Surg Oral Med Oral Pathol Oral Radiol Endod 2009;108(2):270–7.
29. Stavropoulos A, Wenzel A. Accuracy of cone beam dental CT, intraoral digital and conventional film radiography for the detection of periapical lesions. An ex vivo study in pig jaws. Clin Oral Invest 2007;11(1):101–6.
30. Simon JH, Enciso R, Malfaz JM, et al. Differential diagnosis of large periapical lesions using cone-beam computed tomography measurements and biopsy. J Endod 2006;32(9):833 7.
31. Lombardo L. Unexpected artefacts and occult pathologies under CBCT. Oral Implant 2017;10(2):97.
32. Bondemark L, Jeppsson M, Lindh-Ingildsen L, et al. Incidental findings of pathology and abnormality in pretreatment orthodontic panoramic radiographs. Angle Orthod 2006;76(1):98–102.
33. Cha JY, Mah J, Sinclair P. Incidental findings in the maxillofacial area with 3-dimensional cone-beam imaging. Am J Orthod Dentofacial Orthop 2007;132(1):7–14.
34. Carter L, Farman AG, Geist J, Scarfe WC, Angelopoulos C, Nair MK, Hildebolt CF, Tyndall D, Shrout M, American Academy of Oral, Radiology Maxillofacial. American academy of oral and maxillofacial radiology executive opinion statement on performing and interpreting diagnostic cone beam computed tomography. Oral Surg Oral Med Oral Pathol Oral Radiol Endod 2008;106(4):561–2.
35. American College of Radiology: ACR practice parameter for communication of diagnostic imaging findings. Practice Guidelines and Technical Standards (2005). http://www.acr.org Accessed December 29, 2022.

36. European Society of Radiology (ESR). Good practice for radiological reporting. Guidelines from the European Society of Radiology (ESR). Insights Imaging 2011;2(2):93–6.
37. NCRP Report No.160—Ionizing Radiation Exposure of the Population of the United States. Bethesda, MD, National Council on Radiation Protection & Measurements (NCRP), 2009. https://ncrponline.org/publications/reports/ncrp-report-160-2/.
38. Carter JB, Stone JD, Clark RS, et al. Applications of cone-beam computed tomography in oral and maxillofacial surgery: An overview of published indications and clinical usage in United States academic centers and oral and maxillofacial surgery practices. J Oral Maxillofac Surg 2016;74(4):668–79.
39. Loubele M, Bogaerts R, Van Dijck E, et al. Comparison between effective radiation dose of CBCT and MSCT scanners for dentomaxillofacial applications. Eur J Radiol 2009;71(3):461–8.
40. Roberts JA, Drage NA, Davies J, et al. Effective dose from cone beam CT examinations in dentistry. Br J Radiol 2009;82(973):35–40.
41. Ludlow JB, Davies-Ludlow LE, Brooks SL, et al. Dosimetry of 3 CBCT devices for oral and maxillofacial radiology: CB Mercuray, NewTom 3G and i-CAT. Dentomaxillofacial Radiol 2006;35(4):219–26 [published correction appears in Dentomaxillofac Radiol. 2006 Sep;35(5):392].
42. Federal Guidance Report 14: Radiation Protection Guidance for Diagnostic and Interventional X-ray Procedures; 2012. Washing- ton, DC, Interagency Working Group on Medical Radiation, US Environmental Protection Agency (EPA), 2012. http://www.epa.gov/radiation/docs/federal/FGR14%202012-10- 10.pdf Accessed February 17, 2023.
43. Center for Devices and Radiological Health. Dental cone-beam computed tomography: FDA. U.S. Food and Drug Administration. https://www.fda.gov/radiation-emitting-products/medical-x-ray-imaging/dental-cone-beam-computed-tomography. Published September 28, 2020. Accessed February 17, 2023
44. Friedland B. Conebeam computed tomography: legal considerations. Alpha Omegan 2010;103(2):57–61.
45. Dawood A, Patel S, Brown J. Cone Beam CT in dental practice. Br Dent J 2009; 207(1):23–8.
46. Wright B. Contemporary Medico-Legal Dental Radiology. Aust Dent J 2012; 57:9–15.
47. David J. BROOKS, a Minor, by and through His Mother and Next Friend, Leatha Brooks, and Leatha Brooks, Individually, Appellants, v. Ernest SERRANO, Appellee., 279 (https://case-law.vlex.com/vid/brooks-v-serrano-no-892321224 1968).
48. Medical Negligence; Standards of Recovery; Expert Witness.; Fla. Stat. § 766.102; (2011).
49. Maria TORRES, as Parent and Natural Guardian of Luis Torres, Appellant, v. John E. SULLIVAN, Jr., M.D.; John E. Sullivan, Jr., M.D., P.A.; SMH Physician Services, Inc., d/b/a First Physicians Group; Sarasota County Public Hospital Board, d/b/a Sarasota Memorial Hospital; Gary W. Easterling, M.D.; Gary W. Easterling, M.D., P.A.; and Florida Department of Health, Appellees., 1065 (https://caselaw.findlaw.com/fl-district-court-of-appeal/1479410.html 2005).
50. Misch CE. Implant treatment planning. In: Contemporary implant dentistry. 3rd edition. Mosby; 2008. p. 701.

Treatment of Medication-Related Osteonecrosis of the Jaw: Controversies in Causality and Therapy

Leslie Robin Halpern, MD, DDS, PHD, MPH, FICD[a],*,
David Russell Adams, DDS, FICD[b]

KEYWORDS

- Medication-related osteonecrosis of the jaw • MRONJ • Antiresorptive drugs
- Bisphosphonates • Denosumab • Controversy • MRONJ staging • Drug holiday

KEY POINTS

- Medication-related osteonecrosis of the jaw (MRONJ) is a complex and "elusive" condition seen by the oral health care provider and plagued by controversy.
- With the evolution of pharmacologic choices, and debates about staging of disease progression, there is still no uniform agreement on treatment type, duration and resolution of MRONJ.
- It is recommended that all patients who are taking bisphosphonates or antiresorptive therapy for osteoporosis be given an in-depth informed consent of potential risks, although low, of MRONJ as an either early or late causality of implant failure.
- The 2022 AAOMS task force neither supports nor refutes the application of a "drug holiday" and recommends a case-by-case evaluation with respect for applying the principle(s) of a drug holiday.
- Prophylactic dental care, the maintenance of good oral hygiene and good channels of communication among physicians, dentists and patients are essential to decrease the risk of health consequences as a result of MRONJ.

INTRODUCTION

Controversy can be defined as: "a prolonged state of public debate involving conflicting views or opinions."[1] Within everyday practice the oral health care provider is faced with diseases that are at the forefront of controversy and, as such, alternative approaches for treatment of oral disease continue to evolve. Controversy, however,

[a] New York Medical College/NYCHHC, Metropolitan Hospital, 100 Woods Road, Valhalla, NY 10593, USA; [b] Section head, Oral and Maxillofacial Surgery, University of Utah, School of Dentistry, 530 South Wakara Way, Salt Lake City, UT 84108, USA
* Corresponding author.
E-mail address: halpernl@nychhc.org

Dent Clin N Am 68 (2024) 67–85
https://doi.org/10.1016/j.cden.2023.07.005
0011-8532/24/© 2023 Elsevier Inc. All rights reserved.

can be a double-edge sword"; that is, case-by-case clinical decisions may fall into a "gray zone" resulting in a lack of consensus in treatment strategies for disease resolution. Medication-related osteonecrosis of the jaw (MRONJ) is one such disease that is associated with controversy. Since 2003, MRONJ has become a center of discussion with respect to etiology(s), pathologic staging, and algorithms for treatment resolution. Many authors have suggested that MRONJ is refractory to therapy.[2] Evidence-based data supporting this premise lies in the complexity of a pathogenic causation, and in controversies in staging since both play a significant role in treatment algorithms.[2,3]

Over the last few decades, the American Association of Oral and Maxillofacial Surgeons (AAOMS) has worked to develop consensus statements with respect to the management of MRONJ.[3] With the evolution of pharmacologic choices that placed patients at risk and with debates about staging of disease progression, however, there is still no uniform agreement on treatments for the resolution of the various stages of the disease.[4] MRONJ is associated with significant morbidity, adversely affects the health-related quality of life (QoL), and is challenging to treat.[5] Depending on the drug, its dosage, and the duration of exposure, this adverse drug reaction may occur rarely (eg, following the oral administration of bisphosphonate or denosumab treatments for osteoporosis, or antiangiogenic agent-targeted cancer treatment), or commonly (eg, following intravenous bisphosphonate for cancer treatment). This array of pharmacologic therapeutics and more recent drug discoveries with monoclonal antibody development only creates new controversies when deciding which drug therapy will be advantageous to the patient.

As prevention remains the mainstay in treatment of MRONJ, a common wisdom approach may not always follow the strict guidelines for evidence-based outcomes. As such, the surgeon must make his/her clinical decisions within an area of "gray" based upon the existing scientific evidence and clinical experience. The purpose of this article is to explore several controversies associated with the etiology(s), staging, treatments, and long-term resolution of MRONJ in patients who are treated by the oral health care provider team. There are 2 specific aims of this review.

1. Controversies for treatment of MRONJ will be put into context by:
   a. examining the epidemiology of MRONJ due to exposure of pharmacologic agents
   b. hypotheses for its etiologies/causality whether local or systemic
   c. update on the staging of disease
   d. whether a "Drug Holiday" improves treatment outcomes, and
   e. controversies of nonsurgical versus surgical therapy and patient disease resolution.
2. Controversies faced by the oral health care provider in optimizing prevention, and disease control in patients who are at risk for MRONJ.

LITERATURE SEARCH

A literature search was undertaken using Medline within the PubMed Portal, Web of Science Database, and Scopus to choose articles within the last 20 years. Only articles in English were chosen for inclusion. Each article's bibliography was evaluated for relevant publications and reviewed by the authors for inclusion. The keywords chosen included medication-related osteonecrosis of the jaw, MRONJ, bisphosphonate-related osteonecrosis of the jaw (BRONJ), antiresorptive therapy, mechanisms of MRONJ, osteomyelitis of jaw, mandible, surgical therapy for MRONJ, controversies in MRONJ therapy, oral care for MRONJ, MRONJ review, antiresorptive agents for bone disease, drug holiday for MRONJ, nonsurgical treatment for MRONJ. Further articles were extracted from commentaries across the subspecialties of dentistry and oral health. The level of evidence chosen was based upon Sacket's hierarchy of evidence and was predominantly level 1A, 2A, 3A, 4, and 5.[6] Between 30 to 50 articles were chosen that were relevant to this review article.

CONTROVERSIES IN THE EPIDEMIOLOGY OF MEDICATION-RELATED OSTEONECROSIS OF THE JAW

The epidemiologic "database" for MRONJ had its origin in 2003, when Marx and colleagues reported 36 cases of osteonecrosis of the jaw (ONJ) related to the use of the bisphosphonate zoledronate or pamidronate.[7] The patients presented with painful bone exposure in the mandible, maxilla, or both, and were unresponsive to surgical or medical treatment.[7] The disease became known as bisphosphonate-related osteonecrosis of the jaw (BRONJ). From 2004 to 2009, numerous cases began to be seen in the Oral and Maxillofacial Surgery (OMFS) practice, many referred by general dentists and primary care providers, who received notices from the drug companies that patients who were on medications for osteoporosis and osteopenia were at risk for disease within their jaws. A broader drug class warning of this complication for all bisphosphonates including the oral preparations ensued. Novartis, the manufacturer of the IV pamidronate (Aredia) and zoledronic acid (Zometa), notified health care professionals; i.e., "A dental examination with appropriate prevention should be considered prior to treatment with bisphosphonates."[8]

In 2007, the AAOMS appointed a committee composed of clinicians and basic science researchers with extensive experience in caring for these patients.[9] A consensus statement was crafted in 2009 with respect to treatment of patients exposed to bisphosphonates (BRONJ).[9] From 2009 to 2014 pharmacologic therapeutics evolved to not only include bisphosphonates but other antiresorptive agents whose targets were not only for osteoporotic/osteopenia bone but other organ systems under treatment for cancer and other metabolic diseases (**Table 1**). BRONJ evolved into antiresorptive-related ONJ and ultimately medication-related osteonecrosis of the jaw (MRONJ).[3] In 2014 AAOMS developed an updated consensus statement to

Table 1
Bisphosphonates/anti-resorptive/anti-angiogenic/monoclonal preparations for osteoporosis or malignancy

Drug	Primary Indication	Dosing	Route
Alendronate (Fosamax®)	Osteoporosis	70 mg/wk	Oral
Residronate (Actonel®)	Osteoporosis	5 mg/d;35 mg/wk	Oral
Ibandronate (Boniva®)	Osteoporosis	2.5 mg/d; 150 mg/mo	Oral
Pamidronate (Aredia®)	Bone metastasis	90 mg/3 wk	intravenous
Zolendronic acid (Reclast®)	Osteoporosis	5 mg; 1 time/y	Intravenous
Zolendronic acid (Zometa®)	Bone metastasis	4 mg infused/3 wk	Intravenous
Denosumab (Prolia/Xgeva)	Osteoporosis Prolia Xgeva	60 mg/6 mo 120 mg/4 wk	Subcutaneous Subcutaneous
Sunitinib (Sutent®)	Anti-angiogenic tumor	50 mg/d x 4 wk	Oral
Bevasizumab (Avastin ®)	Anti-angiogenic	25 mg; dosing varies	Intravenous
Teriparatide (Forteo)	Osteoporosis	20 µg/d	Subcutaneous
Romosozumab (Evenity)	Osteoporosis	210 mg/mo	Subcutaneous

accommodate the growing number of osteonecrosis cases involving the maxilla and mandible associated with oral and intravenous, as well as other antiresorptive and antiangiogenic agents. This became the 2014 White Paper.[10] The knowledge base, larger population statistics, and experience in addressing MRONJ continued to evolve, necessitating modifications and refinements to the previously published position papers. In 2020, the previous working group returned to appraise the current literature and revise the guidelines to reflect the current knowledge in this field. The 2022 update contained revisions to diagnosis and management strategies for therapy based upon the most current pharmacologic agents, research status, and larger populations.[3] AAOMS maintains that it is vitally important for this information to be disseminated to other relevant health care professionals and organizations both nationally and globally.

With the increase in numbers and types of exposure to the variety of pharmacologic therapies, the epidemiologic prevalence, and cumulative incidence rates of MRONJ as a result of oral, subcutaneous, and intravenous use have changed in terms of risk of MRONJ when the 2014 and 2022 updates are compared (**Table 2**).[3,10,11] A

Table 2
The epidemiology of medication-related osteonecrosis of the jaw with exposure to pharmacologic agents: 2014 AAOMS update compared to 2022 AAOMS update

Pharmacologic Agent	Prevalence/Incidence Rate: 2014 Update[a]	Prevalence/Incidence Rate: 2022 Update[b]
Osteoporosis:		
Alendronate(Fosamax®)	0.1% (10 cases/10,000;< 4 y) 0.21% (21 cases/10,000; > 4 y)	0.02%–0.05% (2–5 cases/ 10,000) (duration of time does not affect rate)
IV Zolendronic acid (Reclast®)	0.017% (1.7 cases/10,000; 3 y)	<0.1%; 0.02 m −0.05 as above
Subcutaneous denosumab (Prolia®)	0.04% (4 cases/10,000; 1–4 y)	0.04%–0.3% (4 cases/10,000– 30/10,000) (duration of time increases the risk)
Teriparatide (Forteo®)	Unknown at this time	Unknown at this time
Romosozumab (Evenity®)	Unknown in 2014	0.03%–0.05% (3–5 cases/ 10,000)
Malignancy/metabolic diseases		
Zolendronate (Zometa®)	1% (100 cases/10,000) Cumulative incidence rate: 0.7%–6.7%	<5.0% to 18% (up to 180/ 10,000 cases) Cumulative incidence rate: up to 18% (duration of time increases risk)
Denosumab	0.7%–1.9% (>190 cases/10,000)	0%–6.9% (most cases < 5% (500/10,000) (duration of time increases risk)
Sunitinib (Sutent®)	Unknown	Unknown
Bevasizumab (Avastin®)	Unknown	0.2% (20 cases/10,000)

[a] *Adapted from* Ruggiero SL, Dodson TB, Fantasia J, et al: American Association of Oral and Maxillofacial Surgeons position paper on medication-related osteonecrosis of the jaw–2014 update. J Oral Maxillofac Surg. 72:1938, 2014.
[b] *Adapted from* Ruggiero SL, Dodson TB, Aghaloo T, Carlson ER, Ward BB, Kademani D. American Association of Oral and Maxillofacial Surgeons' Position Paper on Medication-Related Osteonecrosis of the Jaws-2022 Update Oral Maxillofac Surg 2022 May;80(5):920-943.

systematic review by Cochrane Database in 2022 suggested that 2 related measures are often used to describe the incidence rate of MRONJ: incidence proportion (cumulative incidence) and incidence rate.[12] As incident rate peaks between 2 and 3 years it becomes difficult to maintain a strict selection criterion due to death from disease or patients lost to follow-up. Inconsistencies also exist with follow-up times making it difficult to compare study populations.[12]

A significant controversy relates to the prolonged use of bisphosphonates and denosumab for osteoporosis and risk of hip fractures versus risk of MRONJ.[3] The documented risk for developing MRONJ versus hip fracture is low; however, the patient perceived risk is not.[3,13] As such, patients are unwilling to start or continue antiresorptive medical therapy even though the risk of hip fracture is increased.[3,13,14] Hip fracture carries significant morbidity, with only 40% to 60% of individuals recovering their pre-fracture level of mobility and ability to perform normal activities of daily living.[3] This controversy with respect to risk/benefit analyses is compounded by data confirming a rise in risk of fragility fractures with significant associated morbidity due to patients denying the benefit of antiresorptive therapy to present a significantly decreased risk of developing MRONJ.[13] A study using the HORIZON Pivotal Fracture trial tested 3889 randomized patients given annual zoledronic acid versus placebo for 3 years: 1 patient developed MRONJ in the intervention group and 1 in the placebo group.[15] This study supports evidence of how a controversy can evolve into a true health crisis since the risk of fracture, morbidity, and health care costs outweigh a true risk of MRONJ. Balancing the risks and benefits of treatment in individual cases remain a "cornerstone" of management in this controversial area.[3,11] It is evident from the literature stated that although the incidence rates of MRONJ are higher in patients with cancer the incidence and prevalence rates of MRONJ are relatively low in patients who are being treated for osteoporosis.[3,14-19] Further scrutiny with future position papers can help to develop a more critical lens in examining the epidemiology of MRONJ in the at-risk population to answer the following: *Is the risk of developing MRONJ compatible when a population never exposed to the drug are compared with cohorts that are on anti-resorptive therapy for osteoporosis or other systemic diseases?* .

CONTROVERSIES OF ETIOLOGIES/CAUSALITY OF DISEASE

Box 1 depicts the criteria for diagnosing MRONJ.[13] Studies have shown that patients who present with clinical characteristics of MRONJ may not actually have the disease itself and causality can therefore be challenging (see above). The history of the present illness is most important to discern these disease entities from one another.[3] **Box 2** lists the common misdiagnosed conditions seen. A definitive causality is further based upon the individual patient since clinical presentation can vary (see section on Staging

---

Box 1
Criteria for identification of medication-related osteonecrosis of the jaw

Criterion 1: Current or previous treatment with antiresorptive or antiangiogenic agents.

Criterion 2: Exposed bone or bone that can be probed through an intraoral or extraoral fistula(e) in the maxillofacial region that has persisted for more than 8 weeks of healing.

Criterion 3: No history of radiation therapy to the jaws or obvious metastatic disease to the jaws.

Adapted from Ruggiero S, Drew SJ. Osteonecrosis of the jaw and bisphosphonate therap. J Dent Res 2007;86(11):1013-1021.

Box 2
Conditions often misdiagnosed as medication-related osteonecrosis of the jaw

- Alveolar osteitis
- Sinusitis
- Gingivitis/periodontitis
- Caries
- Periapical pathology
- Fibro-osseous lesion
- Sarcoma
- Acute/chronic osteomyelitis
- Temporomandibular joint (TMJ) disorders
- Osteogenesis imperfecta
- Chronic sclerosing osteomyelitis
- Squamous cell carcinoma of the jaw

Adapted from Ruggiero SL, Dodson TB, Aghaloo T, Carlson ER, Ward BB, Kademani D. American Association of Oral and Maxillofacial Surgeons' Position Paper on Medication-Related Osteonecrosis of the Jaws-2022 Update Oral Maxillofac Surg 2022 May;80(5):920-943.

below). The presentation can be identical to individuals who never been exposed to an antiresorptive agent but are exhibiting necrotic bone due to infections from bacteria, fungi, and deficiencies within their immune-cellular responses, long-term use of steroids, immunocompromised diseases like diabetes, and those being treated for cancer.[3,15–17] These risk predictors support the premise that ONJ can occur without drug exposure. As MRONJ is often clinically similar to osteomyelitis and osteoradionecrosis of the jaw, a good history and clinical evaluation will often avoid "muddy waters" regarding therapeutic intervention.

Triggering factors at the local, systemic, and "other" can serve as major risk predictors for MRONJ (**Box 3**). The following are of most concern in everyday practice and remains a dilemma of controversy when patients require dental rehabilitation.

Dentoalveolar surgery

Tooth extraction

Dentoalveolar surgery (DS) is the most often reported local risk factor for MRONJ with studies characterizing high prevalence rates after tooth extraction.[3,19] The prevalence rate significantly varies when oral bisphosphonate and antiresorptive use for osteoporosis is compared with intravenous bisphosphonate and antiresorptive medication exposure in patients being treated for malignancies.[3,14,19] Most patients who are taking oral bisphosphonates or denosumab for osteoporosis cluster around an MRONJ prevalence rate of 0.15% and 1.0%, respectively, after DS.[3,20] Patients with cancer exposed to intravenous bisphosphonates or denosumab are at risk of MRONJ that can range from 1.6% to 14.8%, respectively, after DS.[3,21,22]

The risk to benefit ratios of the above extend beyond statistical data since these catchments of patients want to know the risks associated with periodontal surgery, endodontic therapy, denture placement, and viability of success after dental implant placement (see below). As there is no consensus on the biologic mechanisms(s), each patient's success with dental rehabilitation is based upon degree of oral disease

---

Box 3
Risk factors associated with medication-related osteonecrosis of the jaw

Local risk factors
  Anatomic: Mandible and maxilla: mandible > maxilla: exostoses, tori, knife edge ridges with lingual area most often violated
  Dental prostheses: ill-fitting dentures and fixed prosthetics that are nonpassive
  Dentoalveolar surgery: tooth extraction, placement of dental implants (controversial), bone augmentation, peri-implantitis, endodontic therapy, other surgeries
  Oral conditions: associated with parafunctional habits

Systemic risk factors:
  Medications: use of corticosteroids, other chemotherapeutic agents for malignant tumors
  Systemic illness: oncology patients receiving IV bisphosphonates or high-dose
    Diabetes
      Osteoporosis/osteopenia
      Rheumatoid arthritis
    Sarcoidosis
    Hypocalcemia hypoparathyroidism renal dialysis anemia Paget's
  Other: tobacco
    Alcohol
    Obesity
    Advanced age/genetic predisposition (single nucleotide polymorphisms, SNP)

Adapted from Kawahara M, Kuroshima S, Sawase T. Clinical considerations for medication-related osteonecrosis of the jaw: a comprehensive literature review. Int J Implant Dent 2021;7(47). https://doi.org/10.1186/s40729-021-00323-0; and Ruggiero SL, Dodson TB, Aghaloo T, Carlson ER, Ward BB, Kademani D. American Association of Oral and Maxillofacial Surgeons' Position Paper on Medication-Related Osteonecrosis of the Jaws-2022 Update Oral Maxillofac Surg 2022 May;80(5):920-943.

---

present either before or during antiresorptive treatment. Systematic reviews indicate that patients who have pre-existing periodontal disease are at a 50% greater risk for MRONJ.[3,21] The assumptions from this review suggest a controversy that is based upon whether preexisting inflammatory sequelae may act as a "confounder" in the correlation of dentoalveolar surgery and risk of MRONJ.[3,21–23]

Future studies may solve this dilemma by examining the association of tooth extraction with risk of MRONJ adjusting for pre-existinginflammatory disease in the oral cavity.[3,14,22,23]

Dental implants

The risk of dental implant placement resulting in acquiring MRONJ is even more controversial.[3,24] Risk for MRONJ after dental implant placement and endodontic or periodontal procedures that require exposure and manipulation of bone is comparable to the risk associated with tooth extraction in osteoporotic patients; that is, 0.5%ˆ (2022 update).[3] Data within the AAOMS 2022 update suggested that "The majority of implant related MRONJ cases were not related to the initial implant surgery but occurred late (>12 months) and often at sites where implants were placed prior to the initiation of BP therapy. The common presentation was an en bloc failure where the osseointegration of implants were maintained within the sequestrum. This is distinct from the peri-implantitis failure and pathognomonic for MRONJ".[3] A systematic review by Sher and colleagues[24] evaluated dental implant placement in patients with a history of MRONJ. A total of 7542 articles were identified using the PRISMA strategy of which 29 studies were included in the qualitative analysis. The premise was that the ability to undergo osseointegration is predicated upon the formation of new bone, blood capillaries, and resorption of old bone by osteoclasts. Drugs that interfere with this process may compromise osseointegration with resultant loss of the implant. Their results indicated that patients who were on oral bisphosphonates for osteoporosis were not at increased risk for implant failure with respect to osseointegration. When compared with patients who were on intravenous therapy for malignancy, both groups were at risk for "implant –triggered" MRONJ. In patients treated with denosumab for osteoporosis results showed a negligible rate of MRONJ. Study limitations included small sample size, no random-control trials for comparison, and therefore, conclusions can be questionable due to a lack statistical validity. A controversy also resides in implant success and implant survival which was not discerned in this study. Longevity of success as compared with radiographic evidence of bone loss was not taken in to account. They did conclude that patients with a history of bisphosphonate use for osteoporosis are not at an increased risk for implant failure when compared to healthy individuals, patients treated with denosumab for osteoporosis have a negligible risk for MRONJ, and there is no evidence of risk based upon use of antiangiogenic medications due to the lack of statistically valid data. A case report by Jung concluded that after placement of dental implants and chemotherapy with pazopanib over 6 months, bone exposure was evident supporting the premise that "implant presence" triggered MRONJ.[24] This supports a contraindication to implant placement in patients who are candidates for antiangiogenic therapy. Future studies are needed to support this premise. Most importantly, it is recommended that all patients who are taking bisphosphonates or antiresorptive therapy for osteoporosis be given an in-depth informed consent of potential risks, although low, in the development of MRONJ as an either early or late causality of implant failure. In addition, patients who already have dental implants in place should be advised of the risk of "spontaneous" MRONJ without identifiable dental etiology(s).[3,14,25]

CONTROVERSIES WITH PATHOPHYSIOLOGY OF MEDICATION-RELATED OSTEONECROSIS OF THE JAW

Current controversies are suggested for the pathogenesis of MRONJ yet the exact mechanism of disease is yet to be elucidated. Although the local factors mentioned above play a major role, that is, extraction of teeth and other dentoalveolar procedures, they are not the only prerequisite for the development of MRONJ. The specificity of disease is unique to the facial skeleton due to the bony physiology of the jaw, specifically the alveolar bone.[26] Healthy alveolar bone is an essential component of an intact dentition. Alveolar bone is a dynamic structure with the bone constantly remodeling and adapting to functional needs. The alveolar bone has a high remodeling rate that is 10 times that of the long bones of the body due to occlusal forces resulting in compression at root apex and furcation, tension on lamina dura, and periodontal ligament and remodeling of lamina dura in response to the forces.[26]

The 2014 AAOMS update on MRONJ identified several evidence-based hypotheses with respect to the pathophysiology of disease.[3,14] **Box 4** characterizes the 4 main hypotheses for the pathophysiology of MRONJ based upon animal and clinical studies.[3,11,14] The following 2 hypotheses are well studied and the reader is referred to the references for further interest.

Inhibition of Bone Remodeling

Suppression of bone turnover has been a most accepted hypothesis for the pathogenesis of MRONJ.[3] Animal studies support the hypothesis that removal of bisphosphonates and other antiresorptive agents will increase the capability of bone remodeling

---

Box 4
Theories of the pathophysiology of medication-related osteonecrosis of the jaw

- *Inhibition of osteoclastic bone resorption and remodeling (turnover):*
  - Bisphosphonates (BP), and other antiresorptive such as denosumab, inhibit osteoclast differentiation and function, increase apoptosis, leading to decreased bone resorption and remodeling
- *Inhibition of angiogenesis:*
  - Osteonecrosis is classically considered an interruption in vascular supply or avascular necrosis. Inhibition of angiogenesis is a leading hypothesis.
- *Genetic predisposition related to occurrence of MRONJ*
  - Specific gene sequences are manifested in diseases; that is, osteoporosis: event rate greater than 50%
- *Inflammation/infection: mucosal biofilms/mucosal toxicity:*
  - Both inflammation or bacterial infection and systemic antiresorptive are sufficient to induce ONJ.
    - *"Outside in effect"*: Effect on mucosa to then invade bone: bone becomes exposed.
    - Biofilms): Development of biofilms are barriers to care well-developed biofilm mucopolysaccharides observed.
    - *Periodontal disease:*

Adapted from Ruggiero SL, Dodson TB, Fantasia J, et al: American Association of Oral and Maxillofacial Surgeons position paper on medication-related osteonecrosis of the jaw–2014 update. J Oral Maxillofac Surg. 72:1938, 2014; and Ruggiero SL, Dodson TB, Aghaloo T, Carlson ER, Ward BB, Kademani D. American Association of Oral and Maxillofacial Surgeons' Position Paper on Medication-Related Osteonecrosis of the Jaws-2022 Update Oral Maxillofac Surg 2022 May;80(5):920-943.

---

by reinstating osteoclastic activity. Oral, subcutaneous, or intravenous administration of bisphosphonates/antiresorptive agents influence bone remodeling suppression and is central to osteoporotic inhibition in addition to an increase in the risk of MRONJ. Their direct effects on osteoclast differentiation and function allow for increased bone mineral density, a decrease in risk of fractures, and a risk of MRONJ. The bisphosphonates and antiresorptive medications, that is, denosumab, are the most commonly approved for both osteoporosis and malignancy with a prevalence of MRONJ stated in the previous section both drugs prevent bone resorption by mechanisms of osteoclast inhibition.[3,11,14]

Despite this evidence, however, other studies have supported an acceleration of bone turnover rather than suppression as a pathologic mechanism for MRONJ.[11,27] Krishnan and colleagues[28] identified the use of MRI with significant tracer uptake in the bone scans and increased numbers of osteoclasts and bone lysis within lesions of patients positive for BRONJ. In patients diagnosed with osteopetrosis whose osteoclasts are absent or nonfunctional, ONJ as a disease complication is absent and there is no evidence of spontaneous bone necrosis at other skeletal sites with bisphosphonates and denosumab.[11,29]

Inflammation/Infection

Infections and inflammation are associated with the pathogenesis of MRONJ and are considered to be susceptible risk factors. The proinflammatory cytokine IL-36a has a key role in the MRONJ incidence and is associated with infected periodontal tissue and gingival crevicular fluid.[3,11,27,30] Further support of inflammatory etiology(s) as a prelude to MRONJ is demonstrated in animal models that, although limited in application to humans, can be "critical to the understanding of disease mechanisms".[3,14] A valid example of the latter is evident in patients who are diagnosed with periodontal disease. Patients with periodontal disease and dental abscesses are at a 7-fold increased risk of MRONJ.[11,29] Their etiologic pathology consists of gram-negative bacteria that stimulate the production of cytokines and lipopolysaccharides that accelerate bone resorption. Other bacteria have the potential to regulate receptor activators of RANKL ligand in human periodontal ligament cells and gingival fibroblasts that also accelerate bone resorption.[3,11,28,29] These findings support the premise that biofilm formation and poor oral hygiene can increase the risk of MRONJ and as such the oral health care provider must be clinically judicious in managing those patients who require pharmacologic management of their systemic illness. This is especially true when surgical management of MRONJ is not advised (see below). Although infection is widely supported as a triggering factor for MRONJ, the above data need to be further scrutinized by larger studies that monitor proper oral hygiene and preventive dental care.[29–31]

CONTROVERSIES IN STAGING OF MEDICATION-RELATED OSTEONECROSIS OF THE JAW

Staging is a rational evidence-based approach to the diagnosis and treatment of MRONJ.[3,9,10] The AAOMS staging system for MRONJ was introduced in the 2009 position paper and modified in 2014 and updated in 2022 (**Box 5**). There are other staging systems that vary somewhat especially in relationship with the early or preclinical manifestations of the condition.[31–33] The 2022 MRONJ Position Paper reiterated the staging from 2014 with the latest documentation and rational. In developing the latest guidelines, the AAOMS authors expressed concern that an overemphasis on radiographic features often attributed to MRONJ may result in false positives. Some of these cases may be radiographically suggestive of MRONJ but the patients otherwise do not fit the criteria for the diagnosis of MRONJ. The authors also discussed treatment planning for patients at risk for MRONJ should include a thorough examination and radiographic assessment when indicated.[3]

Other studies have argued radiographic criteria as controversial. Drs Campisi, Mauceri, and colleagues argued that clinical examination was insufficient and that a CT is an essential tool of the diagnostic algorithm of MRONJ.[31] They felt that radiographic evidence of bone necrosis can be present in patients at risk for MRONJ well before clinical signs. They urged imaging in the diagnostic work-up to exclude dental and bone diseases with similar clinical manifestations which would facilitate the adoption of a broader definition of MRONJ. Fusco, Santini, and colleagues discussed that a purely clinical definition of MRONJ without CT radiographic evidence could place patients with nonbone exposure symptoms as described in the AAOMS stage 0 in a wait-and-see situation that might delay diagnosis and the start of appropriate treatments.[33] They advocated for earlier surgical treatment of MRONJ quoting "a growing body of knowledge that surgery performs better than conservative treatments in all stages of the disease in terms of both symptom control and disease resolution". Future prospective analyses with larger sampling may help to allow for more clarity when staging cases for MRONJ, but for now, the AAOMS staging approach is still used when patient workup is required to formulate a treatment plan.

CONTROVERSIES WITH DRUG HOLIDAYS AND MEDICATION-RELATED OSTEONECROSIS OF THE JAW

Consensus opinions vary significantly with regard to the benefit of a "drug holiday", that is, temporarily pausing treatment with bisphosphonates, denosumab, and other

---

Box 5
Staging of disease state of medication-related osteonecrosis of the jaw

Stage 0
  History of oral or IV antiresorptive therapy
  No clinical evidence of necrotic bone
  Nonspecific symptoms and/or radiographic findings
    Symptoms
    • Ondontalgia not explained by odontogenic cause
    • Dull, aching jaw pain that may radiate to TMJ
    • Sinus pain that may be associated with inflammatory sinus membrane thickening
    • Altered neurosensory function
    Clinical findings
    • Loosening of teeth associated with periodontal disease
    • Intraoral or extraoral swelling
    Radiographic findings
    • Alveolar bone loss not associated with chronic periodontal disease
    • Increased bone sclerosis of alveolar or basilar bone
    • No new bone in extraction sockets
    • Changes in trabecular pattern
    • Thickening or obscuring of periodontal ligament

Stage 1
  Asymptomatic patient
  Exposed/necrotic bone or fistula that tracks to bone
  No evidence of inflammation or infection
  Radiographic changes localized to alveolar bone

Stage 2
  Symptomatic patient
  Exposed/necrotic bone or fistula that tracks to bone
  Evidence of inflammation or infection
  Radiographic changes localized to alveolar bone

Stage 3
  Exposed/necrotic bone or fistula which tracks to bone
  Evidence of inflammation or infection plus one or more of following:
  • Exposed bone extending beyond alveolar bone
  • Pathologic fracture
  • Extraoral fistula
  • Oral antral/nasal communication
  • Osteolysis extending to inferior border of mandible or sinus floor

Adapted from Ruggiero SL, Dodson TB, Aghaloo T, Carlson ER, Ward BB, Kademani D. American Association of Oral and Maxillofacial Surgeons' Position Paper on Medication-Related Osteonecrosis of the Jaws-2022 Update Oral Maxillofac Surg 2022 May;80(5):920-943.

---

antiresorptive therapy in patients who require invasive dental procedures. Historically, a drug holiday was thought to decrease the prevalence of MRONJ subsequent to dentoalveolar surgery.[3] Both the 2014 and 2022 AAOMS task force reiterate that this is a controversial debate due to a lack of evidence that can neither support nor refute the benefit of a drug holiday.[3,14] The basis of this controversy lies in the rarity of MRONJ in the patient populations treated and the lack of high-level A evidence with random-controlled trials. There is therefore insufficient data to arrive at a consensus for valid treatment protocols.[3,10,34,35]

Studies have been undertaken across other specialties globally that support a drug holiday.[3,31,32] In Denmark and other European countries it is a "gold standard" to discontinue drug therapy in relation to tooth extraction although high level evidence is lacking.[35] A study from Japan, however, suggested that drug holidays did not decrease the risk of MRONJ in patients receiving oral bisphosphonate therapy.[31,34] Adding to the controversy is the type of antiresorptive therapy being used.[35] Although all antiresorptive agents modify bone remodeling by inducing apoptosis and inhibiting osteoclast mediated bone resorption, bisphosphonates and denosumab behave differently due to the different mechanisms of action and pharmacokinetic properties of the 2 agents.[3,10,35] A bisphosphonate drug holiday may be ineffective due to the long half-life of the drugs.[3,10] Oral bisphosphonates remain in the bone for 8 to 10 years after patients have stopped receiving them. A temporary discontinuation of denosumab could be favorable due to denosumab's short half-life.[3,10] A denosumab drug holiday, however, may also increase the risk of SREs including recurrence of bone pain and possibly progression of bone metastases in the patient.[3,10,36]

Campisi and colleagues[36] in a commentary hypothesized of a "window of opportunity" to minimize the risk for MRONJ development in patients who are prescribed denosumab for osteoporosis. The premise resides in the pharmacokinetics and pharmacodynamics of denosumab whose serum concentration becomes undetectable by 6 months as compared with the pharmacokinetics and pharmacodynamics of bisphosphonates whose serum levels remain elevated for up to 8 to 10 years.[3,10,36] The window of opportunity for denosumab between post-dose month 5 and 7 allows for recovery of bone turnover and supports dentoalveolar manipulation. The authors, however, are cautious and recommend larger well-designed clinical trials are required to prove this hypothesis of a low risk of MRONJ in this population.[36] The 2022 AAOMS task force has evaluated these and other studies and recommended a case-by-case evaluation with respect for applying the principle(s) of a drug holiday. A risk to benefit analysis must be offered as a discontinuation of denosumab in osteoporotic patient will increase their susceptibility to multilevel vertebral fractures. With this as a concern they suggest "that any planned dentoalveolar surgery can be completed 3–4 months following the last does of Denosumab and reinstitute it 6–8 weeks post-surgery".[3]

CONTROVERSIES WITH NONSURGICAL VERSUS SURGICAL MANAGEMENT FOR MEDICATION-RELATED OSTEONECROSIS OF THE JAW

Decisions on operative versus nonoperative therapies should continue to be predicated upon a case-to-case basis with a thorough discussion of risks to benefit when considering any invasive treatment. The AAOMS position papers of 2014 and 2022 continue to address the management strategies of MRONJ based upon the staging criteria (see section on controversies in staging of MRONJ). The staging of disease has been at the forefront and sets the tone for treatment guidelines (see above). Staging as a criterion for disease treatment continues to form the mainstay of the AAOMS update. Other societies in the international arena have also created their own staging criteria and controversy still exists especially with radiographic imaging criteria and staging. The latter 2 risk predictors have reframed treatment alternatives.[3,10]

Several systematic reviews have been published that characterize the controversy of operative versus nonoperative therapy.[3,19,38] Rupel and colleagues [37] demonstrated that conservative and extensive surgical approaches improved the healing rate of MRONJ when compared with a nonsurgical intervention. The study reported that the healing rates of stages 1, 2, and 3 with nonsurgical therapy was 33%, 24%, and 0%, respectively. The authors, however, have also demonstrated that the healing rates of MRONJ with conservative surgical and extensive surgical approaches were 72% and 87% for stage 1, 79% and 96% for stage 2, and 27% and 81% for stage

3, respectively. Therefore, a surgical approach, rather than a nonsurgical approach, may be considered first if the patient's systemic condition permits. Kawahara and colleagues[19] in their systematic review support a case-by-case approach with respect to patients receiving antiresorptive therapy for cancer since complete healing of MRONJ may only be at 50% with surgical intervention. The authors conclude that caution should be taken with limited data and larger sample sizes are needed to support the findings above. The 2022 update has developed several algorithms based upon the latest nonoperative and surgical therapies. The following are a portion of strategies (the reader is referred to reference 3 for an in-depth discussion):

Nonsurgical Treatment

Decisions on whether to treat MRONJ nonsurgically must be predicated on a case-to-case basis and not necessarily on the stage of disease (see above and below). QoL issues and a patient's ability to maintain good oral hygiene are essential to prevent infection and loss of bone. The oral health care provider must educate the patient on the benefits of good oral hygiene and have scheduled recall follow-up from 8 to 12 week intervals (see below). Yearly radiographic imaging is of the utmost importance in evaluating new or existing bony lesions of MRONJ.[3] Refillable prescriptions of .12% chlorhexidine rinses (Peridex) will aid in wound care and removal of biofilm. Patients with stage 2 or 3 disease and wounds that are refractory to this therapy are candidates for antibiotics to aid in management of symptoms not resolving with more palliative methods. Bony sequestrum can exfoliate often without any surgical manipulation with resultant mucosal healing. Nonresolution with any of the above therapy warrants surgical intervention.

Medication, which may be referred to as conservative medical treatment, is the primary method currently available in the early stages of MRONJ.[2,3] According to the position paper of AAOMS in 2014,[2] patients with MRONJ stage 0 and 1 can benefit from medical treatments such as systematic antibiotics and/or antimicrobial rinse. It can also be applied as adjuvant therapy in stages 2 and 3 when evidence of infection begins to appear.[10] However, the conservative medical treatment may take the lead even in later stages that require surgical treatment despite these recommendations creating a controversy in therapeutic management.[2] Further controversy comes about on whether conservative medical treatment can be applied at all stages.[2] Ramaglia and colleagues[38] recommended starting with 2 weeks of conservative medical treatment for the management of MRONJ in their systematic review and meta-analysis because it showed effectiveness at all stages although the medical treatment had a lower treatment success rate in the advanced stages, that is, success rates of 63.6% to 100% in stage 2 and 73% in stage 3. The most widely used antibiotics for the systematic medication in patients with MRONJ appear to be penicillin, amoxicillin, amoxicillin/clavulanate, metronidazole, or a combination of each.[2,3] These drugs are also used as medications for common oral infections. Studies have indicated that these drugs are being applied because bacterial migration in the progression of MRONJ can cause inflammation or infection.[2,3] Local antimicrobial rinses potentiate these antibiotics and chlorhexidine is most chosen as an adjunct to antibiotic therapy.[3,10] Medication therapy, however, is not without controversy due to a lack of consensus on which antibiotic is the most effective. Dosing schedules vary depending upon the study read, and disagreement on whether there is a true resolution of disease.[2,38] Many studies support eventual surgical treatment for the complete healing of the necrotic presentation of MRONJ.[2,3,38]

Surgical Therapy

Numerous reports in the literature support high success rates with surgical intervention in MRONJ lesions.[3,39,40] Surgical resection in early stage MRONJ was a controversial issue in the 2014 update.[10,41] Data from 2014 to 2022 now support that early surgical intervention can result in a more beneficial patient outcome regardless of stage of disease.[3,39–41] With the wealth of studies undertaken since then, bony resection of tissue can cause disease resolution even in a stage 1 and asymptomatic stage 2 patients (**Fig. 1**).[3] Surgical resections in patients with malignant disease can also determine whether the necrotic bone is a metastasis of disease itself and aid in further reassessment of therapeutic intervention.[41] Recent use of adjuvant therapies has added to the controversy of type of surgical intervention and resolution of MRONJ.[40]

A systematic review by Govaerts and colleagues[42] suggests that laser ablation and fluorescence-guided surgery may have the potential to enhance the bony and mucosal healing process in patients with MRONJ. The authors, however, do caution that larger random-controlled trials are needed to validate this hypothesis. The evidence above supports a surgical model that demonstrates a maintenance of wound healing, an increased health-related QoL, and a resumption of drug therapy in patients at all stages of disease. The controversy of nonoperative versus operative therapy

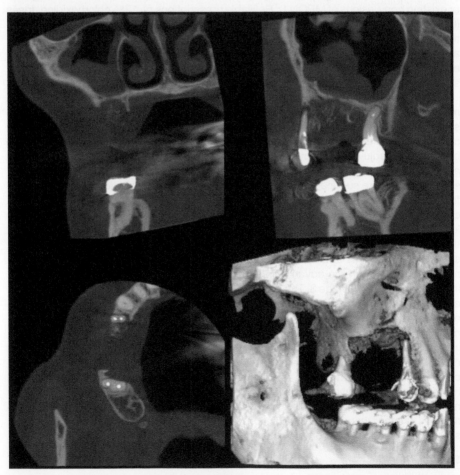

Fig. 1. CT scan depicting areas of necrotic bone along the floor of the sinus adjacent to teeth #2, 5, 12 and 15.

remains a debate due to the complexity of MRONJ. Further studies are required with a higher level of evidence to support or refute the studies presented above.

CONTROVERSIES IN CLINICAL MANAGEMENT OF MEDICATION-RELATED OSTEONECROSIS OF THE JAW BY THE ORAL HEALTH CARE PROVIDER

Numerous studies have supported the premise that preventive strategies for decreasing risk of MRONJ not only allow for disease resolution but more importantly contribute to better oral and overall health of the population.[3,43] The role of the oral health care provider is pivotal in minimizing a patient's risk for developing MRONJ. Controversies arise, however, based upon whether dental rehabilitation should precede commencement of pharmacotherapy for patients with osteoporosis, malignancies, and other metabolic diseases, or, whether dental rehabilitation should occur concomitantly while patients are on oral or intravenous antiresorptive therapies. **Box 6** depicts the strategies crafted by the 2022 AAOMS Task Force on prevention to minimize the risks of MRONJ in patients either about to start, or those who are already on regimens of either oral or intravenous pharmacologic therapies.[3]

These findings, however, continue to require strong clinical research with prospective studies to support this standard of care. Most importantly, the oral health care

---

Box 6
Medication-related osteonecrosis of the jaw oral health care strategies

Pretherapy (nonmalignant disease)	Educate patient about the potential risks associated with long-term ART
	Optimization of the dental health can occur with ART
Pretherapy (malignant disease)	Educate the patient about the higher risk of MRONJ and the importance of regimented dental care
	Optimization of the dental health prior to the initiation of ART if systemic conditions permit (extraction of nonrestorable teeth or teeth with a poor prognosis)
During antiresorptive therapy (nonmalignant disease)	No alteration of operative plan for most
	Drug holidays are controversial
	Dental implant risk to benefit needs discussion; that is, early vs late failures
	Dental follow-up 10–12 wk intervals; perio/restorative/endodontic therapies
During antiresorptive therapy/targeted Therapies (malignant disease)	Dental follow-up 8–12 wk intervals
	Educate patients about the higher MRONJ risk in the setting of malignant disease
	Educate the patient about the importance of regimented dental care and prevention:
	Avoid dentoalveolar surgery if possible
	Consider root retention techniques to avoid extractions
	Dental implants are contraindicated

Abbreviation: ART: antiresorptive therapy.

Adapted from Ruggiero SL, Dodson TB, Aghaloo T, Carlson ER, Ward BB, Kademani D. American Association of Oral and Maxillofacial Surgeons' Position Paper on Medication-Related Osteonecrosis of the Jaws-2022 Update Oral Maxillofac Surg 2022 May;80(5):920-943.

provider should ascertain the following information during initial discussions with the physician: "why is the patient on therapy of bisphosphonates or denosumab; is there prior exposure; how long has the patient been on therapy; are there other pharmacologic agents being taken concomitantly; what are the risks of dental therapy and MRONJ; and timeline of follow up of oral care since it can vary between 10 weeks to 3 month recalls".[3,10,32,43] An interdisciplinary approach must be considered with the oral health care provider, the primary care provider, the oncologist (if needed) and an oral and maxillofacial surgeon to provide a team approach in the management of patients at risk or already suffering from MRONJ. Good channels of communication are essential since data suggest that a lack of cooperation between physicians and dentists is related to an increased rate of bony fractures and other health consequences as a result of MRONJ.[3,32,44]

SUMMARY/FUTURE DIRECTIONS

MRONJ is a most interesting, complex and "elusive" condition seen by the oral health care provider. It is plagued by controversy and although a wealth of research has created preclinical and clinical databases, there is no "gold standard" algorithm to be applied for true resolution of disease. Controversies with respect to therapeutic options remain since although numerous treatment modalities exist all appear insufficient to heal disease in all cases presented. The latter may be due to small sample sizes and require larger prospective population studies over a longer period of time. Studies are underway to use mesenchymal stem cell therapies, platelet concentrates with bone morphogenetic proteins, and monoclonal antibodies to parathyroid hormone; that is, teriparatide, a drug already being used to treat osteoporosis refractory to other anti-resorptive agents.[2] The latter is being applied in larger clinical trials to determine if it can be an option for standard treatment across the board.[2,43,44] Another approach for the use of medications as a clinical tool in the treatment of MRONJ is the combination of pentoxifylline and tocopherol.[45,46] This combination of therapy is based upon their use in the management of osteoradionecrosis with success.[45,46] A systematic review by Heifetz-Li and colleagues[45] concluded that pentoxifylline and tocopherol were associated with subjective and objective improvement in disease resolution. They do caution, however, that larger clinical trials are needed to determine a statistically valid conclusion in its application as a nonsurgical approach for MRONJ. These innovative strategies, however, have the potential to be combined with treatments already successful on a case to case comparison and provide a promising "roadmap" for therapeutic approaches in the treatment of MRONJ.

The future of prevention is just as important as disease resolution. The oral health care provider must be judicious in educating their patient community. Patients scheduled to be administered antiresorptive or antiangiogenic agents should undergo thorough intraoral screening and appropriate dental care including strategies for patient motivation and education to maintain good oral hygiene, and strict treatment recall on a regular basis (see **Box 6**). To optimize these strategies an interprofessional collaborative should be in place among dentists, oral and maxillofacial surgeons, physicians, oncologists, and other ancillary health care providers to avoid any gaps in communicating risks to benefits of antiresorptive therapy. This will avoid a patient's lack of adherence to treatment and enhance why their oral health affects their health-related QoL. The authors agree that further research and studies to develop effective treatment strategies for MRONJ can increase the potential for consensus and decrease the controversy in the management of MRONJ.

CLINICS CARE POINTS

- There is no "gold standard" algorithm to be applied in a universal fashion to resolve the risk for MRONJ.

- Dentists have a pivotal role to play in patient care with respect to thorough assessment, and prophylactic dental treatment, in the successful management of patients predisposed to the risk of MORONJ.

- The risk of implant failure , although low ,exists in the development of MRONJ In.

- Patients who already have dental implants in place should be advised of the risk of "spontaneous" MRONJ without identifiable dental etiology(s).

- AAOMS neither supports or refutes the application of a "drug holiday" and recommends a case by case evaluation with respect for applying the principle(s) of a drug holiday.

DISCLOSURE

The authors disclose no commercial or financial conflicts of interest or any funding resources for this Dental Clinics article.

REFERENCES

1. Vega LG, Meara DJ. Controversies in oral and maxillofacial surgery: Preface. Oral Maxillofac Surg Clin NA 2017;29(4):IX.
2. On S-W, Cho S-W, Byun S-H, et al. Various therapeutic methods for the treatment of medication-related osteonecrosis of the jaw (MRONJ) and their limitations: A narrative review on new molecular and cellular therapeutic approaches. Antioxidants (Basel) 2021;10:680.
3. Ruggiero SL, Dodson TB, Aghaloo T, et al. American Association of Oral and Maxillofacial Surgeons' Position Paper on Medication-Related Osteonecrosis of the Jaws-2022 Update. Oral Maxillofac Surg 2022;80(5):920–43.
4. Campisi G, Mauceri R, Bedogni A, et al. Comment Re: AAOMS position paper on Medication-related osteonecrosis of the jaw-2022 update. J Oral Maxillofac Surg 2022;80(11):1723–4.
5. Beth-Tasdogan NH, Mayer B, Hussein H, et al. Interventions for managing medication-related osteonecrosis of the jaw (Review). Cochrane Database Syst Rev 2022;7(7):CD012432.
6. Sackett DL, Rosenberg WMC, Muir Gray JA, et al. Evidence-based medicine: what it is and what it isn't. BMJ 1996;312:71–2.
7. Marx RE. Pamidronate (Aredia) and zoledronate (Zometa) induced avascular necrosis of the jaws: A growing epidemic. J Oral Maxillofac Surg 2003;61:1115–7.
8. Available at: https://news.bloomberglaw.com/product-liability-and-toxics-law/novartis-wins-judgment-in-jaw-decay-suit-allegedly-faulty-warning-didnt-cause-harm.
9. Ruggiero SL, Dodson TB, Assael LA, et al. American Association of Oral and Maxillofacial Surgeons position paper on bisphosphonate-related osteonecrosis of the jaw - 2009 update. J Oral Maxillofac Surg 2009;67. Supp 1.
10. Ruggiero SL, Dodson TB, Fantasia J, et al. American Association of Oral and Maxillofacial Surgeons position paper on medication-related osteonecrosis of the jaw–2014 update. J Oral Maxillofac Surg 2014;72:1938.
11. Wat WZM. Current controversies on the pathogenesis of medication-related osteonecrosis of the jaw. Dent J 2016;4(38):1–9.

12. Beth-Tasdogan NH, Mayer B, Hussein H, et al. Interventions for managing medication-related osteonecrosis of the jaw. Cochrane Database Syst Rev 2022;7: CD012432.
13. Lewiecki EM, Wright NC, Curtis JR, et al. Hip fracture trends in the United States, 2002 to 2015. Osteoporosis Int 2018;29:717.
14. Ruggiero SL, Drew SJ. Osteonecrosis of the jaw and bisphosphonate therapy. J Dent Res 2007;86(11):1013–21.
15. Black DM, Delmas PD, Eastell R, et al. Once-yearly zoledronic acid for treatment of postmenopausal osteoporosis. N Engl J Med 2007;356:1809.
16. Friel P, Macintyre DR. Bone sequestration from lower 3rd molar region. Br Dent J 2002;193:366.
17. Huang JS, Kok SH, Lee JJ, et al. Extensive maxillary sequestration resulting from mucormycosis. Br J Oral Maxillofac Surg 2005;43:532.
18. Peters E, Daley T. American Academy of Oral and Maxillofacial Pathology. Persistent painful ulcer of the posterior lingual mandibular mucosa. J Contemp Dent Pract 2003;4:71.
19. Kawahara M, Kuroshima S, Sawase T. Clinical considerations for medication-related osteonecrosis of the jaw: a comprehensive literature review. Int J Implant Dent 2021;7(47). https://doi.org/10.1186/s40729-021-00323-0.
20. Watts NB, Grbic JT, Binkley N, et al. Invasive oral procedures and events in postmenopausal women with osteoporosis treated with denosumab for up to 10 years. J Clin Endocrinol Metab 2019;104:2443.
21. Yamazaki T, Yamori M, Ishizaki T, et al. Increased incidence of osteonecrosis of the jaw after tooth extraction in patients treated with bisphosphonates: A cohort study. Int J Oral Maxillofac Surg 2012;41:1397.
22. Bodem JP, Kargus S, Eckstein S, et al. Incidence of bisphosphonate-related osteonecrosis of the jaw in high-risk patients undergoing surgical tooth extraction. J Cranio-Maxillofacial Surg 2015;43:510.
23. Saad F, Brown JE, Van Poznak C, et al. Incidence, risk factors, and outcomes of osteonecrosis of the jaw: Integrative analyses from three-blinded active-controlled phase III trials in cancer patients with bone metastases. Ann Oncol 2012;23:1341.
24. Sher J, Kirkham-Ali K, Luo JD, et al. Dental implant placement in patients with a history of medication related osteonecrosis of the jaw: A systematic review. J Oral Implantol 2021;67(3):249–68.
25. Mcgowan K, McGowan T, Ivanovski S. Risk factors for medication-related osteonecrosis of the jaws: A systematic review. Oral Dis 2018;24:527.
26. Cheng A, Daly CG, Logan RM, et al. Alveolar bone and the bisphosphonates. Aust Dent J 2009;54(1 Suppl):851–61.
27. Kim S, Williams DW, Lee C, et al. IL-36 induces bisphosphonate-related osteonecrosis of the jaw- Like lesions in mice by inhibiting TGF-b-mediated collagen expression. J Bone Miner Res 2017;32:309–18.
28. Krishnan A, Arslanoglu A, Yildirm N, et al. Imaging findings of bisphosphonate-related osteonecrosis of the jaw with emphasis on early magnetic resonance imaging findings. J Comput Assist Tomogr 2009;33:298–304.
29. Belibasakis GN, Meir M, Guggenheim B, et al. Oral biofilm challenge regulates the RANKL-OPG system in periodontal ligament and dental pulp cells. Microb Pathog 2011;50:6–11.
30. Dodson TB, Raje NS, Caruso PA, et al. Case records of the Massachusetts General Hospital Case-9-2008. A 65-year-old woman with a nonhealing ulcer of the jaw. N Engl J Med 2008;358:1283–91.

31. Campisi G, Mauceri R, Bertoldo E, et al. Medication-related osteonecrosis of jaws (MRONJ) prevention and diagnosis: Italian consensus update 2020. Int J Environ Res Public Health 2020;17.
32. Nicolatou-Galitis O, Schiadt M, Mendes RA, et al. Medicaiotn- related osteonecrosis of the jaw: definition and best practice for prevention, diagnosis, and treatment. Oral surg Oral Path Oral Med Oral Radiol 2019;127(3):117–35.
33. Fuco V, Santini D, Campisi G, et al. Comment on medication-related osteonecrosis of the jaw: MASCC/ISOO/ASCO clinical Practice Guideline summary. JCO Oncol Pract 2020;16:142–5.
34. Hasegawa T, Kawakita A, Ueda N, et al. A multicenter retrospective study of the risk factors associated with medication-related osteonecrosis of the jaw after tooth extraction in patients receiving oral bisphosphonates therapy: Can primary wound closure and a drug holiday really prevent MRONJ? Osteoporos Int 2017; 28:2465–73.
35. Ottesen C, Schiodt M, Gotfredsen K. Efficacy of a high-dose antiresorptive drug holiday to reduce the risk of medication-related osteonecrosis of the jaw (MRONJ): A s systematic review. Heliyon 2020;6:e03795.
36. Campisi G, Maucen R, Bertoldo F, et al. a pragmatic window of opportunity to minimize the risk of MRONJ development in individuals with osteoporosis on Denosumab therapy: a hypothesis. Head Face Med 2021;75(25):1–4.
37. Rupel K, Ottaviani G, Gobbo M, et al. A systematic review of therapeutic approaches in bisphosphonates-related osteonecrosis of the jaw (BRONJ). Oral Oncol 2014;50(11):1049–57.
38. Ramaglia L, Guida A, Iorio-Siciliano V, et al. stage-specific therapeutic strategies of medication-related osteonecrosis of the jaws: A systematic review and meta- analysis of the drug suspension protocol. Clin Oral investigat 2018;22: 597–615.
39. Carlson ER, Basile JD. The role of surgical resection in the management of bisphosphonate-related osteonecrosis of the jaws. J Oral Maxillofac Surg 2009; 67:85.
40. Wilde F, Heufelder M, Winter K, et al. The role of surgical therapy in the management of intravenous bisphosphonates-related osteonecrosis of the jaw. Oral Surg Oral Med Oral Pathol Oral Radiol Endod 2011;111:153.
41. Carlson ER, Fleisher KE, Ruggiero SL. Metastatic cancer identified in osteonecrosis specimens of the jaws in patients receiving intravenous bisphosphonate medications. J Oral Maxillofac Surg 2013;71:2077.
42. Govaerts D, Piccart F, Ockerman A, et al. Adjuvant therapies for MRONJ: A systematic review. Bone 2020. https://doi.org/10.1016/j.bone.2020.115676.
43. Bonacina R, Mariani U, Villa F, et al. Preventive strategies and clinical implications for bisphosphonate-related osteonecrosis of the jaw: A review of 282 patients. J Can Dent Assoc 2011;77:b147.
44. Silverman S, Langdahl BL, Fujowara S, et al. Reduction in hip and other fractures on patients receiving Teriparatide in real-world clinical practice : Integratedb analysis of four prospective observational studies. Calcif Tissue Int 2019;104: 193–200.
45. Heifetz-Li JJ, Abdelsamie S, Campbell CB, et al. Systematic review of the use of pentoxifylline and tocopherol for the treatment of medication -related osteonecrosis of the jaw. Oral Surg Oral Med Oral Pathol Oral Radiol 2019;128:491–7.
46. Delfrate G, Mroczek, Mecca LEA, et al. Effect of pentoxifylline and alpha-tocopherol on medication-related osteonecrosis of the jaw in rats: Before and after dental extraction. Arch Oral Biol 2022;137:1–8.

One Provider Anesthesia Model in Oral and Maxillofacial Surgery

Anh Thieu Nguyen, DMD[a],*, Earl Clarkson, DDS, FACS[a,b]

KEYWORDS

- One provider anesthesia model • Oral and maxillofacial surgery (OMS)
- Dental Anesthesia Assistants (DAAs) • Patient safety • Mortality rates
- Centers for Medicare and Medicaid Services (CMS) • Anesthesiologists
- OMS team anesthesia model

KEY POINTS

- Historical aspect: OMS specialists have made significant contributions to modern anesthesia, dating back to the discovery of nitrous oxide.
- Recent Centers for Medicare and Medicaid Services (CMS) changes: Increased scrutiny of the OMS anesthesia model has arisen due to policy changes in the CMS.
- Arguments for the model: Proponents highlight the safety and effectiveness of the OMS model, supported by well-trained Dental Anesthesia Assistants and the experience of OMS surgeons.
- Arguments against the model: Critics question the adequacy of OMS surgeons' anesthesia training compared with anesthesiologists.
- Conclusion: Studies demonstrate the safety and effectiveness of the OMS anesthesia model, debunking concerns and supporting the role of OMS professionals in providing exceptional anesthesia services.

INTRODUCTION

The delivery of anesthesia in oral and maxillofacial surgery (OMS) has been a topic of much debate and controversy in recent years. Specifically, the use of the one provider anesthesia model has generated much discussion and concern. In this model, the surgeon is responsible for administering anesthesia to the patient, in addition to performing the surgery. This differs from the traditional model of having a separate anesthesia provider, such as an anesthesiologist or a nurse anesthetist, who works alongside the

[a] Oral and Maxillofacial Surgery, The Brooklyn Hospital Center, 155 Ashland Plc, Brooklyn, NY 11201, USA; [b] Oral and Maxillofacial Surgery, Woodhull Medical Center and Attending, The Brooklyn Hospital Center, 760 Broadway, Brooklyn, New York City, NY, USA
* Corresponding author.
E-mail address: Bruceng9218@gmail.com

Dent Clin N Am 68 (2024) 87–98
https://doi.org/10.1016/j.cden.2023.07.006
0011-8532/24/© 2023 Elsevier Inc. All rights reserved.

surgeon. The one provider anesthesia model has been proposed as a mean to increase efficiency, decrease costs, and expedite the surgical process. However, the model is not without its critics, who question its safety, ethical implications, and overall effectiveness.

Historical Aspect

To gain a comprehensive perspective on the ongoing dispute, it is imperative to comprehend the profound historical relationship between anesthesiology and OMS. In his 2017 publication, Dr King succinctly elucidated this rich history.[1]

The history of anesthesiology is abundant with significant contributions from dentistry in general and OMS in particular. The early history and "discovery" of anesthesiology are intrinsically linked to dentistry, with pioneers like Horace Wells and William T Morton among the first clinicians to demonstrate and promote anesthetic techniques for surgical procedures. From Wells' promotion of nitrous oxide/oxygen anesthesia in 1844 to the 1940s, the trajectories of dentistry and anesthesiology were closely intertwined. In the late 1800s, dentistry was a leader in anesthesia provision, both qualitatively and quantitatively.[2] The strong connection between dentistry and anesthesia was evident in contemporary literature, with The Dental and Surgical Microcosm, published in 1891, claiming to be the world's first journal dedicated primarily to the science of anesthesia and anesthetics.[3]

During this era, only a few hundred medical anesthesia providers existed in the United States, whereas numerous dentists administered thousands of anesthetics annually in their offices.[4] Charles Teeter, DDS, an early innovator of anesthesia equipment and designer of the first nasopharyngeal tubes for clinical use, was elected an early President of the American Society of Anesthesiologists (ASA).[2] Even during the 1940s and particularly during World War II, anesthesia for general surgical procedures was often administered by dentist anesthetists, who were usually OMS-trained practitioners.[4]

Although the American Board of Oral Surgery and the American Board of Anesthesiology were established only a year apart, in 1940 and 1941, respectively, it is clear that from the early 1900s onward, medical anesthesiology began to experience significant growth in practitioners focusing exclusively on anesthesia. In 1911, there were 23 members of the ASAs precursor, which increased to 487 members in 1936 and over 50,000 in 2012.[2] In comparison, in 2012, the American Society of Oral and Maxillofacial Surgeons had just over 9000 members.[1]

Anesthesiology's rapid growth as an independent medical specialty led to the first significant "turf war" in the 1950s. In 1951, the ASA revoked unrestricted membership for dentists, effectively excluding dentist anesthetists and many OMS members from its ranks.[1] The American Medical Association has twice published documentation attempting to directly define or refute the "scope of practice" for OMS, once in the early 1950s and again in 2009.[5,6] This controversy, where attempts have been made by practitioners outside of dentistry to limit the scope of practice for dentists and specifically OMS providers, has manifested in various forms over the years. The term "dentist" can be easily and convincingly used to mislead the uninformed, as most medical professionals and laypeople have a preconceived notion of what a dentist is, which usually aligns with the general dentist's practice rather than the surgeon's scope of practice.

Furthermore, multiple studies have shown that there is a general lack of recognition and understanding of the overall scope of practice of the OMS, further confusing both medical professionals and the general public.[7] Even senior dental students have demonstrated a clear lack of understanding of the scope of training and expertise of the oral and maxillofacial surgeons.[8] In addition, there are numerous well-documented instances where the lay press deliberately uses the term "dentist" instead of the appropriate specialist title to sensationalize a story, making it seem as though "dentists" are practicing well beyond their scope of expertise. Consider the 2004 New York Times article titled "A Nip and Tuck With That Crown?" which exemplifies the issue of negligent omission and general misunderstanding regarding oral and maxillofacial surgeons, their training, and their scope of practice. The article erroneously stated that "an oral surgeon has a DDS or a DMD degree, which is conferred after a 4-year course of study limited to oral health, followed by another 4-year period of study in dental surgery, of which only 18 months are usually spent in surgical rotation."[9] This kind of misleading public information, ignorance, and downright disrespect can only harm our specialty as a whole. There is a pressing need to rectify public misconceptions to preserve our practice autonomy before it is irreversibly compromised.

Recent Centers for Medicare and Medicaid Services Changes

Some recent changes from Centers for Medicare and Medicaid Services (CMS) also greatly affected our specialty in hospital setting. Dr King in his publication laid out the changes clearly.[1]

In 2010, the CMS issued a memorandum clarifying and adding new requirements and interpretive guidelines for anesthesia services in Medicare-certified hospitals, which took effect in 2011. The new rules explicitly mandated the establishment of a single anesthesia service or department responsible for developing policies and procedures for all anesthesia services, including sedation and analgesia. This department would also determine the minimum qualifications for each practitioner permitted to provide anesthesia services of all forms in all locations within the hospital. The new regulations required that anesthesia services be under the direction of one individual who is a qualified doctor of medicine (MD) or doctor of osteopathic medicine (DO).[10,11]

As a result of these rule changes, many hospitals experienced a shift in the dynamics of their OMS departments or divisions and dental departments, causing them to lose their autonomy and control over the anesthesia services that they had previously provided in their hospital-based clinics. Many non-anesthesiologist physicians, such as gastroenterologists, provide sedation for their procedures. However, unlike dental/OMS providers, they typically do not require additional state licensing or training documentation.

In many institutions, the overarching policies that anesthesia departments created to oversee the delivery of anesthesia services, as required by CMS, neglected the fact that oral and maxillofacial surgeons and dental providers are specifically licensed by their state boards to provide various levels of anesthesia depending on their training. As anesthesia departments assumed the role of gatekeeper for their institutions, they gained control and oversight of the anesthetics and sedations performed in clinics previously beyond the scope of the anesthesia department. In the process of creating blanket policies for all sedation, analgesia, and anesthesia, OMS providers were often grouped with other non-anesthesiologist providers, despite their varying levels of training, and subsequently lost significant autonomy.

Consequently, hospital-based OMS departments faced several challenges, including losing the ability to perform single-provider anesthetist–operator procedures, the ability to use specific anesthesia medications in the clinic (such as propofol, ketamine, and sevoflurane), and occasionally losing the ability to provide anything beyond conscious or moderate sedation.

These new rules created significant obstacles regarding the training and accreditation of OMS residents, particularly in meeting the specific Commission on Dental Accreditation (CODA) requirements for anesthesia training. In some cases, these rules essentially doubled the number of cases residents needed to perform, placing an additional burden on their training. The policies also limited the use of certain anesthesia medications and procedures in outpatient OMS surgery centers, further affecting the quality of training and patient care.

These alarming and counterproductive changes serve as a wake-up call for our entire specialty. It is crucial for us to be more vocal and proactive in engaging with the public, and we must strive to have a voice in determining the future and survival of our specialty as it exists today.

In the following section, we explore the arguments both in favor of and against the single provider model, which is currently the standard practice within OMS.

Arguments for the Model

Proponents of the one provider anesthesia model argue that it can reduce costs and streamline the surgical process. Several studies have examined the benefits of this model and have provided evidence to support these claims. Here are some of the pros of the one provider anesthesia model supported by the most current research.

Lower cost and better convenience for the patient

Advocates of the one provider anesthesia model assert that it can help reduce costs associated with using an additional, separate anesthesia provider. Multiple studies have examined the financial impact of the one provider anesthesia model, and the evidence supports the potential benefits. It is widely recognized that the average cost of intravenous (IV) sedation in an OMFS office typically ranges from $250 to $700, with an average of approximately $482.[12] In contrast, the fee for a separate anesthesiologist's presence is usually between $500 and $3500, exceeding the expenses associated with the one provider model.[13]

Besides cost reduction, patient convenience is another advantage of the one provider anesthesia model. Patients who desire anesthesia can typically receive the service on the same day or the next available day, without having to depend on a third-party provider whose schedule may be restricted or limited. Moreover, the third-party anesthesia provider might often be in-network with different insurance providers than the surgeon, requiring patients to undertake the extra hassle of verifying if the anesthesia portion of the procedure is covered by their insurance. Given the complex landscape of insurance in the contemporary United States, this additional step can frequently cause delays and complications in patients' much-needed treatments.

Comparative patient satisfaction

Proponents of the one provider anesthesia model argue that it can improve patient satisfaction by reducing anxiety and providing a more comfortable surgical experience. Although there have been no comparative studies between the different models, a study by Coyle and colleagues has found that 95.8% of patients who received deep sedation/general anesthesia (DS/GA) in OMFS offices were extremely or moderately satisfied, whereas only 1.1% were moderately or extremely dissatisfied. Factors predicting satisfaction included increased age, memory of postoperative instructions, and the addition of nitrous oxide to some regimens. On the other hand, predictors of dissatisfaction were young age, anxiety, pain, vomiting, and being awake during the procedure. The study concluded that patients are generally satisfied with DS/GA provided in an office-based setting, although some factors, such as anxiety, pain, and vomiting, can lead to dissatisfaction.[14]

Another study by Perrott and colleagues used a prospective cohort design and a sample composed of patients undergoing procedures in the office-based ambulatory setting of oral and maxillofacial surgeons practicing in the United States who received local anesthesia (LA), conscious sedation (CS), or DS/GA. The results showed that the sample comprised 34,191 patients, with 71.9% receiving DS/GA, 15.5% receiving CS, and 12.6% receiving LA. The complication rate was 1.3 per 100 cases, which were minor and self-limiting. Two patients had complications requiring hospitalization. Most patients (80.3%) reported some degree of anxiety before the procedure. After the procedure, 61.2% of patients reported having no anxiety about future operations. Overall, 94.3% of patients reported satisfaction with the anesthetic, and more than 94.7% of all patients would recommend the anesthetic technique to a loved one. The study concluded that the office-based administration of LA, CS, or DS/GA delivered via OMS anesthesia teams was safe and associated with a high level of patient satisfaction.[15]

On the other hand, a retrospective study by Okuda and colleagues investigated the dissatisfaction rate for anesthesia and the contributing factors for it using a questionnaire that included anesthesia-related adverse events and a simplified patient satisfaction scale. The study analyzed an institutional registry containing 21,606 anesthesia cases and conducted multivariate logistic analysis in 9429 patients. In the study population, 549 patients rated the anesthesia service as dissatisfactory (a rate of 5.8%).[15]

As noted, the rate of patient dissatisfaction is comparable or lower for the OMFS one provider anesthesia model compared with the service provided by MD anesthesiologist. Even though the studies are not direct comparison, one could see that the one provider anesthesia model has a comparable, if not better, patient satisfaction.

Increased surgeon control

Advocates of the one provider anesthesia model contend that it offers surgeons enhanced control over anesthesia administration, which may contribute to more successful outcomes. Although no scientific studies currently substantiate this claim, anecdotal evidence and the authors' personal experience seem to support it.

In the single provider model for DS, surgeons can more precisely manage the timing and depth of sedation while also facilitating improved patient communication throughout the procedure. In addition, when administering anesthesia in this manner, surgeons are ideally positioned to manage airway complications and maintain patient safety. Being in close proximity to the patient's airway allows the surgeon to quickly detect and address any potential risks, ensuring a safer surgical experience.

The surgeon's familiarity with their trained staff, equipment, and room layout further enhances their control over the sedation process. Efficient communication, equipment retrieval in emergencies, and streamlined logistics are facilitated by this consistency. Having a stable surgical environment with the same staff and equipment each time is beneficial for the surgeon and the patient, rather than introducing variability by changing the anesthesiologist for each procedure.

Arguments Against the Model

Although the one provider anesthesia model has some potential benefits, there are also several concerns and disadvantages associated with this approach. Here are some of the cons of the one provider anesthesia model supported by the most current research.

Inadequate training

One of the main concerns associated with the one provider anesthesia model is the potential for inadequate training of surgeons in administering anesthesia. To look further into this issue, it is important to understand the current anesthesia training of a typical oral maxillofacial surgeon during residency.

In 2012, the CODA extended the required duration of the dedicated anesthesia rotation for OMS residents from 4 to 5 months. However, this 5-month period does not fully represent the comprehensive anesthesia experience and training OMS residents receive during their residency, and this is what most other anesthesia providers and outside observers do not understand: The anesthesia exposure for OMS residents is designed to accumulate over the course of their 4 to 6 years of training, as it is an essential component of numerous standard OMS office and clinic-based procedures. The training in any specific procedure or technique is a result of a combination of experiences over time. OMS residents' anesthesia training not only includes general anesthesiology training during their formal anesthesia rotation but also encompasses administering anesthesia for OMS-specific office-based outpatient procedures. This often involves serving as the sole provider of both anesthesia and surgical services, which frequently occurs throughout the entire 4- to 6-year training program. It is safe to say that OMFS residents are trained in anesthesia for a much longer time than the critiques of the model expected, and the initial required 5 months rotation in GA is just the start of their comprehensive anesthesia training.[16]

Compare this with the training for an MD anesthesiologist, the training for an MD anesthesiologist during residency typically lasts 4 years, including a 1-year internship (in either medicine, surgery, or a transitional year) followed by 3 years of anesthesiology training. During this time, anesthesiology residents are required to complete a minimum number of cases and gain experience in various anesthesia subspecialties, including pediatric, obstetric, neurosurgical, and cardiac anesthesia.

According to the Accreditation Council for Graduate Medical Education Program Requirements for Graduate Medical Education in Anesthesiology (effective July 1, 2021), anesthesiology residents must complete at least 850 anesthetic cases, with a minimum of 200 cases in the Clinical Anesthesia first year (CA-1 year) and 250 cases in each of the CA-2 and CA-3 years. The requirements also specify the minimum number of cases in different subspecialty areas and clinical experiences, such as 40 cases in pediatric anesthesia, 30 cases in obstetric anesthesia, and 20 cases in cardiac anesthesia. In addition, residents are required to complete a minimum number of regional anesthesia procedures, pain management experiences, and critical care rotations.[1]

The training for an MD anesthesiologist is undeniably rigorous and comprehensive, encompassing a wide range of requirements. However, it is important to note that there are no specific mandates for MD anesthesiologists to gain experience in sedating OMFS patients within an ambulatory office setting. Most of an anesthesia resident's time is dedicated to the operating room, which is understandable considering what the anesthesia residency is meant for. In fact, anesthesiology residency programs have themselves recognized the inadequacy of their training in providing exposure to office-based anesthesia (OBA) during residency.[17] Given the general unfamiliarity of MD anesthesiologists with OMFS procedures, environments, and equipment, and considering the extensive 4- to 6-year training of OMFS in administering anesthesia using the one provider anesthesia model, it would be unreasonable to argue that oral and maxillofacial surgeons are ill-equipped to provide anesthesia under this model.

A closer examination of the American Association of Oral and Maxillofacial Surgeons' requirements for graduating OMFS residents reveals the extensive and rigorous training involved in their education. The anesthesia training program encompasses a comprehensive curriculum, addressing pain and anxiety control, outpatient surgery experience, and airway management competence. Each graduating resident must administer GA/DS to a minimum of 300 patients, including 150 ambulatory cases and 50 pediatric cases. In addition, the program features a core didactic component that highlights patient evaluation, risk assessment, anesthesia techniques, monitoring, and complication management. To complete their training, residents must obtain and maintain advanced cardiac life support (ACLS) certification and acquire pediatric advanced life support (PALS) certification.[18] On graduation, surgeons must apply for a GA permit from their practicing state, which mandates the maintenance of both ACLS and PALS permits to uphold the anesthesia permit.[19] Contrary to the "wild west" portrayal often depicted by the media, the existing anesthesia model is, in fact, stringently regulated and demanding.

Inadequate attention to the patient while performing surgery

A common concern regarding the one provider anesthesia model is the perceived lack of attention given to the patient, whereas the surgeon performs surgery. However, in reality, surgeons are supported by highly trained staff who are always present during the surgery. These team members assist in monitoring the patient, performing emergency maneuvers when necessary and acting as a second or even third layer of safety for the patient. The term "one-provider-anesthesia" is a misnomer that fails to accurately represent the practice model often used in an OMS practice. A more suitable description would be the "OMS team anesthesia model" or the "OMS staff anesthesia model." It is not only the surgeon overseeing the patient but also the entire team working together. This level of attentiveness may not be present in a standard operating room, where only an anesthesiologist or a Certified Registered Nurse Anesthetist (CRNA) might be trained to monitor the patient, unless, of course, an OMS specialist is also in the room.

It is crucial to note that the specialized assistants supporting the OMS are not ordinary dental assistants. These professionals, known as "Dental Anesthesia Assistants" (DAA), are highly trained members of the OMS team who focus on monitoring anesthesia. Many providers outside the specialty, including general dentists and other specialized dentists, may be unaware of the extensive training and expertise that DAAs possess, ensuring their competence in assisting with anesthesia during surgery.

Again, a review of the current requirements of the DAAs will reveal a rigorous certification program. To become a DAA, one must pass the Dental Anesthesia Assistant National Certification Examination (DAANCE) administered by the American Association of Oral and Maxillofacial Surgeons (AAOMS). The DAANCE is a comprehensive two-part continuing education program for OMS assistants or those used by dental professionals with valid anesthesia permits. Consisting of around 36 hours of self-study material, quizzes, and a standardized computer-based examination, the program is recognized by the American Association of Oral and Maxillofacial Surgeons as an ADA Continuing Education Recognition Program (CERP) provider, offering 36 continuing education credits. On successfully completing the final examination, assistants receive certification proof and a program completion lapel pin. To participate in DAANCE, candidates must meet certain eligibility requirements; they must have at least 6 months of employment with an AAOMS fellow or member oral and maxillofacial surgeon or a dental professional holding a valid anesthesia permit, and non-AAOMS offices must submit a copy of their anesthesia permit with each application. In addition, candidates must provide a current Cardiopulonary Resuscitation (CPR) or basic life support certification with their registration form to receive study materials, and this certification must remain valid through their examination date, with a minimum of 6 months. If a new CPR card is not received within 6 months of notification, candidates must submit a new application and fee to qualify for the examination.

On completing the DAANCE course, dental anesthesia assistants should be able to demonstrate a comprehensive understanding of various aspects of anesthesia and patient care. This includes describing the basic anatomy and physiology of the cardiovascular and respiratory systems as well as the vascular anatomy of the forearm and the divisions of the central nervous system. Assistants should be proficient in discussing components of the medical history and reviewing systems, differentiating between GA, DS, CS, nitrous oxide analgesia, and LA. They must be familiar with the drugs and techniques used by OMS anesthesia teams to achieve the various levels of anesthesia or sedation. In addition, they should be capable of identifying and treating basic office emergencies, such as cardiovascular, respiratory, allergic, and convulsive emergencies. They must also be proficient in monitoring blood pressure, pulse, and oxygen saturation and can recognize normal electrocardiograph waves and serious abnormal variations from the normal rhythm. Last, dental anesthesia assistants should understand the essentials and importance of maintaining complete and accurate medical records. The program consists of a self-study component with quizzes and a final examination, allowing participants to customize their study schedules based on their learning pace. Sponsoring surgeons should be available to address questions and discuss module content during the study period. Candidates have 6 months from their activation date to take the DAANCE test, ensuring ample time for preparation and mastery of the material.

The comprehensive training required for DAAs ensures that patients are under the care of highly skilled and capable professionals. It is a significant misrepresentation to suggest that a seasoned surgeon, supported by well-trained, certified, and competent staff in a strictly regulated environment, provides "inadequate" care. Patients can be confident that they are in expert hands throughout the procedure.[20]

Safety and mortality

The primary and most significant concern regarding the current OMS anesthesia model is its safety and potential impact on mortality rates. Critics argue that this model is inherently unsafe and could potentially result in higher mortality rates compared with a two-provider anesthesia model. However, such arguments lack solid evidence and have been repeatedly debunked in numerous studies. Comparative analyses of mortality rates consistently show that the existing OMFS anesthesia model, when executed correctly, can be deemed exceptionally safe, if not even safer than the current GA model used in the operating room nationwide.

According to a study conducted by D'Eramo and colleagues focused on the incidence of specific complications and mortality rates for office anesthesia administered by fully qualified oral and maxillofacial surgeons in Massachusetts, concluding that outpatient anesthesia in the OMS office continues to be a safe therapeutic modality with a mortality rate of one in 1,733,055.[21] The latest and most extensive analysis can be found in the 2003 anesthesia study conducted by the Oral and Maxillofacial Surgery National Insurance Company (OMSNIC), which insures approximately 80% of practicing OMFS in the United States.[15,22] This research examined negative outcomes associated with outpatient anesthesia during a decade, spanning from 1994 to 2003. Findings from the study indicated that for ASA I/II patients, the intrinsic mortality risk linked to outpatient anesthesia was roughly one in 800,000. A more recent OMSNIC report from 2000 to 2013 including a total of 39,392,008 cases reveals one occurrence of death or brain injury per 348,602 sedation procedures.[23] Another study from the AAOMS Insurance Company released data from 1988 to 1999. In an analysis of insurance claims, Deegan and colleagues revealed that the mortality risk in oral surgery offices was 19 out of 14,206,923 anesthetics administered (a rate of 1:748,000).[22] In 2003, D'Eramo and colleagues published the third part of this series, which reported two anesthesia-related fatalities in 1,706,100 anesthetics, resulting in a mortality rate of 1:853,000.[24] Hunter and Molinaro shared the findings of a retrospective study on outpatient mortality within the Boston University Oral Surgery training program, which revealed zero fatalities in 1126 anesthetic cases.[25] The Mayo Clinic published a report on 17,634 sedations from 2004 to 2019 that was done at the Mayo Clinic's OMFS division which found that the mortality rate is 0% and the adverse reaction rate to medication is 0.1%.[26]

In comparison, in GA literatures, it is found that the mortality rate due to GA complications overall in the United States range from one in 100,000 to 200,000 cases, which is much higher than that of current OMFS numbers.[27,28] Dr King in his article also pointed out that in a study by Lee and colleagues named "Trends in death associated with pediatric dental sedation and general anesthesia" that included cases from 1980 to 2011, 56.8% of the deaths occurred when a general or pediatric dentist administered anesthesia. There were eight deaths when an OMS-provided anesthesia and seven deaths when an anesthesiologist was the provider. Although the number of deaths involving oral and maxillofacial surgeons and anesthesiologists was almost identical, the data do not take into account the probable higher number of OBA cases performed by the surgeons compared with medical anesthesiologists within this patient population. The study did not report the overall number of cases or rate. This also pointed to the fact that dental anesthesia cases performed by oral and maxillofacial surgeons routinely have lower mortality rates than those performed by the anesthesiologists.[1,29]

It is essential to clarify that the authors of this article do not assert that oral and maxillofacial surgeons have superior anesthesia training compared with anesthesiologists, as evidenced by lower mortality rates across the board. Such a comparison would be akin to comparing apples and oranges. The likely reason for lower mortality rates among OMSs anesthesia cases are their careful patient selection (primarily ASA I/II, often young and healthy) and their extensive familiarity and experience with dental anesthesia cases, alongside their well-trained staff. Although oral and maxillofacial surgeons may not be experts in GA, we are unparalleled experts in dental and oral–maxillofacial OBA.

SUMMARY

In conclusion, the one provider anesthesia model used in OMS practices has been a subject of debate due to concerns about patient safety, inadequate attention, and mortality rates. However, these concerns have been largely addressed and debunked by studies and analyses that demonstrate the safety and effectiveness of the OMS anesthesia model when executed correctly.

The well-trained and certified DAAs play a crucial role in supporting OMS surgeons during surgery, ensuring that patients receive attentive care throughout the procedure. The term "one-provider-anesthesia" may be misleading, as the model relies on an entire OMS team, which includes DAAs and other staff members who work together to provide a safe environment for patients.

Furthermore, studies have consistently shown that the OMS anesthesia model has lower mortality rates compared with the GA model used in operating rooms nationwide. This can be attributed to careful patient selection, the extensive experience of OMS surgeons in dental anesthesia cases, and the support of well-trained staff.

It is essential to recognize the expertise of OMS surgeons in dental and oral–maxillofacial OBA, rather than comparing their training to that of anesthesiologists. The OMS anesthesia model, supported by rigorous training and certification programs for DAAs, offers a safe and effective option for patients undergoing oral and maxillofacial procedures.

In closing this article, the authors would like to emphasize that OMS professionals have been at the forefront of modern anesthesia, making significant contributions to its development and shaping the field as we know it today. OMS specialists have a long and distinguished history in anesthesia, dating back to the discovery of nitrous oxide by Dr Horace Wells and Dr Morton. They have been providing safe, efficient, and high-quality office-based dental and maxillofacial surgery anesthesia services for longer and safer than any other medical field, including anesthesiology.

To suggest that OMS specialists should be restricted from providing their patients with exceptional anesthesia services based on unfounded fears and allegations is not only unreasonable but potentially harmful. Imposing limitations on the current OMS anesthesia model could adversely impact the training of future OMS professionals and compromise the safety and effectiveness of their services. This could subsequently result in increased accident rates, which would likely become sensational stories in the mainstream media. The ASA might seize this opportunity to further advocate for restrictions on the current OMS practice model. As a result, patients might end up receiving inferior anesthesia care from anesthesiologists or CRNAs who lack the experience and expertise in dental and maxillofacial surgery anesthesia as they admitted themselves.

The potential consequences of adopting a subpar anesthesia model include increased mortality rates, patient inconvenience, longer wait times, and higher costs, all without any proven benefits. In a time when health care costs and waiting times are escalating, it would be unwise to transition to such a model that offers reduced quality of care.

The authors advocate for more rigorous training for residents in both GA and the OMS team anesthesia model, increased public awareness of the scope of OMS specialty services, enhanced public education and outreach, greater representation of the field in legislative bodies, and continued research demonstrating the safety of the current OMS anesthesia practice. The OMS specialty faces challenges from various quarters, making it crucial for professionals and peers to educate themselves on this pressing issue and proactively address these concerns. In summary, the debate surrounding the OMS anesthesia model should not be a controversy at all.

CLINICS CARE POINTS

- The oral and maxillofacial surgery team anesthesia model holds a superior record of safety, offering numerous advantages to patients.
- We should amplify our focus on the comprehensive anesthesia training of emerging oral and maxillofacial surgeons.
- It is imperative for established practices to perpetually engage in continuing education, emphasizing in-office anesthesia for both surgeons and their supporting staff. A minimum requirement should be compliance with basic life support, advanced cardiac life support, and pediatric advanced life support. Regular medical emergency drills involving the entire office team are recommended for optimal preparation.

> • The presence of highly trained dental anesthesia assistants and adherence to all safety standards for in-office anesthesia are paramount to perpetuating the high standard of care in our specialty.

DISCLOSURE

The authors have nothing to disclose.

REFERENCES

1. King BJ, Levine A. Controversies in Anesthesia for Oral and Maxillofacial Surgery. Oral Maxillofac Surg Clin North Am 2017;29(4):515–23.
2. Orr DL 2nd. The development of anesthesiology in oral and maxillofacial surgery. Oral Maxillofac Surg Clin North Am 2013;25(3):341.
3. Wood Library-Museum of Anesthesiology. History of Anesthesia. Wood Library-Museum of Anesthesiology. https://www.woodlibrarymuseum.org/history-of-anesthesia/. Accessed April 8, 2023.
4. Diaz JH. Calling all anesthetists to service in World War II. Anesthesiology 2002; 96(3):776–7.
5. Lynch DF. Are You Interested in the Definition of Oral Surgery? Newsmonthly 1957;4(6):7–8.
6. American Medical Association. AMA scope of practice data series: oral and maxillofacial surgeons. Chicago, IL: American Medical Association; 2009.
7. Hunter MJ, Rubeiz T, Rose L. Recognition of the scope of oral and maxillofacial surgery by the public and health care professionals. J Oral Maxillofac Surg 1996;54(10):1227–33.
8. Guerrero AV, Elo JA, Sun HB, et al, OMS Versus OFS Workgroup. What Name Best Represents Our Specialty? Oral and Maxillofacial Surgeon Versus Oral and Facial Surgeon. J Oral Maxillofac Surg 2017;75(1):9–20.
9. Kuczynski A. A nip and tuck with that crown? New York Times. 2004. Correction published May 30, 2004.
10. Rosing JR. CMS anesthesia rules are stiffened. OR Manag 2010;26(3):20–1.
11. Department of Health & Human Services (DHHS). Certification Centers for Medicare & Medicaid Services (CMS). CMS Manual System, Pub. 100-107 State Operations Provider Certification. Transmittals 59 and 74. May 21, 2010 and December 2, 2011.
12. Sedation Dentistry Cost" Cost of Dental Sedation: General Anesthesia, IV Sedation. Accessed April 8, 2023. https://health.costhelper.com/dental-sedation.html.
13. CostHelper. Anesthesia cost. Accessed April 8, 2023. https://health.costhelper.com/anesthesia.html.
14. Coyle TT, Helfrick JF, Gonzalez ML, et al. Office-based ambulatory anesthesia: Factors that influence patient satisfaction or dissatisfaction with deep sedation/general anesthesia. J Oral Maxillofac Surg 2005;63(2):163–72.
15. Perrott DH, Yuen JP, Andresen RV, et al. Office-based ambulatory anesthesia: outcomes of clinical practice of oral and maxillofacial surgeons. J Oral Maxillofac Surg 2003;61(9):983–96.
16. Okuda C, Inoue S, Kawaguchi M. Anesthesia-related care dissatisfaction: a cohort historical study to reveal related risks. Braz J Anesthesiol 2021;71(2): 103–9.
17. Accreditation Council for Graduate Medical Education. ACGME Program Requirements for Graduate Medical Education in Anesthesiology. Effective July

1, 2021. https://www.acgme.org/Portals/0/PFAssets/ProgramRequirements/040_Anesthesiology_2021.pdf?ver=2021-06-28-145121-637. Accessed April 2023.

18. Accreditation Standards for Advanced Specialty Education Programs in Oral and Maxillofacial Surgery. 2022.

19. New York State Education Department, Office of the Professions. Dental Anesthesia/Sedation Certification. Available at: https://www.op.nysed.gov/professions/dentists/dental-anesthesia-sedation-certification. Accessed April 8, 2023.

20. American Association of Oral and Maxillofacial Surgeons. Dental Anesthesia Assistant National Certification Examination (DAANCE) Handbook. https://www.aaoms.org/docs/cont_education/daance/daance_handbook.pdf. Accessed April 8, 2023.

21. D'Eramo EM, Bontempi WJ, Howard JB. Anesthesia morbidity and mortality experience among Massachusetts oral and maxillofacial surgeons. J Oral Maxillofac Surg 2008;66(12):2421–33.

22. Deegan AE. Anesthesia morbidity and mortality, 1988-1999: claims statistics from AAOMS National Insurance Company. Anesth Prog 2001;48(3):89–92.

23. Bennett JD, Kramer KJ, Bosack RC. How safe is deep sedation or general anesthesia while providing dental care? J Am Dent Assoc 2015;146(9):705–8.

24. D'eramo EM, Bookless SJ, Howard JB. Adverse events with outpatient anesthesia in Massachusetts. J Oral Maxillofac Surg 2003;61(7):793–800.

25. Hunter MJ, Molinaro AM. Morbidity and mortality with outpatient anesthesia: the experience of a residency training program. J Oral Maxillofac Surg 1997;55(7):684–8.

26. Wiemer SJ, Nathan JM, Heggestad BT, et al. Safety of Outpatient Procedural Sedation Administered by Oral and Maxillofacial Surgeons: The Mayo Clinic Experience in 17,634 Sedations (2004 to 2019). J Oral Maxillofac Surg 2021;79(5):990–9.

27. Bainbridge D, Martin J, Arango M, et al. Perioperative and anaesthetic-related mortality in developed and developing countries: a systematic review and meta-analysis. Lancet 2012;380(9847):1075–81.

28. Bhananker SM, Posner KL, Cheney FW, et al. Injury and liability associated with monitored anesthesia care: a closed claims analysis. Anesthesiology 2006;104(2):228–34.

29. Lee HH, Milgrom P, Starks H, et al. Trends in death associated with pediatric dental sedation and general anesthesia. Paediatr Anaesth 2013;23(8):741–6.

Indications for Antibiotic Prophylaxis for Dentoalveolar Procedures

Chad Dammling, DDS, MD[a],*, Evan M. Gilmartin, BS[b],
Shelly Abramowicz, DMD, MPH[c], Brian Kinard, DMD, MD[a]

KEYWORDS

• Antibiotic • Prophylaxis • Maxillofacial surgery • Dentoalveolar

KEY POINTS

- Antibiotic prophylaxis should be used to protect at-risk patients from microbial infection.
- Most dentoalveolar procedures do not require antibiotic prophylaxis. Patients with specific cardiac comorbidities or procedures involving implants or grafts may necessitate antibiotic prophylaxis.
- Localized infection and alveolar osteitis can be decreased with prophylactic antibiotics during extraction of third molars.
- Amoxicillin and other penicillin derivatives have the highest efficacy on oral cavity flora and can be effective when given as a single preoperative dose.
- Providers must consider the potential for increased microbial antibiotic resistance and an increase in treatment costs when prescribing antibiotics.

INTRODUCTION

Most oral and maxillofacial surgery (OMS) procedures have a risk of a transient bacteremia from exposure to oral cavity flora. Antibiotic prophylaxis is the use of antibiotics perioperatively to *prevent* potential infections at the surgical site or at a distant location by providing adequate blood levels of a medication before surgical incision.[1] Antibiotic prophylaxis is *not* used for therapeutic purposes as the goal of therapeutic antibiotics is to treat active infection—often over an extended period of time.[2]

According to the American Society of Health System Pharmacists, the goals of antimicrobial prophylaxis are to prevent surgical site infections, prevent morbidity and mortality, reduce the duration and cost of health care, and produce no adverse effects and have no

[a] Department of Oral and Maxillofacial Surgery, School of Dentistry, University of Alabama at Birmingham, 1919 7th Avenue South- Room 406, Birmingham, AL 35233, USA; [b] School of Dentistry, University of Alabama at Birmingham, 1919 7th Avenue South, Birmingham, AL 35233, USA; [c] Division of Oral and Maxillofacial Surgery, Department of Surgery, Emory University School of Medicine, Oral and Maxillofacial Surgery, Children's Healthcare of Atlanta, 1365 Clifton Road, Building B, Suite 2300, Atlanta 30322, Georgia, USA
* Corresponding author.
E-mail address: Dammling@gmail.com

Dent Clin N Am 68 (2024) 99–111
https://doi.org/10.1016/j.cden.2023.07.004
0011-8532/24/© 2023 Elsevier Inc. All rights reserved.

adverse consequences to the flora of the hospital or of the patient.[3] The decision to provide antibiotic prophylaxis must balance the risks of antibiotic resistance, adverse drug reactions, and increased health care costs with the benefit of decreasing infection.

Established guidelines have been created and should be observed to avoid the risk of antibiotic toxicity, microbial resistance, and excess health care costs.[4,5] Recently, these guidelines have become more stringent and narrow due to an increased risk to benefit ratios.[6]

Multiple patient-based and health care system risks exist. They must be minimized and evaluated before prescribing. Patient-specific adverse risks are life-threatening anaphylaxis, *Clostridium difficile* colitis, and/or gastrointestinal side effects. These adverse drug reactions can occur in 6% to 7% of patients who are taking antibiotics.[7] Of all antibiotics, clindamycin carries the highest risk of *C difficile* colitis with a risk of 2% to 10% even with a single dose.[8–11] In the United States, dentists are the number one prescriber of clindamycin.[12] Amoxicillin, the most frequently used antibiotic overall, commonly can cause a rash, gastrointestinal effects, and/or hematologic complications.[13]

At a health care system level, antibiotic stewardship is critical to prevent multiple drug-resistant bacteria that can evolve even with a single dose of antibiotics.[1,14] The Global Antimicrobial Surveillance Program of the World Health Organization has identified over 500,000 people in 22 countries with antibiotic-resistant organisms.[5] Further, a significant health care system cost exists to patient and hospitals in the management of drug-resistant bacteria.[15] Infections from resistant bacteria are more difficult to treat, require prolonged courses of expensive antibiotic regimens, and have potential to cause a high number of deaths per year.[5] The cost per patient of an antibiotic-resistant infection ranges from $18,588 to $29,069 and has been estimated to be as high as $20 billion in health care costs.[15]

Overprescribing and misuse of antibiotics causes increased cost and antimicrobial resistance.[16] It is estimated that dentists prescribe 10% of all antibiotic prescriptions and 80% of these prescriptions are unnecessary.[5,17] In dentistry, there are limited indications for antibiotics as most periodontal and dental diseases can be managed with improved oral hygiene, local measures, and/or minor operative interventions.[18,19] Similarly, in a previous health care survey, 88% of orthopedic surgeons have been found to prescribe antibiotic prophylaxis as a "defensive medicine" rather than by following the standard of care.[5,20]

The determination for which procedures require perioperative prophylaxis has been studied extensively. This decision is often based on procedure and patient-specific factors. Inherently, the insertion of foreign bodies such as bone grafts or dental implants has the potential to cause an infection. In addition, patient-related factors (ie, immune status, diabetes, nutritional status) exist that must be taken into consideration when stratifying the risk of postoperative complications.[3] There also are critical steps within OMS procedures that fundamentally decrease the risk of infection (ie, clean incisions, hemostasis, and/or copious and adequate irrigation).[21]

This article discusses the indications for antibiotic prophylaxis during dentoalveolar procedures. For the majority of these procedures on healthy patients, guidelines are limited and are at the discretion of the provider. As a result, it is critical that the surgeon takes into consideration multiple factors (ie, overall health of the patient and complexity of the procedure).

INFECTIVE ENDOCARDITIS PROPHYLAXIS

In patients presenting with specific cardiac conditions (**Box 1**), the use of prophylactic antibiotics for dentoalveolar procedures can decrease the risk of infective endocarditis

---

Box 1
Cardiac conditions for which infective endocarditis prophylaxis is indicated[24]

Cardiac Conditions for Which Prophylaxis with Dentoalveolar Procedures is Indicated
- Prosthetic cardiac valve or prosthetic material used for cardiac valve repair
- Previous infective endocarditis
- Unrepaired cyanotic congenital heart disease including palliative shunts and conduits
- Completely repaired congenital heart defect with prosthetic material or device during the first 6 months after the procedure
- Repaired congenital heart disease with residual defects at the site or adjacent to the site of a prosthetic patch or prosthetic device (which inhibit endothelialization)
- Cardiac transplant recipients who develop cardiac valve regurgitation

---

(IE). IE is a rare infection of the inner lining of the heart with a high morbidity. IE is most often caused by *S aureus,* viridans group streptococci, and enterococcus species.[6,22,23] Guidelines by the American Heart Association (AHA) indicate the use of prophylactic antibiotics for patients undergoing select dental procedures that pierce the oral mucosa or involve manipulation of gingival tissue/periapical region of teeth. Guidelines attempt to manage patients with risk factors for IE (**Box 2**).[22,24] Examples of dentoalveolar procedure that require prophylaxis are tooth extraction/s, implants, grafts, and/or abscess drainage.[25] Prophylactic antibiotics are not indicated for use during the administration of routine anesthetic injections through healthy tissue, radiographic examinations, prosthodontic or orthodontic procedures, and/or during exfoliation of deciduous teeth. It is imperative that health care providers promote the maintenance of oral health and hygiene as the main effective means of prevention of IE as daily activities such as chewing and tooth brushing produce a greater cumulative risk of bacteremia compared with dental procedures.[4,22,25]

If a patient meets the above criteria for cardiac antibiotic prophylaxis, a single preoperative dose of antibiotic 30 to 60 minutes before the procedure should be administered to reduce bacteremia caused by bacteria in the oral cavity (**Table 1**). If the preoperative dose is inadvertently missed, the medication can be administered up to 2 hours postoperatively.[22,26] For patients taking an antibiotic for another reason, it is recommended that a medication from a different class be used for prophylactic coverage.[27] Patients may also delay treatment for 10 days following the completion of the antibiotic course to reestablish the oral flora and then proceed with IE prophylaxis.[26]

The AHA guidelines for antibiotic prophylaxis were first published in 1955 and have had multiple revisions—most recently in 2021. Of note, it was not until 1997 that the guidelines for postoperative antibiotics were removed and only preoperative doses were recommended.[20] Further, antibiotic choices for patients with penicillin allergies

---

Box 2
Dental procedures requiring infective endocarditis prophylaxis[24]

Dental Procedures Requiring Endocarditis Prophylaxis
- All dental procedures that involve manipulation of gingival tissue or the periapical region of teeth or perforation of the oral mucosa
- The following do not need prophylaxis: routine anesthetic injections through noninfected tissue, dental radiographs, placement of removable prosthodontic or orthodontic appliances, adjustment of orthodontic appliances, placement of orthodontic brackets, shedding of deciduous teeth, and bleeding from trauma to the lips or oral mucosa

Table 1
Antibiotic regimens for a dental procedure regimen: single dose 30 to 60 minutes before procedure

Situation	Agent	Adults	Children
Oral	Amoxicillin	2g	50 mg/kg
Unable to take oral medication	Ampicillin OR	2 g IM or IV	50 mg/kg IM or IV
	Cefazolin or ceftriaxone	1 g IM or IV	50 mg/kg IM or IV
Allergic to penicillin or ampicillin—oral	Cephalexin[a] OR	2g	50 mg/kg
	Azithromycin or	500 mg	15 mg/kg
	clarithromycin OR	100 mg	<45 kg, 2.2 mg/kg >45 kg,
	Doxycydine		100 mg
Allergic to penicillin or ampicillin and unable to take oral medication	Cefazolin or ceftriaxone[b]	1 g IM or IV	50 mg/kg IM or IV

have recently transitioned away from clindamycin to cephalexin, azithromycin, clarithromycin, or doxycycline.

PROSTHETIC JOINTS

Evidence supports that patients with prosthetic joints do not require prophylactic antibiotics for dentoalveolar procedures as there is no increased risk to cause prosthetic joint infection (PJI).[26,28–31]

In 2014, the American Dental Association (ADA) found no relationship between PJI and dental procedures. Further, in a population-based cohort of 255,568 Taiwanese patients, the correlation of PJI and previous invasive dental treatment was evaluated for 2 years.[32] PJI occurred in 0.61% of the non-dental treatment group and 0.57% of the dental treatment cohort. An association between PJI and antibiotic prophylaxis did not exist.

In a case-crossover study with over 9000 patients in England with PJI (where no prophylactic antibiotics were used), Thornhill and colleagues determined that no infection was caused by an invasive dental procedure.[33] A similar observational study in the United States completed in 2023 with over 2300 late infection cases also showed no correlation to invasive dental treatment and further support no antibiotic prophylaxis.[34]

Despite the above literature, many orthopedic surgeons and dentists continue to prescribe antibiotic prophylaxis for PJI.[20] This may be due to "defensive" medicine or lack of knowledge about the literature changes. Before 2013, the American Academy of Orthopedic Surgeons (AAOS) reported that "clinicians should consider AP for all total joint replacement patients before any invasive procedure that may cause a bacteremia".[35] Along with help from the ADA, this decision was reversed in 2013 by the AAOS.[36]

As previously discussed, when improperly prescribed, the use of prophylactic antibiotics for patients with prosthetic joints can lead to an increased risk of adverse drug reactions, treatment costs, and antibiotic resistance. The only times that an antibiotic prophylaxis is recommended for joint prophylaxis is in the setting of significant immunodeficiency (cancer, acquired immunodeficiency syndrome, or solid organ transplant on immunosuppression).[37]

When patients present following a total temporomandibular joint (TMJ) replacement, standard guidelines on recommendations for joint prophylaxis do not exist. Despite this, anecdotally, patients with TMJ prosthesis are recommended to receive prophylactic antibiotics to cover oral flora if they are to receive an inferior alveolar nerve injection during the procedure.[38] This is due to the potential close contact of the needle tip and the condylar component fixation screws of the TMJ prosthesis near the pterygomandibular space.[39] A need for long-term studies on the risk of potential seeding of bacteria at the site of the joint prosthesis exists.

THIRD MOLARS

Aside from third molar extractions by OMS, there remains little evidence of antibiotic prophylaxis for dental extractions by general dentists in the literature. As a result, the following section focus on third molar removal by specialists. Antibiotic prophylaxis for simple dental extractions should only be provided by the criteria above or if the patient is in an immunocompromised state. This discussion will also include review risks of both alveolar osteitis and local wound infection.

Alveolar osteitis (dry socket) is the most common sequelae of third molar extractions with an estimated rate of 6% to 30% of cases.[40–45] Localized wound infection is a far less common complication and is reported in 2% to 12% of patients.[41,46–48] Alveolar osteitis is not considered a bacterial infection and is instead a healing disturbance. Bacteria likely contribute to a loss of blood clot; however, there are several other factors that can contribute to this delayed healing (ie, smoking, oral contraceptives, or excessive rinsing).[49]

Historically, the initial investigation of antibiotic prophylaxis was completed by Kay and colleagues.[50] During this study, it was found that preoperative penicillin could reduce alveolar osteitis by 21% in patients without pericoronitis and by 63% in patients with pericoronitis. As a result, this study was a likely impetus for prescribing antibiotics for third molar extractions. An additional landmark paper by Dr Peterson conversely references the need for antibiotic prophylaxis for third molars *only* in the setting of an immunocompromised state or poorly controlled metabolic disease.[51]

Recently published data remain similarly conflicting regarding antibiotic prophylaxis during third molar extractions. In a Cochrane review by Lodi and colleagues, there was a statistically significant decrease in localized infection risk and alveolar osteitis with prophylactic antibiotics.[52] Sixteen trials were evaluated; they showed a decrease in infectious complications by 66%. The number needed to treat to prevent one episode of infection was 19 patients. Further, these investigators found a reduction in dry socket by 34% with a number needed to treat 46 patients. All adverse effects of antibiotics were transient and there was no difference if antibiotics were provided preoperatively, postoperatively, or both.

In a meta-analysis completed by Ren and colleagues, the investigators showed that systemic antibiotics given before surgery helped reduce the frequency of alveolar osteitis and local wound infection.[49] In this study, a total of 2932 patients saw a decrease in alveolar osteitis by 8.2% with a number needed to treat 13. In addition, a total of 2396 patients saw a decreased risk of wound infection by 2.1% with a number needed to treat 25. Antibiotics provided *after* surgery were not effective in decreasing alveolar osteitis or localized infection.

Similarly, in a study by Morrow and colleagues, a total of 1877 patients were evaluated prospectively after extractions of their third molars.[53] Sixty-one percent of patients received only preoperative antibiotics. The frequency of complications (eg, alveolar osteitis, localized infection) was 4.3% in the antibiotic cohort and 7.5% in the placebo cohort. Overall, there was a 40% decrease in inflammatory complications with marginal statistical significance. Similar findings were found by Lacasa and colleagues where the postsurgical infection rates for preoperative, postoperative, and placebo groups were 9%, 4%, and 24%. When bone removal was not required, these rates dropped to 2%, 1%, and 7%, respectively.[54]

Conversely, there are various studies that demonstrate no difference in morbidity following third molar extractions without antibiotics. Poeschl and colleagues evaluated almost 300 patients prospectively after treatment with amoxicillin–clavulanic acid, clindamycin, or a placebo.[55] No difference was found in wound healing, pain, or maximum incisal opening at 1 month postoperatively.

It is recommended that the provider evaluate the patient to determine specific comorbidities and if patient has risk factors for infection. Given that alveolar osteitis can be locally treated, it is important that the provider understand the risks of prescribing antibiotics such as allergic reactions and antimicrobial resistance.[49] Further, one must weigh the benefit of antibiotic prophylaxis with the risk of adverse side effects. Postoperative infection following third molar removal has been estimated at 2%, whereas the risk of adverse drug effects from antibiotics has been stated to occur in 6% to 7% of patients.[56]

If an antibiotic is chosen then generally a single preoperative dose is preferred.[11,57] One preoperative dose 1 hour before surgery has been shown to have similar effects on alveolar osteitis compared with 3 to 5 day postoperative therapy or combined pre-op and post-op therapy.[11,49] By prolonging therapy, it has been found that this leads to an increased risk of side effects especially nausea, vomiting, and stomach pain. In addition, similar to dental implant placement, amoxicillin and other penicillin derivatives have the highest effect on oral cavity flora.[49,58,59] If antibiotic prophylaxis is chosen for third molars, amoxicillin has been shown to be equivalent to amoxicillin–clavulanic acid with less gastrointestinal side effects.[60]

DENTAL IMPLANTS

Infections following dental implant placement are difficult to eradicate and many times require removal of the implant.[61] Following removal, there is significant difficulty in replacement due to the hard and soft tissue changes that can occur.[62] Previous studies and Cochrane reviews have shown that preoperative doses of antibiotics are beneficial, although more recent publications are changing this notion and not recommending prophylaxis if the patient is healthy.[61,63]

An initial Cochrane review by Esposito and colleagues summarized these findings and recommended 2 g or 3 g of amoxicillin 1 hour preoperatively to reduce the failure rate of implants caused by infection.[61] Four randomized controlled trials were evaluated in this review and determined that 33 patients are needed to prevent one failure. Similar to the aforementioned Cochrane review on prophylaxis for third molars, only mild adverse side effects were reported and all were transient. Without antibiotics, the success rate of implants is approximately 92%. When preoperative antibiotics are used the results are 96% to 97%.[11] In a separate retrospective analysis, no differences were noted between clindamycin, amoxicillin, or cephalosporins when given preoperatively.[1]

Kim and colleagues found that similar beneficial results from preoperative antibiotics with a number needed to treat of 35 and that prophylaxis decreased implant failure by 53%.[62] Roca-Millan and colleagues in a systematic review and meta-analysis of 11 articles determined that antibiotic prophylaxis is indicated in patients having implants placed.[63] The investigators specifically evaluated patients who were "healthy" and noted a statistically significant improvement in implant failure. All studies evaluated in their review received amoxicillin, or if allergic to penicillin, clindamycin.

Despite the results of these reviews, Singh Gill and colleagues discuss the overall health care costs and risks of antibacterial resistance with such a high number needed to treat.[5] The investigators mention that the provider must carefully consider the increase in resistant organisms and the overall cost: almost $150 for 33 to 35 patients to receive a 2-g prophylactic dose. In a prospective clinical trial in 2021 by Momand and colleagues, a group of 474 healthy patients were evaluated with 2 g of amoxicillin or a placebo before surgical implant placement. A significant number of their cohort also received multiple implants and simultaneous grafting procedures. These patients were followed for 3 to 6 months and antibiotic prophylaxis was not shown to be statistically beneficial.[64] The absolute risk reduction for implant failure or postoperative infection was 0.46% with a number needed to treat in this study was 219 patients.

Further, in a complex systematic review by Lund and colleagues, the investigators estimated that the number needed to treat for implant failure was much higher due to previous studies with risks of bias. As a result of antibiotic risk and clinical heterogeneity in previous reviews, these investigators did not recommend prophylaxis for "straightforward" implant placement in healthy patients.[65] These results were backed by a consensus report from the European Association for Osseointegration in 2015 that antibiotics had no role in "straightforward" cases.[66] To add to the controversy, an additional consensus report by the Italian Academy of Osseointegration responded with recommendations of a single dose of antibiotics, chlorhexidine before and after surgery, and continued antibiotics in "complex cases" (eg, long surgical time or regenerative procedures).[67] These conclusions leave to the decision regarding antibiotic prophylaxis to the prescriber.

When antibiotics are indicated, *postoperative* regimens have not been shown to aid in decreasing infection or failure of dental implants.[16,62,68,69] A study by Braun and colleagues notes that there was no difference between 1 g amoxicillin preoperatively or an extended post-op regimen. However, the side effects were present whenever a post-op regimen was provided.[69] Arduino and colleagues also noted increased side effects postoperatively, further justifying the need to limit antibiotics following treatment.[70] When indicated, the best regimen remains the one referenced by Esposito and colleagues with preoperative 2 to 3 g of amoxicillin 1 hour before surgery.[16]

In actual practice, Deeb and colleagues found no consensus among OMS regarding their use of antibiotic regimen for dental implants.[71] Seventy-one percent of OMS prescribed antibiotics postoperatively and 51.6% prescribed antibiotics preoperatively despite the above findings that preoperative treatment is the main beneficial modality. Seventy-two percent indicated that they use both preoperative and postoperatively. The results of this study show that there is not a definitive consensus and there remains a need for specific published guidelines.

When it comes to bone grafting without implant placement, there remain little data in the literature. A meta-analysis by Khouly and colleagues found that there are insufficient data to support the use of prophylactic antibiotics for bone grafting when there is no implant placed during same procedure.[72] Similarly, Klinge and colleagues found a lack of evidence in the literature.[73] A need for an adequate randomized controlled trial to evaluate prophylaxis when bone grafts are placed independent of dental implants remains.

SUMMARY

Aside from a few exceptions, most dentoalveolar procedures do not require antibiotic prophylaxis. It is critical to recognize which patients require prophylaxis and to follow the established guidelines referenced above. Approximately 77% of unnecessary antibiotic prophylaxis was prescribed by general dentists with the highest risk of unnecessary prophylaxis in patients with prosthetic joints.[74]

When an antibiotic is required, amoxicillin is the primary choice for dentoalveolar procedures unless otherwise stated by the IE guidelines. Clindamycin and amoxicillin–clavulanic acid have high gastrointestinal adverse effects and, if prescribed, should be also provided with a probiotic.[11] In support of the Therapeutic Guidelines, antibiotic prophylaxis should not be used unless there is a proper indication, given within 60 minutes before incision, and provided a single preoperative dose.[56] As with all procedures, clinical judgment and evaluation of the patient's medical status must be evaluated.[75]

Our goal for limiting antibiotic resistance must be aligned with all facets of health care. As providers we should not use "defensive medicine" and provide antibiotics based on the approved guidelines above. In studies by McHenry, Knolle, and Zeitler, each author references surgeons that want to be on the "safe side," although this should never be a reason to deviate from established guidelines.[76–78] It is critical to see the larger picture as antibiotic resistance and health care costs continue to worsen.

There exists a clear need for standardization of antibiotic prophylaxis with a well-designed randomized and placebo-controlled multicenter study for both dental implants and dental extractions.[49] Further, OMS must develop goals of treatment. Additional options including topical therapy with antiseptics (chlorhexidine) or local antibiotics (intrasocket tetracycline) must be evaluated to decrease the use of systemic therapy. We all must continue to regulate antibiotic use through established guidelines and continue to investigate the risks and benefits of prophylaxis.

CLINICS CARE POINTS

- When indicated, prophylactic antibiotics administered perioperatively can prevent surgical site infection, reduce the duration and cost of healthcare, and limit adverse effects to the patient.

- Within the dental field, there are limited indications for antibiotics as most periodontal and dental diseases are adequately managed via oral hygiene, local therapies, and/or minor surgical interventions. Dentists account for an estimated 10% of all antibiotic prescriptions while 80% of prescriptions are unnecessary.

- The decision to provide prophylactic antibiotics should be based on procedure and patient specific factors.

- Patients with an increased risk for infective endocarditis are candidates for antibiotic prophylaxis. Patient risk factors include prosthetic cardiac valves, previous or recurrent infective endocarditis, unrepaired congenital heart defects or repaired defects with residual deficits, and cardiac transplant recipients with cardiac valvulopathies.

- Prophylactic antibiotics are not indicated for use during administration of routine anesthetic injections through healthy tissue, radiographic examinations, prosthodontic or orthodontic procedures, and/or during primary tooth exfoliation.

- The American Dental Association determined that no relationship exists between prosthetic joint infections and dental procedures.

- Postoperative infection rate following extraction of third molars is estimated to be 2%. A 6-7% risk of adverse drug effects from antibiotics has been observed in patients.

- For patients undergoing dental implant procedures, postoperative antibiotic regimens have not been shown to decrease infection rates or failure rates of dental implants.

- Amoxicillin is the primary choice for dentoalveolar procedures.
- The risk for infection during OMS procedures can be decreased via clean incisions, hemostasis, and/or copious and adequate irrigation.

DISCLOSURE

The authors have nothing to disclose.

REFERENCES

1. Blatt S, Al-Nawas B. A systematic review of latest evidence for antibiotic prophylaxis and therapy in oral and maxillofacial surgery. Infection 2019;47(4):519–55.
2. Sancho-Puchades M, Herráez-Vilas JM, Berini-Aytés L, et al. Antibiotic prophylaxis to prevent local infection in Oral Surgery: use or abuse? Med Oral Patol Oral Cir Bucal 2009;14(1):E28–33.
3. Dammling C, Abramowicz S, Kinard B. Current Concepts in Prophylactic Antibiotics in Oral and Maxillofacial Surgery. Oral Maxillofac Surg Clin North Am 2022; 34(1):157–67.
4. Enzler MJ, Berbari E, Osmon DR. Antimicrobial prophylaxis in adults. Mayo Clin Proc 2011;86(7):686–701.
5. Singh Gill A, Morrissey H, Rahman A. A Systematic Review and Meta-Analysis Evaluating Antibiotic Prophylaxis in Dental Implants and Extraction Procedures. Medicina (Kaunas) 2018;54(6):95.
6. Hafner S, Albittar M, Abdel-Kahaar E, et al. Antibiotic prophylaxis of infective endocarditis in oral and maxillofacial surgery: incomplete implementation of guidelines in everyday clinical practice. Int J Oral Maxillofac Surg 2020;49(4):522–8.
7. Macy E. Penicillin and beta-lactam allergy: Epidemiology and diagnosis. Curr Allergy Asthma Rep 2014;14:476.
8. Vardakas KZ, Trigkidis KK, Boukouvala E, et al. Clostridium difficile infection following systemic antibiotic administration in randomised controlled trials: a systematic review and meta-analysis. Int J Antimicrob Agents 2016;48(1):1–10.
9. Deshpande A, Pasupuleti V, Thota P, et al. Community-associated Clostridium difficile infection and antibiotics: a meta-analysis. J Antimicrob Chemother 2013;68(9):1951–61.
10. Brown KA, Khanafer N, Daneman N, et al. Meta-analysis of antibiotics and the risk of community-associated Clostridium difficile infection. Antimicrob Agents Chemother 2013;57(5):2326–32.
11. Azher S, Patel A. Antibiotics in Dentoalveolar Surgery, a Closer Look at Infection, Alveolar Osteitis and Adverse Drug Reaction. J Oral Maxillofac Surg 2021;79(11): 2203–14.
12. Suda KJ, Roberts RM, Hunkler RJ, et al. Antibiotic prescriptions in the community by type of provider in the United States, 2005-2010. J Am Pharm Assoc (2003) 2016;56(6):621–6.e1.
13. Farbod F, Kanaan H, Farbod J. Infective endocarditis and antibiotic prophylaxis prior to dental/oral procedures: latest revision to the guidelines by the American Heart Association published April 2007. Int J Oral Maxillofac Surg 2009;38(6): 626–31.
14. Naimi-Akbar A, Hultin M, Klinge A, et al. Antibiotic prophylaxis in orthognathic surgery: A complex systematic review. PLoS One 2018;13(1):e0191161.

15. Ventola CL. The antibiotic resistance crisis: part 1: causes and threats. P T 2015; 40(4):277–83.

16. Romandini M, De Tullio I, Congedi F, et al. Antibiotic prophylaxis at dental implant placement: Which is the best protocol? A systematic review and network meta-analysis. J Clin Periodontol 2019;46(3):382–95.

17. Suda KJ, Henschel H, Patel U, et al. Use of Antibiotic Prophylaxis for Tooth Extractions, Dental Implants, and Periodontal Surgical Procedures. Open Forum Infect Dis 2017;5(1):ofx250.

18. Scottish Dental Clinical Effectiveness Programme. Drug Prescribing for Dentistry. Dental Clinical Guide. https://www.sdcep.org.uk/media/2wleqlnr/sdcep-drug-prescribing-for-dentistry-3rd-edition.pdf.

19. Swift JQ, Gulden WS. Antibiotic therapy managing odontogenic infections. Dent Clin N Am 2002;46:623–33 [CrossRef].

20. Goff DA, Mangino JE, Glassman AH, et al. Review of Guidelines for Dental Antibiotic Prophylaxis for Prevention of Endocarditis and Prosthetic Joint Infections and Need for Dental Stewardship. Clin Infect Dis 2020;71(2):455–62.

21. Salmeron-Escobar JI, del Amo-Ferna'ndez deVelasco A. Antibiotic prophylaxis in Oral and Maxillofacial Surgery. Med Oral Patol Oral Cir Bucal 2006;11(3): 292–6.

22. Wilson W, Taubert KA, Gewitz M, et al. Prevention of infective endocarditis: guidelines from the American Heart Association: a guideline from the American Heart Association Rheumatic Fever, Endocarditis, and Kawasaki Disease Committee, Council on Cardiovascular Disease in the Young, and the Council on Clinical Cardiology, Council on Cardiovascular Surgery and Anesthesia, and the Quality of Care and Outcomes Research Interdisciplinary Working Group. Circulation 2007;116(15):1736–54 [published correction appears in Circulation. 2007 Oct 9;116(15):e376-7].

23. American Academy of Pediatric Dentistry. Antibiotic pro- phylaxis for dental patients at risk for infection. The reference Manual of Pediatric dentistry. Chicago, III: American Academy of Pediatric Dentistry; 2022. p. 500–6.

24. Wilson WR, Gewitz M, Lockhart PB, et al. Prevention of Viridans Group Streptococcal Infective Endocarditis: A Scientific Statement From the American Heart Association. Circulation 2021;143(20):e963–78 [published correction appears in Circulation. 2021 Aug 31;144(9):e192] [published correction appears in Circulation. 2022 Apr 26;145(17):e868].

25. Chu VH, Otto CM, Edwards MS, et al. Prevention of endocarditis: Antibiotic prophylaxis and other measures. UpToDate 2023.

26. American Association of Endodontists. Antibiotic prophylaxis 2017 update. Supplement 2017. p. 1–3. Available at: https://www.aae.org/specialty/wp-content/uploads/sites/2/2017/06/aae_antibiotic-prophylaxis-2017update.pdf.

27. Halpern LR, Adams DR. The Dentoalveolar Surgical Patient: Perioperative Principles Based on Contemporary Controversies. Oral Maxillofac Surg Clin North Am 2020;32(4):495–510.

28. Sollecito TP, Abt E, Lockhart PB, et al. The use of prophylactic antibiotics prior to dental procedures in patients with prosthetic joints: Evidence-based clinical practice guideline for dental practitioners–a report of the American Dental Association Council on Scientific Affairs. J Am Dent Assoc 2015;146(1):11–6.e8.

29. Baddour LM, Spelman D, Hall KK. Prevention of prosthetic joint and other types of orthopedic hardware infection. UpToDate 2023.

30. Alao U, Pydisetty R, Sandiford NA. Antibiotic prophylaxis during dental procedures in patients with in situ lower limb prosthetic joints. Eur J Orthop Surg Traumatol 2015;25:217–20.
31. Berbari EF, Osmon DR, Carr A, et al. Dental procedures as risk factors for prosthetic hip or knee infection: a hospital-based prospective case-control study [published correction appears in Clin Infect Dis. 2010 Mar 15;50(6):944]. Clin Infect Dis 2010;50(1):8–16.
32. Kao FC, Hsu YC, Chen WH, et al. Prosthetic Joint Infection Following Invasive Dental Procedures and Antibiotic Prophylaxis in Patients With Hip or Knee Arthroplasty. Infect Control Hosp Epidemiol 2017;38(2):154–61.
33. Thornhill MH, Crum A, Rex S, et al. Analysis of Prosthetic Joint Infections Following Invasive Dental Procedures in England. JAMA Netw Open 2022;5(1): e2142987.
34. Thornhill MH, Gibson TB, Pack C, et al. Quantifying the risk of prosthetic joint infections after invasive dental procedures and the effect of antibiotic prophylaxis. J Am Dent Assoc 2023;154(1):43–52.e12.
35. Little JW, Jacobson JJ, Lockhart PB, et al. The dental treatment of patients with joint replacements: a position paper from the American Academy of Oral Medicine. J Am Dent Assoc 2010;141:667–71.
36. Watters W 3rd, Rethman MP, Hanson NB, et al. American Academy of Orthopedic Surgeons; American Dental Association. Prevention of orthopaedic implant infection in patients undergoing dental procedures. J Am Acad Orthop Surg 2013;21: 180–9.
37. Quinn RH, Murray JN, Pezold R, et al. Members of the Writing and Voting Panels of the Appropriate Use Criteria for the Management of Patients with Orthopaedic Implants Undergoing Dental Procedures. The American Academy of Orthopaedic Surgeons appropriate use criteria for the management of patients with orthopaedic implants undergoing dental procedures. J Bone Joint Surg Am 2017;99: 161–3.
38. Mercuri LG. Prophylaxis after total joint replacement. J Oral Maxillofac Surg 2010; 68(7):1702–3.
39. Mercuri LG. Prevention and detection of prosthetic temporomandibular joint infections—update. Int J Oral Maxillofac Surg 2019;48(2):217–24.
40. Blum IR. Contemporary views on dry socket (alveolar osteitis): A clinical appraisal of standardization, etiopathogenesis and management: A critical review. Int J Oral Maxillofac Surg 2002;31:309.
41. Chiapasco M, De Cicco L, Marrone G. Side effects and complications associated with third molar surgery. Oral Surg Oral Med Oral Pathol 1993;76:412.
42. Parthasarathi K, Smith A, Chandu A. Factors affecting incidence of dry socket: A prospective community-based study. J Oral Maxillofac Surg 2011;69:1880.
43. Sigron GR, Pourmand PP, Mache B, et al. The most common complications after wisdom tooth removal: Part 1: A retrospective study of 1,199 cases in the mandible. Swiss Dent J 2014;124:1042.
44. Pourmand PP, Sigron GR, Mache B, et al. The most common complications after wisdom tooth removal: part 2: A retrospective study of 1,562 cases in the maxilla. Swiss Dent J 2014;124:1047.
45. Bui CH, Seldin EB, Dodson TB. Types, frequencies, and risk factors for complications after third molar extraction. J Oral Maxillofac Surg 2003;61:1379.
46. Goldberg MH, Nemarich AN, Marco WP 2nd. Complications after mandibular third molar surgery: A statistical analysis of 500 consecutive procedures in private practice. J Am Dent Assoc 1985;111:277.

47. Happonen RP, Backstrom AC, Ylipaavalniemi P. Prophylactic use of phenoxyme-thylpenicillin and tinidazole in mandibular third molar surgery, a comparative placebo controlled clinical trial. Br J Oral Maxillofac Surg 1990;28(12).

48. Osborn TP, Frederickson G Jr, Small IA, et al. A prospective study of complications related to mandibular third molar surgery. J Oral Maxillofac Surg 1985; 43:767.

49. Ren YF, Malmstrom HS. Effectiveness of antibiotic prophylaxis in third molar surgery: a meta-analysis of randomized controlled clinical trials. J Oral Maxillofac Surg 2007;65(10):1909–21.

50. Kay LW. Investigations into the nature of pericoronitis—II. Br J Oral Surg 1966;4(52).

51. Peterson LJ. Antibiotic prophylaxis against wound infections in oral and maxillofacial surgery. J Oral Maxillofac Surg 1990;48(6):617–20.

52. Lodi G, Azzi L, Varoni EM, et al. Antibiotics to prevent complications following tooth extractions. Cochrane Database Syst Rev 2021;2(2):CD003811.

53. Morrow AJ, Dodson TB, Gonzalez ML, et al. Do Postoperative Antibiotics Decrease the Frequency of Inflammatory Complications Following Third Molar Removal? J Oral Maxillofac Surg 2018;76(4):700–8.

54. Lacasa JM, Jimenez JA, Ferras V, et al. Prophylaxis versus pre-emptive treatment for infective and inflammatory complications of surgical third molar removal: a randomized, double-blind, placebo-controlled, clinical trial with sustained release amoxicillin/clavulanic acid (100/62.5 mg). Int J Oral Maxillofac Surg 2007;36:321.

55. Poeschl PW, Eckel D, Poeschl E. Postoperative prophylactic antibiotic treatment in third molar surgery–a necessity? J Oral Maxillofac Surg 2004;62(1):3–9.

56. Milic T, Raidoo P, Gebauer D. Antibiotic prophylaxis in oral and maxillofacial surgery: a systematic review. Br J Oral Maxillofac Surg 2021;59(6):633–42.

57. Polk HC Jr, Lopez-Mayor JF. Postoperative wound infection: A prospective study of determinant factors and prevention. Surgery 1969;66(97).

58. Sixou JL, Magaud C, Jolivet-Gougeon A, et al. Microbiology of mandibular third molar pericoronitis: Incidence of beta-lactamase-producing bacteria. Oral Surg Oral Med Oral Pathol Oral Radiol Endodont 2003;95:655.

59. Roberts GJ, Watts R, Longhurst P, et al. Bacteremia of dental origin and antimicrobial sensitivity following oral surgical procedures in children. Pediatr Dent 1998;20:28.

60. Iglesias-Martin F, Garcia-Perla-Garcia A, Yanez-Vico R, et al. Comparative trial between the use of amoxicillin and amoxicillin clavulanate in the removal of third molars. Med Oral Patologia Oral y Cirugia Bucal 2014;19:e612–5.

61. Esposito M, Grusovin MG, Worthington HV. Interventions for replacing missing teeth: antibiotics at dental implant placement to prevent complications. Cochrane Database Syst Rev 2013;7:CD004152.

62. Kim AS, Abdelhay N, Levin L, et al. Antibiotic prophylaxis for implant placement: a systematic review of effects on reduction of implant failure. Br Dent J 2020; 228(12):943–51.

63. Roca-Millan E, Estrugo-Devesa A, Merlos A, et al. Systemic Antibiotic Prophylaxis to Reduce Early Implant Failure: A Systematic Review and Meta-Analysis. Antibiotics (Basel) 2021;10(6):698.

64. Momand P, Becktor JP, Naimi-Akbar A, et al. Effect of antibiotic prophylaxis in dental implant surgery: A multicenter placebo-controlled double-blinded randomized clinical trial. Clin Implant Dent Relat Res 2022;24(1):116–24.

65. Lund B, Hultin M, Tranæus S, et al. Complex systematic review - perioperative antibiotics in conjunction with dental implant placement. Clin Oral Implants Res 2015;26:1–14.
66. Klinge B, Flemming T, Cosyn J, et al. The patient undergoing implant therapy. Summary and consensus statements. The 4th EAO consensus conference 2015. Clin Oral Implants Res 2015;26(Suppl 11):64–7.
67. Caiazzo A, Canullo L. Consensus Meeting Group, Pesce P. Consensus Report by the Italian Academy of Osseointegration on the Use of Antibiotics and Antiseptic Agents in Implant Surgery. Int J Oral Maxillofac Implants 2021;36(1):103–5.
68. Ireland RS, Palmer NO, Lindenmeyer A, et al. An investigation of antibiotic prophylaxis in implant practice in the UK. Br Dent J 2012. https://doi.org/10.1038/sj.bdj.2012.960.
69. Braun RS, Chambrone L, Khouly I. Prophylactic antibiotic regimens in dental implant failure: A systematic review and meta-analysis. J Am Dent Assoc 2019; 150:61–91.
70. Arduino PG, Tirone F, Schiorlin E, et al. Single preoperative dose of prophylactic amoxicillin versus a 2-day postoperative course in dental implant surgery: A two-centre randomised controlled trial. Eur J Oral Implantol 2015;8:143–9.
71. Deeb GR, Soung GY, Best AM, et al. Antibiotic Prescribing Habits of Oral and Maxillofacial Surgeons in Conjunction With Routine Dental Implant Placement. J Oral Maxillofac Surg 2015;73(10):1926 31.
72. Khouly I, Braun RS, Silvestre T, et al. Efficacy of antibiotic prophylaxis in intraoral bone grafting procedures: a systematic review and meta-analysis. Int J Oral Maxillofac Surg 2020;49(2):250–63.
73. Klinge A, Khalil D, Klinge B, et al. Prophylactic antibiotics for staged bone augmentation in implant dentistry. Acta Odontol Scand 2020;78(1):64–73.
74. Hubbard CC, Evans CT, Calip GS, et al. Appropriateness of Antibiotic Prophylaxis Before Dental Procedures, 2016-2018. Am J Prev Med 2022;62(6):943–8.
75. Bennett-Guerrero E. Postoperative surgical site infection: risk factors and prevention. Rev Mex Anestesiol 2008;31:S90–2.
76. McHenry MC, Weinstein AJ. Antimicrobial drugs and infections in ambulatory patients: Some problems and perspectives. Med Clin North Am 1983;67(3).
77. Knolle G. Kritik an der lokalen Antibiotika-Anwendung in der Zahnheilkunde. Dtsch Zahnarztebl 1968;22:263.
78. Zeitler DL. Prophylactic antibiotics for third molar surgery: A dissenting opinion. J Oral Maxillofac Surg 1995;53:61.

Management of Burning Mouth Syndrome

Jaykrishna Thakkar, DDS*, Harry Dym, DDS

KEYWORDS

• Burning mouth syndrome • Neuropathic pain • Dysphagia • Sialorrhea

KEY POINTS

- Burning mouth syndrome (BMS) is defined in the International Association for the Study of Pain as "burning pain in the tongue or other oral mucous membrane associated with normal signs and laboratory findings lasting at least 4 to 6 months."
- The most common affected areas are the anterior two-thirds, tip, the dorsum, and the anterior lateral margins of the tongue.
- Causes that have been linked to BMS include hormonal, smoking, medications, xerostomia, and salivary gland hypofunction, nutritional deficiencies, and candidiasis.
- BMS can be classified as type 1, type 2, type 3, primary, and secondary.
- Treatment includes topical medication, systemic medication, and behavioral therapy.

INTRODUCTION

Encountering a patient with BMS can be devastating and difficult to treat without appropriate guidance from the literature. In this article, we provide an update to the practicing dentist and/or oral and maxillofacial surgeon on the recognition, identification, and treatment of burning mouth syndrome (BMS). BMS is defined in the International Association for the Study of Pain as "burning pain in the tongue or other oral mucous membrane associated with normal signs and laboratory findings lasting at least 4 to 6 months[1]." BMS has been referred to with different names based on the location and quality of pain; burning mouth condition, burning lips syndrome, scalded mouth syndrome, stomatodynia, oral dysesthesia, glossopyrosis, and stomapyrosis. The International classification of Headache Disorders describes it as an intraoral burning sensation for which there are no medical or dental-related causes.[2]

Oral and Maxillofacial Surgery, The Brooklyn Hospital Center, 155 Ashland Place, Brooklyn, NY 11201, USA
* Corresponding author. 1761 Ebenezer Road, Rock Hill, SC 29732.
E-mail addresses: jpthakka@umich.edu; jthakkarta@gmail.com

Dent Clin N Am 68 (2024) 113–119
https://doi.org/10.1016/j.cden.2023.07.007
0011-8532/24/Published by Elsevier Inc.

EPIDEMIOLOGY

Higher incidence in women than men. The ratio between women and men varies from 3:1 to 16:1. Postmenopausal women aged 50 to 89 years had the highest disease incidence, with the maximum rate in women aged 70 to 79 years.[2]

CLINICAL FINDINGS

The most common affected areas are the anterior two-thirds, tip, the dorsum, and the anterior lateral margins of the tongue. Other areas include the anterior hard palate, mucosal aspect of the lip, and mandibular alveolar regions. BMS is typically bilateral and symmetric. Most patients with BMS will subjectively report xerostomia, dyspepsia, sialorrhea, halitosis, and dysphagia.[2,3]

BMS patients will also often report subjective conditions such as xerostomia and dysgeusia, as well as sialorrhoea, globus hystericus, halitosis, or dysphagia.[4,5] Most patients suffering from BMS experience their symptoms without any known triggering factor. Clinical signs of BMS include[3] the following:

1. Frothy saliva indicating a parotid hypofunction and dominance of mucoid subman-dibular saliva over the serous parotid saliva (anxiety is the most common cause of both acute and chronic xerostomia).
2. Dryness of the inner aspect of the lower lip from minor labial gland hypofunction
3. Scalloping of the lateral lingual margins secondary to habitual pressure against the adjacent teeth
4. Buccal mucosal irregularity often with leukoedema, translucent keratosis and linea alba, also due to pressure against the adjacent teeth
5. Low-grade erythema of the anterior dorsum of the tongue because of traumatic abrasion of the filiform papillae against the adjacent teeth and palate and exposure of the sensitive fungiform papillae
6. Low-grade erythema and often slight sensitivity of the coincident anterior hard palate
7. Low-grade linear erythema of the inner aspect of the lip coincident with the edges of the incisor teeth, mainly on the lower lip.[4]

CAUSES

1. Hormonal—Studies found that among menopausal women with BMS, follicle-stimulating hormones higher, whereas estradiol was significantly lower.[2]
2. Smoking—There is a significant link between cigarette smoking and patients with BMS. Some report that benzopyrene and polycyclic aromatic hydrocarbons are harmful substances in cigarette smoke that may correlate the incidence of BMS and cigarette smoking.[6]
3. Medications—Many medications can alter salivary flow, these medications have also been found in patients with BMS by sympathomimetic and parasympathomimetic actions on the salivary cellular processes.[4]
4. Xerostomia and salivary gland hypofunction—Xerostomia and SGH is multifacto-rial, comprising both physiologic and psychological reasons.
5. Nutritional deficiencies—BMS has links to nutritional deficiencies including vitamins and minerals, more specifically those associated with anemia: iron and vitamin B12 deficiency. Others include zinc and vitamin B complexes.[2]
6. Candidiasis—Candidiasis has been linked to BMS very closely due to similar predisposing factors such as nutritional deficiency, diabetes, and change in salivary function[7] **(Fig. 1).**

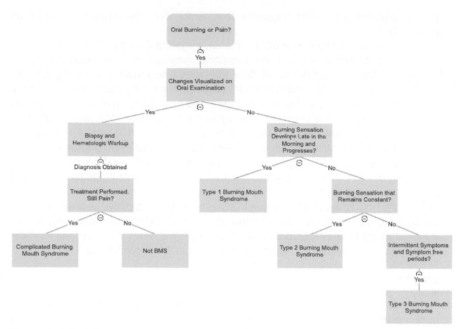

Fig. 1. BMS flowchart.

CLASSIFICATION

Type 1—Characterize day burning sensation that is not present on waking but develops late in the morning and progress throughout the day with greatest discomfort in the evening (see flowchart above).

Type 2—A burning sensation that remains constant throughout the day and prevents the patient from falling asleep.

Type 3—Characterize day intermittent symptoms and symptom-free periods with variable presence between days and may experience the symptoms at unusual sites (floor of mouth and buccal mucosa).

Primary BMS—When no clinical or laboratory test abnormalities are present.

Secondary BMS—There is an identifiable underlying cause for BMS.

PATHOPHYSIOLOGY

Neuropathic—Dysfunction in the trigeminal nerve and chorda tympani induces an alteration of the sensitivity threshold and reflection in the trigeminal area. Neural alterations reduce the threshold of pain transmission and transmit an ascending nociceptive signal that is not transmitted under healthy conditions. In BMS, alteration of gray matter is recognized in the prefrontal cortex, anterior cingulate gyrus, and hippocampus. Thus, it is proposed that central sensitization is one of the many entities that plays a role in BMS.[2] A case report by Gautam discusses dopaminergic pathway alterations, specifically a disruption in striatal dopamine regulation.[8]

Endocrine—Decreased synthesis of ovarian steroids after menopause induces deficiency or dysfunction in adrenal steroids, which abolishes the neuroprotective effects of steroids on neural tissues.[2]

A proposed hypothesis included the increase of mucosal blood flow of the oral cavity when stimulated was increased in patients that suffered from BMS when compared with controls. This suggests that BMS may be related to disturbed vasoreactivity.[9]

Another hypothesis proposes a comprehensive mechanism for BMS, taste disturbances, and / or xerostomia based on a regional neuropathy. The mechanism suggested is via either a regional small-fiber idiopathic neuropathy affecting salivary secretion and oral sensation, or a primary idiopathic neuropathy causing sensory neural dysfunction at the receptor level by changing the oral cavity environment. Sensory changes in the tongue and changed salivary composition with normal salivary flow rates have been demonstrated in patients with BMS, xerostomia, and dysgeusia.[10]

Psychological—Several studies suggest link between anxiety and depressive disorders in unexplained somatic symptoms. BMS patients have self-reported poorer health and complain of more illnesses, gastrointestinal problems, chronic fatigue, disturbed sleep patterns, and headaches, are anxious, and have low self-esteem. BMS have higher levels of neuroticism in all facets: anxiety, anger, hostility, depression, self-consciousness, impulsiveness, and vulnerability. To support this somatoform pain disorder model of BMS anxiolytic drugs, such as selective serotonin reuptake inhibitor (SSRI) and amisulpride, can cause an improvement in BMS symptoms.[2]

TREATMENT

Even though the mechanism of BMS is not fully understood and no standard treatment protocol is present, there are topical medications, systemic medications, and behavioral therapy, which can be used in the treatment of BMS as seen in **Table 1**. These treatments have been agreed on among the scientific community, which can alleviate the symptoms of BMS.

TOPICAL MEDICATION

Clonazepam—It is a benzodiazepine that acts as an agonist on the *gamma*-aminobutyric acid (GABA) receptor. It was found to be efficacious in reducing symptoms of BMS. Protocols required patients to suck on a 1-mg tablet of clonazepam for 3 minutes, holding the saliva near the pain sites and then spitting out the excess saliva (tid × 14 days).[11] Other protocols included a similar method using 0.5 mg tablets up to 4 times a day. Patients were instructed to suck on a clonazepam tablet for 3 minutes, spit out excess saliva, and hold their saliva near the pain sites. It was found to be effective both short term (<10 weeks) and long term (>10 weeks), showing a 50% reduction in symptoms for most patients; however, people may develop dependence as symptoms can return when medication is not continued. Common side effects include xerostomia, lethargy, and fatigue.[12]

Table 1			
Treatment of burning mouth syndrome			
Drug Name	**Drug Category**	**Mechanism**	**Topical or Systemic**
Clonazepam	Benzodiazepine	Agonist of GABA receptor	Topical and systemic
Capsaicin	Topical analgesic	TRPV1 agonist	Topical
Alpha-lipoic acid	Antioxidant	Debated in literature	Systemic
Gabapentin	Anticonvulsant	GABA agonist	Systemic
Nystatin	Antifungal	Binds to ergosterol	Topical
Vitamin B complex	Multivitamin	Cofactor	Systemic
Magic mouthwash	Combination therapy	Multiple mechanisms	Topical

CAPSAICIN

This topical analgesic, given as an oral gel 0.01% and 0.025% on the dorsal tongue 3 times daily for 14 days, has shown to be efficacious.[13] Prolonged used of this analgesic causes depletion of TRPV1, the afferent receptor responsible for transmitting heat sensation, therefore desensitizing this pain receptor.[13] About 0.01% or 0.025% oral capsaicin gel on the dorsal part of tongue 3 times daily for 14 days has shown to be efficacious. However, patient history of gastric-related disorders must be considered because side effects include increased sensation of burning immediately after application.[14]

Lactoperoxidase (Biotine mouthwash) and topical lidocaine has not shown to be effective due to their short duration of action.[15]

SYSTEMIC MEDICATION
Clonazepam

Treatment varied from 0.25 to 2 mg daily with an overall increasing dosage being positively correlated to efficacy; however, some instances presented in which patients stopped treatment using less than 1 mg daily due to negative side effects.[12] Some studies show that it is not effective in improving mood, xerostomia, and taste dysfunction[9] but works best when normal salivary flow is present and in those beginning with severe initial symptoms or do not use psychotropic medications.[16]

ALPHA LIPOIC ACID

A coenzyme shown to have neuroprotective and antioxidant properties and which is thought to exert neuroregenerative actions. Current literature has conflicting evidence for improvement of symptoms and the proposed side effects of gastrointestinal upset and headaches when compared with placebo; therefore, further research is indicated to determine its effectiveness when used in isolation.[14]

GABAPENTIN

An anticonvulsant commonly used for neuropathic pain that is a GABA agonist. Although effective when used alone, GABA in combination with alpha lipoic acid (300 mg Gabapentin + 600 mg alpha lipoic acid per day × 60 days) showing a 70% success rate in the reduction of burning sensation.[17]

CATUAMA

An herbal product from Brazil composed of 4 extracts of medicinal plants (catuaba, ginger, guarana, and muira puama) is sought after for supposed improvement of physical and mental fatigue. Its components have demonstrated antinociceptive, antidepressant, and vasorelaxant effects in addition to affecting dopaminergic and serotonergic pathways in animal studies. Three hundred milligram Catuama capsules bid × 8 weeks resulted in 51.5% reduction in symptoms.[18]

BEHAVIORAL THERAPY
Cognitive Behavioral Therapy

Relaxation and cognitive restructuring are 2 specific techniques relevant to the management of BMS. As the name implies, relaxation techniques include progressive muscle relaxation and focused breathing to alleviate discomfort, whereas cognitive restructuring seeks to identify and modify destructive thoughts related to emotional and behavioral problems.[19] In patients with resistant BMS after receiving pharmacologic treatment, patients who received additional cognitive therapy for 12 to 15 sessions had decreased symptoms compared with a placebo group after 6 months. This further strengthens the argument that part of BMS has a psychological component.[20]

Clinical management is complex and there is no uniform treatment protocol but in each case, both the physiologic and psychological components of the patient's symptoms must be addressed. The acceptance of psychological factors by the patient is often an important element of BMS management but this in itself can present a clinically challenging situation.[4] As BMS is regarded as a multifactorial condition, refraining from bad oral habits, removing local irritating factors, stopping smoking, keeping good mental health status may help in the prevention of BMS.[6]

CLINICS CARE POINTS

- BMS is defined in the International Association for the Study of Pain as "burning pain in the tongue or other oral mucous membrane associated with normal signs and laboratory findings lasting at least 4 to 6 months."
- The most common affected areas are the anterior two-thirds, tip, the dorsum, and the anterior lateral margins of the tongue.
- The majority of patients suffering from BMS experience their symptoms without any known triggering factor.
- Even though the mechanism of BMS is not fully understood and no standard treatment protocol is present, there are topical medications, systemic medications, and behavioral therapy, which can be used in the treatment of BMS.

DISCLOSURE

The authors have nothing to disclose.

REFERENCES

1. Merskey H, Bogduk N. Descriptions of chronic pain syndromes and definitions of pain terms. Classification of chronic pain. 2nd edition. Seattle (WA): IASP Press; 1994. p. 74.
2. Dym H, Lin S, Thakkar J. Neuropathic Pain and Burning Mouth Syndrome: An Overview and Current Update. Dental Clinics 2020;64(2):379–99.
3. Thakkar JP, Lane CJ. Hyposalivation and xerostomia and burning mouth syndrome: medical management. Oral and Maxillofacial Surgery Clinics 2022;34(1):135–46.
4. Abetz LM, Savage NW. Burning mouth syndrome and psychological disorders. Aust Dent J 2009;54:84–93.
5. Bergdahl M, Bergdahl J. Low unstimulated salivary flow and subjective oral dryness: association with medication, anxiety, depression, and stress. J Dent Res 2000;79:1652–8.
6. Gao J, Chen L, Zhou J, et al. A Case-control study on etiological factors involved in patients with burning mouth syndrome. J Oral Pathol Med 2008;38:24–8.
7. Terai H, Shimahara M. Tongue pain: burning mouth syndrome vs Candida-associated lesion. Oral Dis 2007;13(4):440–2.
8. Gautam M, Patel S, Sablaban I, Sivananthan M. Burning Mouth Syndrome: Case Report. J Clin Psychopharmacol 2021;41(4):499–500.

9. Heckmann SM, Heckmann JG, Hilz MJ, et al. Oral mucosal blood flow in patients with burning mouth syndrome. Pain 2001;90(3):281–6.

10. Granot M, Nagler R. Association between regional idiopathic neuropathy and salivary involvement as the possible mechanism for oral sensory complaints. J Pain 2005;6:581–7.

11. Gremeau-Richard C, Dubray C, Aublet-Cuvelier B, et al. Effect of lingual nerve block on burningmouth syndrome (stomatodynia): a randomized crossover trial. Pain 2010;149:27–32.

12. Cui Y, Xu H, Chen FM, et al. Efficacy evaluation of clonazepam for symptom remissionin burning mouth syndrome: a meta-analysis. Oral Dis 2016;22:503–11. https://doi.org/10.1111/odi.12422.

13. Kisely S, Forbes M, Sawyer E, et al. A systematic review of randomized trials for the treatment of burning mouth syndrome. J Psychosom Res 2016;86:39–46.

14. Ritchie A, Kramer JM. Recent Advances in the Etiology and Treatment of Burning Mouth Syndrome. J Dent Res 2018;97(11):1193–9.

15. Femiano F. Burning mouth syndrome (BMS): An open trial of comparative efficacy of alpha- lipoic acid (thioctic acid) with other therapies. Minerva Stomatol 2002; 51:405–9.

16. Ko JY, Kim MJ, Lee SG, et al. Outcome predictors affecting the efficacy of clonazepam therapy for the management of burning mouth syndrome (BMS). Arch Gerontol Geriatr 2012;55(3):755–61.

17. López-D'alessandro E, Escovich L. Combination of alpha lipoic acid and gabapentin, its efficacy in the treatment of Burning Mouth Syndrome: a randomized, double-blind, placebo controlled trial. Med Oral, Patol Oral Cirugía Bucal 2011; 16(5):e635–40.

18. Spanemberg JC, Cherubini K, de Figueiredo MA, et al. Effect of an herbal compound for treatment of burning mouth syndrome: randomized, controlled, double-blind clinical trial. Oral Surg Oral Med Oral Pathol Oral Radiol 2012;113:373–7.

19. Tu TTH, Takenoshita M, Matsuoka H, et al. Current management strategies for the pain of elderly patients with burning mouth syndrome: a critical review. Biopsychosoc Med 2019;13:1.

20. Bergdahl J, Anneroth G, Perris H. Cognitive therapy in the treatment of patients with resistant burning mouth syndrome: a controlled study. J Oral Pathol Med 1995;24:213–5.

Medication Management of Neuropathic Pain Disorders

Rebecca Fisher, DMD[a],*, Earl Clarkson, DDS, FACS[b]

KEYWORDS

- Neuropathic pain disorders • Orofacial pain • Trigeminal neuralgia
- Postherpetic neuralgia

KEY POINTS

- Many patients can be affected by neuropathic pain disorders of the orofacial region. Chronic pain conditions have severe effects on patient quality of life. Many neuropathic disorders are difficult to adequately treat due to their poorly understood pathophysiology.
- Various treatment modalities exist and have been shown to be effective in neuropathic pain. Specific medications have been shown more effective in particular subsets of neuropathic pain.
- Appropriate treatment depends on the ability of the clinician to be able to carefully diagnose the appropriate neuropathic pain disorder. Therefore, Oral and Maxillofacial Surgeons and dentists must be familiar with the various neuropathic pain disorders and the pharmacologic treatments available to treat these conditions.

INTRODUCTION

Often, patients may present with no clear odontogenic source to their orofacial pain. Neuropathic pain syndromes in the craniofacial region are common and often difficult to diagnose and manage. Many times, patients with neuropathic pain disorders have seen multiple providers and have had numerous unnecessary treatments prior to correct diagnosis and treatment to alleviate their symptoms. Therefore, extensive history and proper head and neck exam are crucial. This should include nature of pain, intensity, location, duration, aggravating or alleviating factors. Dentists and oral and maxillofacial surgeons should always consider neuropathic pain disorders in their differential diagnoses. Prompt and accurate diagnosis will allow for appropriate treatment. This can improve patient quality of life and hopefully yield complete resolution of symptoms.

[a] Department of Oral and Maxillofacial Surgery, Woodhull Medical Center, 760 Broadway, Brooklyn, NY 11206, USA; [b] Oral and Maxillofacial Surgery, Woodhull Medical Center, 760 Broadway, Brooklyn, NY 11206, USA
* Corresponding author. Woodhull Medical Center, Room 2C-319, 760 Broadway, Brooklyn, NY 11206.
E-mail address: fisherr2@nychhc.org

Dent Clin N Am 68 (2024) 121–131
https://doi.org/10.1016/j.cden.2023.07.010
0011-8532/24/© 2023 Elsevier Inc. All rights reserved.

When conducting a full history and physical examination specific symptoms will allow the characterization of neuropathic pain in two categories: episodic or continuous. Episodic neuropathic pain syndromes are characterized by severe, paroxysmal, electric shock-like, and/or lancinating pain with short duration. Examples of episodic neuropathic pain disorders are trigeminal neuralgia and glossopharyngeal neuralgia. Continuous neuropathic pain syndromes are characterized by aching, burning, throbbing, stabbing pain for longer duration. Continuous neuropathic pain disorders include idiopathic trigeminal neuropathic pain, post-herpetic neuralgia, central post-stroke pain, and complex regional pain syndrome (CRPS).[1] The goal of this article is to discuss the medication management of these various neuropathic pain disorders.

NEUROPATHIC PAIN PATHOPHYSIOLOGY

The International Association for the Study of Pain (IASP) defines neuropathic pain as pain caused by a lesion or disease of the somatosensory nervous system.[2] The physiologic experience of pain involves the processes of transduction, transmission, and modulation. First, a stimulus activates free nerve endings of nociceptors. Then, a-delta and c-fibers are activated and transmit information to the spinal cord and information finally reaches the central nervous system and thalamus. Cortical centers process this sensory information and pain is experienced.[1] Many neurochemicals are involved with pain transmission but most commonly involve glutamate and substance P.[1] Although the pathophysiology of many chronic pain conditions remains poorly understood, endogenous opioids, serotonin, norepinephrine, and alteration in receptor function are thought to be involved.[1]

EPISODIC NEUROPATHIC PAIN
Trigeminal Neuralgia

Trigeminal neuralgia is a disorder characterized by short bouts of excruciating shock-like facial pain in the distribution of the trigeminal nerve. Trigeminal neuralgia is also known as "tic douloureux" due to the nature of facial spasms during attacks and was described during the late first century.[3] This pain is unilateral, affecting the right side more than left and usually with the maxillary (second) and mandibular (third) division of the trigeminal nerve. Patients usually endorse triggers that cause attacks such as brushing teeth, talking, smiling, chewing, or shaving.[3] These painful attacks are usually followed by periods of time that are pain free. Before establishing a diagnosis of trigeminal neuralgia, multiple sclerosis and intracranial tumors of posterior and middle fossa must be ruled out. MRI imaging should be completed to rule out multiple sclerosis or tumors.[4] These diagnoses would need prompt referral to neurology or neurosurgery. Trigeminal neuralgia effects 4 in 100,000 people and usually occurs in the fifth decade of life and older. Women have slightly higher incidence than men. Diagnosis depends on the clinician's ability to recognize the disorder's specific signs and symptoms. International Headache Society characterizes trigeminal neuralgia into classical, secondary trigeminal neuralgia, and idiopathic trigeminal neuralgia.[3]

Classical trigeminal neuralgia refers to the disorder characterized by recurrent paroxysmal episodes of unilateral facial pain and nerve root atrophy or neurovascular compressions within the trigeminal nerve distribution.[4] Secondary or symptomatic trigeminal neuralgia is associated with an underlying disease such multiple sclerosis, tumor of cerebellopontine angle, or AV malformation.[4]

The pathophysiology of trigeminal neuralgia is believed to be caused by the demyelination of the trigeminal nerve which leads to ephaptic transmission.[3] Ephaptic transmission causes electrical impulse by one neuron to alter the excitability of neighboring neurons. The cause of this demyelination is hypothesized to be caused by compression of the nerve root by aberrant or torturous vessels.[3] Trigeminal neuralgia usually more commonly affects the right side of the face possibly due to a more narrow foramen rotundum and foramen ovale where the second and third divisions of the trigeminal nerve exit the skull respectively.[3]

Pharmacologic Therapy of Trigeminal Neuralgia

It is important to note in the discussion of medication management of TN that there are few studies with high level of evidence supporting the particular treatments for trigeminal neuralgia. Chole and colleagues completed a systematic review of the literature evaluating drug treatments for trigeminal neuralgia and found that although anticonvulsants were found effective in treating trigeminal neuralgia there are few studies with high level of evidence.[5] As always, clinicians strive to have their treatment be evidence based. The lack of high level evidence for the treatment of trigeminal neuralgia illuminates the need for randomized controlled studies with larger patient populations.

Historically, treatment for trigeminal neuralgia usually includes antiepileptic drugs such as carbamazepine and phenytoin. These medications are often started at small dose and increased until relief of symptoms. Many patients experience complete relief of symptoms and can be titrated down or off medications completely. According to Zakrzewska and colleagues and their review of four systematic reviews with metanalysis in British Journal of Neurosurgery, carbamazepine is still first-line treatment for trigeminal neuralgia.[6] However, evidence suggests that this should be changed to oxcarbazepine if poor response or undesirable side effects are observed.[6] When treatment with carbamazepine or oxcarbazepine fails, second-line treatment can include carbamazepine with lamotrigine or baclofen. The evidence supporting these combinations however, is weak.[6]

CARBAMAZEPINE

Carbamazepine is considered first-line treatment in classical trigeminal neuralgia and Cochrane review has established that carbamazepine is an effective treatment.[7] Carbamazepine is an antiepileptic drug that inactivates voltage gated sodium channels and decreases transmission of postsynaptic reflex arcs in the spinal cord. Carbamazepine requires cautious dosing due to numerous side effects associated with this treatment. Side effects include leukopenia, agranulocytosis, aplastic anemia, drowsiness, and ataxia. Carbamazepine doses range from 100 to 2400 mg per day. Most patient respond positively with 200 mg to 800 mg per day in two to three divided doses.[3] If treatment alone with carbamazepine fails, alternative drugs can be prescribed or additional drugs can be added. Medications that have been reported to successfully treat trigeminal neuralgia with lower-level evidence include baclofen, phenytoin, lamotrigine, gabapentin, topiramate.[3] Oxcarbazepine is a newer agent similar to carbamazepine with fewer severe side effects. Phenyoin mechanism of action is an anticonvulsant drug that blocks voltage-dependent sodium channels responsible for increasing action potentials and was historically thought to be second-line treatment for trigeminal neuralgia. However, Chole and colleagues found no studies with a high level of evidence that phenytoin is an effective treatment of trigeminal neuralgia.[5]

GABAPENTIN AND PREGABALIN

Other anticonvulsant agents used in the treatment of trigeminal neuralgia include gabapentin and pregabalin. These medications increase GABA in the brain and inhibit pain sensors and have been prescribed for many neuropathic pain disorders. Merren suggested that gabapentin proves as an effective therapy or co therapy particularly in peripherally mediated neuropathic pain.[8] Although these medications are contraindicated in kidney disease they have fewer side effects than previously mentioned anticonvulsants.

Lamotrigine

Lamotrigine is an anticonvulsant that blocks voltage-sensitive sodium channels and inhibits the release of neurotransmitters, glutamate, and aspartate. Zakrzewska and colleagues suggest that in combination with carbamazepine or phenytoin that lamotrigine has antineuralgia properties due to decreased pain scores in refractory trigeminal neuralgia in a double blind placebo-controlled trial.[9] Lamotrigine has been reported as a potential cause of Steven-Johnson Syndrome so should be used with caution.

Baclofen

Baclofen is muscle relaxant drug that is a GABA agonist that reduces release of excitatory neurotransmitters in presynaptic neurons and stimulates inhibitory signals in postsynaptic neurons. Baclofen has less effect on blood cells than other treatment modalities but side effects include GI upset including vomiting and cramping. Fromm and colleagues exhibited in a double-blind study that showed baclofen decreased number of painful episodes in 7 out of 10 patients suffering from trigeminal neuralgia.[10] Another study illustrated patients with refractory trigeminal neuralgia that 74% of patients were relived of pain with baclofen either alone or in combination with ineffective dose of carbamazepine.[10] Dosages of 10 to 80 mg per day have been shown to help in trigeminal neuralgia.[3]

Topiramate

Topiramate acts on voltage gated sodium channels and modulates GABA. Side effects of topiramate include nephrolithiasis, somnolence, anxiety, and drowsiness. Gilron and colleagues showed topiramate reduced pain by up to 64% in a small study of 3 patients but was unable to confirm results in follow up study.[11]

OTHER AGENTS

Tricyclic antidepressants have also been used in the treatment of trigeminal neuralgia with limited efficacy supported with studies. These agents should be used with caution due to potential side effects such as anticholinergic effects, cardiac side effects, xerostomia, constipation, and urinary retention.[10] Amitriptyline is an antidepressant that has been effective in treating atypical trigeminal neuralgia due to its ability to increase endogenous serotonin and norepinephrine at the synaptic cleft. Carraso and colleagues compared amitriptyline and clomipramine, both serotonin reuptake blockers, and found clomipramine is better at treating trigeminal neuralgia.[12] Recently, selective serotonin reuptake receptor inhibitors (SSRIs) have been employed to treat trigeminal neuralgia. SSRIs such as fluoxetine, paroxetine as well as selective norepinephrine receptor inhibitors (SNRIs) such as duloxetine have been effectively used to treat trigeminal neuralgia. Adverse effects of these medications include nausea, loss of appetite, constipation, sedation, dry mouth, hyperhidrosis, and anxiety.[6] Chung-Chih et al. reported rapid relief in patients with TN treated with 40 mg duloxetine.[5] One small study has shown success of treatment of trigeminal neuralgia with botulinum toxin A.[13] Topical capsaicin has been used to treat neuropathic pain and was shown to be help in to a lesser extent in trigeminal neuralgia in one study.[14] Common medications used to treat trigeminal neuralgia and their dosages are summarized in **Table 1**. Due to limited large scale high level of evidence of the effectiveness of these drugs in the treatment of trigeminal neuralgia this an important area of future research. Clinicians should proceed with caution and consider patient comorbidities and side effect profile of each drug before proceeding with specific treatment.

Glossopharyngeal Neuralgia

Glossopharyngeal neuralgia is a rare pain disorder affecting the distrubtuion of the ninth cranial nerve, the glossopharyngeal nerve.[1] Glossopharyngeal neuralgia is marked by brief unilateral severe, sharp, and stabbing pain near the angle of mandible, ear, tonsillar fossa, and base of tongue.[15] These painful episodes are usually stimulated by coughing, talking or swallowing.[1] The underlying mechanism of glossopharyngeal neuralgia is not known.[15] Similar to trigeminal neuralgia, glossopharyngeal neuralgia can be caused by vascular compression at the nerve root, multiple sclerosis, or space occupying lesions such as tumors in central pontine angle.[15] Eagle syndrome or calcification of stylohyoid ligament can also be a cause of glossopharyngeal neuralgia.[15] Thus, CT and MRI are often employed to evaluate stylohyoid ligament and identify tumors or vascular compression.[15] Painful attacks of glossopharyngeal neuralgia have sometimes been reported, in the literature, accompanied by syncopal episodes, transient or persistent bradycardia, and even seizures.[15] This condition is referred to vagoglossopharyngeal neuralgia and is likely due to the communication of glossopharyngeal nerve with the vagus nerve.[15] Glossopharyngeal neuralgia has been shown to respond well to treatment with carbamazepine or oxcarbazepine.[16] Carbamazepine dosage for glossopharyngeal neuralgia is 200 mg per day in a single extended release dose or two divided doses of immediate release tablets. The dose can be gradually increased by 200 mg per day as needed until the relief of symptoms to a maximum 1200 mg per day. If pain is not resolved by carbamazepine alone, supplementation with other agents such as gabapentin, valproic acid, lamotrigine, baclofen, phenytoin, pregabalin, or topiramate can be successful.

Gabapentin can be added with a dosage of 100 to 500 mg per day in one to four divided doses. Duloxetine, an SNRI, may be added at a dose of 20 to 90 mg per day and valproic acid, an anticonvulsant, can be added at a dose of 125 to 2500 mg per day in one to two divided doses.[16] Other drugs that can be supplemented are lamotrigine at dose of 50 to 500 mg per day in one to two divided doses, baclofen at a dose of 10 to 80 mg per day in one to two divided doses, phenytoin 200 to 600 mg per day in one to three divided doses, pregabalin 75 to 500 mg per day in one to two divided doses, or topiramate 50 to 1000 mg per day in one to two divided doses.[16] Medications should be prescribed at low doses and increased as needed based on relief of

Table 1
Common medication dosages for the treatment of trigeminal neuralgia[1]

	Initial	Maximum
Carbamazepine	100–300 mg tid	1200–2400 mg
Baclofen	10 mg tid	60–80 mg
Oxcarbazepine	150–300 mg tid	1500–3000 mg
Gabapentin	300 mg tid	2400–4800 mg
Lamotrigine	25 mg bid	300–600 mg
Topirimate	25 mg tid	100–300 mg

symptoms and side effects experienced by patients. Usually, doses can be decreased over time to lower maintenance dose.[16]

CONTINUOUS NEUROPATHIC PAIN
Idiopathic Trigeminal Neuropathic Pain

Idiopathic trigeminal neuropathic pain is defined by the International Classification of Headache Disorders by "recurrent paroxysms of unilateral facial pain fulfilling criteria of trigeminal neuralgia with concomitant continuous of near-continuous pain between attacks in the affective trigeminal distribution."[17] This pain can be unilateral or bilateral in the distribution of one or more branches of trigeminal nerve of unknown etiology.[17] This pain can be unilateral or bilateral with associated hyperalgesia, allodynia, hypoesthesia, hypoalgesia.[17] Treatment is similar to that of trigeminal neuralgia as discussed above.[17]

Post-Herpetic Neuralgia

Postherpetic neuralgia is a potential sequelae of shingles, also known as herpes zoster, which is a reactivation of latent varicella zoster virus(VZV).[18] VZV is a highly contagious virus responsible for chicken pox usually experienced in childhood. VZV remains latent within sensory ganglia following infection.[1] Herpes zoster is a reactivation of the virus which travels along affected neurons and propagates to the epidermis.[1] Herpes zoster is unilateral and usually only affects a single dermatome and involves an erythematous maculopapular rash accompanied by pain and dysesthesia.[18] The characteristic rash begins as clear vesicles that ulcerate and scab over.[18] Postherpetic neuralgia occurs in the same dermatomes as the original herpes zoster rash. This painful syndrome can last for months to years after the resolution of the initial rash.[18] It is estimated that 1 in every 3 people will develop herpes zoster in their life time and 5% to 20% of these people will develop postherpetic neuralgia. However, due to the creation of vaccination against varicella and shingles these numbers are expected to decline in future years.[18] Postherpetic neuralgia usually occurs in elderly over 65 years and is more common in immunocompromised individuals.[1] Patients with postherpetic neuralgia usually experience constant burning, aching, throbbing pain or pain.[1] Postherpetic neuralgia is diagnosed when pain occurs for 3 months or longer after the resolution of rash.[18] The first approach to managing postherpetic neuralgia is prevention through vaccination or antiviral treatment.[18] Children should now be vaccinated against VZV and adults over 50 years of age should be vaccinated with live attenuated shingles vaccine as recommended by their primary care physicians.[18] The vaccine has been effective at decreasing infection with herpes zoster, lessening the burden of illness due to infection with herpes zoster, and minimizing incidence of postherpetic neuralgia.[18] If diagnosed with herpes zoster, prompt treatment with oral virals (acyclovir, famiciclovir, or valcyclovir) slow the production of the virus and decreases the viral load present in the dorsal root ganglia.[18]

Postherpetic neuralgia is challenging to treat due to patient population of elderly individuals usually with multiple comorbidities and tendancy for postherpetic neuralgia pain to persist for years.[1] The first choices for the treatment of postherpetic neuralgia are calcium channel α2-δ ligands, tricyclic antidepressants, or topical lidocaine patches.[18] Calcium channel α2-δ ligands such as gabapentin or pregabalin are considered best initial treatment due to limited side effects. These side effects include dizziness, somnolence, and GI disturbances. Calcium channel α2-δ ligands are also not metabolized by cytochrome P450 system and therefore have a lower incidence of drug-drug interactions.[18] Initial dosing of gabapentin of post-herpetic neuralgia is

100 to 300 mg at bedtime or 100 to 300 mg three times daily. If symptoms do not improve, clinicians can increase the doseby 100 to 300 mg three times every 1 to 7 days as tolerated to maximum 3600 mg.[18] Studies have shown it can take up to 10 weeks with the treatment of gabapentin to reach therapeutic effective dose.[18] Pregabalin can be dosed at 150 to 600 mg/day taken in two to three divided doses and has been shown to take 1 week to reach effective dose.[18] Pregabalin and gabapentin are excreted by the kidney and doses should be adjusted in patients with reduced renal function.[18] Tricyclic antidepressants (TCAs) such as nortriptyline, desipramine, and amitriptyline should be used with caution in elderly patients due to anticholinergic side effects and cardiotoxicity. The starting dose for nortriptyline or amitriptyline is 25 mg at bedtime with increase by 25 mg/day for 3 to 7 days as tolerated to a maximum of 150 mg per day.[18] Lidocaine 5% topical patch has been shown to reduce pain and improve quality of life in patients with postherpetic neuralgia but no high-quality evidence studies have been completed. Lidocaine 5% patch has less severe side effects than other treatment modalities and include application site reaction, dizziness, and headache.[18] Second or third line medications for postherpetic neuralgia can include opioid analgesics. Opioids must be used with caution due to potential side effects and possible misuse.[18]

Central Post-Stroke Pain

Central Post-Stroke pain (CPSP) is a pain disorder that is difficult to diagnose and treat that can occur in up to 14% of patients who suffer from stroke.[19] Central Post-Stroke pain (CPSP) is defined as "pain resulting from a primary lesion or dysfunction of the central nervous system after a stroke."[19] Most patients with CPSP experience pain such as burning, aching, pricking, lacerating, shooting, squeezing, or throbbing.[20] Most patients with CPSP are found to have multiple lesions on MRI. These patients may experience severe extremity pain with supratentorial lesions and severe facial pain with infratentorial lesions.[19] Patients with infratentorial central post-stroke pain usually have a defect in c fiber mediated temperature sensation.[19] Medullary infarctions are associated with numbness, burning and sensation of cold on the face. The pathophysiology of central post-stroke pain is poorly understood but thought to involve "central disinhibition between relay cells that project cerebral cortex and GABAergic inter-neurons that produce local inhibition."[19] First-line treatments for central post-stroke pain include amitriptyline and lamotrigine and second-line treatments include fluvoxamine and gabapentin.[20] Amitriptyline up to 75 mg daily was found effective and well tolerated compared to placebo in patients with CPSP.[21] Lamotrigine 50 mg per day, increased to up to 200 mg per day, was found to decrease pain in central post-stroke pain.[21] Lamotrigine is a triazine derivative antiepileptic drug that inhibits release glutamate and inhibits voltage sensitive sodium channels that stabilize neuronal membranes.[19] Fluvoxamine, a selective serotonin reuptake inhibitor, up to 125 mg daily showed to reduce pain mildly in central post-stroke pain.[21] Gabapentin has been tried in patients with central post-stroke pain up to 2400 mg daily and results in the reduction of pain in only about 20% of patients.[19] Further larger patient population studies are needed to define appropriate treatment for central post-stroke pain.

Complex Regional Pain Syndrome

Complex Regional Pain Syndrome is a regional neuropathic pain disorder that involves "allodynia, hyperalgesia, motor abnormalities, and skin changes usually affecting extremities."[22] However, rarely Complex Regional Pain Syndrome can affect the face.[22] Complex Regional Pain Syndrome is characterized into CRPS I and CRPS II. CRPS I

Table 2
Drugs therapy for common neuropathic pain disorders[3,15,18,20,22]

	Treatment	Maximum Dose	Refractory
Trigeminal Neuralgia	Carbamazepine 200–800 mg in 2–3 divided doses[3]	1200–2400 mg	Add baclofen: 10–80 mg daily Add: lamotrigine, gabapentin, topiramate.
Glossopharyngeal Neuralgia	Carbamazepine 200 mg/day[15]	1200 mg/day	Alternative or add: gabapentin 100–500 mg/day in 1–4 divided doses.
Postherpetic Neuralgia	Gabapentin 100–300 mg nightly or tid Pregabalin 50 mg tid or 75 mg twice daily. increase dose to 300 mg/day after 3–7 d TCAs (nortriptyline, amitriptyline) 25 mg nightly[18]	3600 mg/day 600 mg/day 150 mg/day	Add lidocaine 5% patch every 4–12 h up to three patches daily
Central Poststroke Pain	Amitriptyline 75 mg daily Lamotrigine 50 mg daily[20]	75 mg/day 200 mg/day	
Complex Regional Pain Syndrome	Short course of oral Prednisone 30 mg daily[22] Alendronate 40 mg daily for 8 wk	n/a	
Burning Mouth Syndrome	Amitriptyline 5–10 mg daily[26] Clonazepam 1 mg tab dissolved intraorally and held in mouth[26]	50 mg daily	

was historically referred to as sympathetic dystrophy and occurs in the absence of nerve trauma.[23] CRPS II also known as causalgia occurs in known nerve trauma.[22] The mechanism of CRPS is not known but thought to involve neuropathic inflammation and activation of c fibers and local hyperactivity of sympathetic nervous system.[24] CRPS is difficult to diagnose and treat. Usually, CRPS must be a diagnosis of exclusion and is treated similar to other neuropathic pain disorders.[24] Diagnosis of CRPS is further complicated by being associated with patients who have suffered stroke similar to central post-stroke pain.[23] However, CRPS is also associated with trauma, fracture, or surgery.[22] CRPS must include a multidisciplinary approach with neurology, physical therapy, psychotherapy, and primary care. Successful treatments for CRPS have included systemic steroids, bisphosphonates, and antiepileptic drugs such as gabapentin. Studies have shown that short course prednisone 30 mg per day illustrated significant improvement in pain.[22] The mechanism of use of bisphosphonates in CRPS is poorly understood but alendronate-treated patients have been found to have marked improvement levels in pain.[22] Gabapentin has been shown to have only a mild improvement in pain in patients who suffer from CRPS.[22]

Burning Mouth Syndrome

Burning mouth syndrome does not fall into the traditional categories of episodic or continuous neuropathic pain. In this condition patients experience a burning sensation in the oral cavity most commonly, on the tongue.[1] This pain can be intermittent or continuous.[25] The cause of Burning Mouth Syndrome is poorly understood but through to be multifactorial.[25] These factors could be local factors, systemic, or psychological factors. Local factors include such as ill fitting dentures, allergic reactions, infections.[25] Systemic factors include vitamin deficiencies (iron, B complex, zinc), anemia, Sjogren's syndrome, and esophageal reflux disease.[25] Psychological factors include anxiety, depression, and compulsive disorders.[25] Patients often report decreased pain with eating, dry mouth, and abnormal taste.[25] Treatment for burning mouth syndrome include topical medications, tricyclic antidepressants, and selective serotonin receptors. Topical medications such as clonazepam 1 mg dissolvable tabs and 0.025% capsaicin cream have been reported with some success in the treatment of burning mouth syndrome.[26] Tricyclyic antidepressants such as nortriptyline 5 to 10 mg per day with gradual increase has shown improvement in burning mouth syndrome however it is best avoided in patients who also suffer from dry mouth.[26] Selective serotonin reuptake inhibitors such as sertraline 50 mg/day and duloxetine at a dose of 30 to 60 mg per day have been used to effectively treat burning mouth syndrome.[26] An initial dose of 300 mg per day of gabapentin increased gradually to a maximum of 2400 mg has been shown to have mixed results in the treatment of burning mouth syndrome.[26] Treatment of burning mouth syndrome remains difficult due to poorly understood pathophysiology of the disease.[26]

SUMMARY

Neuropathic pain disorders remain to be a challenging to treat. The first step to helping our patients who suffer from neuropathic pain disorders is recognizing specific signs and symptoms of the specific neuropathic pain disorder they experience. Such as trigeminal neuralgia, glossopharyngeal neuralgia, idiopathic trigeminal neuropathic pain, post-herpetic neuralgia, central post-stroke pain, complex region pain syndrome, or burning mouth syndrome. Each specific disorder has pharmacologic management best tailored to that specific disorder. A summary of first line and refractory treatments are summarized in **Table 2**. However, many studies have included small patient populations with low level evidence. This exemplifies the importance of future studies in neuropathic pain disorders in order to improve the treatment of these patients.

CLINICS CARE POINTS

- A thorough history and, dental/head and neck physical exam are crucial to establishing adequate diagnosis in all of our patients but especially patients who suffer from neuropahic pain.

- Often, a multidisciplinary teamapproach is beneficial to patients who suffer from neuropathic pain including but not limited to primary care physicians, psychiatrists, neurology specialists.

- Many patients who suffer from neuropathic pain may not respond to medication management upon initiation of treatment. Patients typically do not respond to medication management before 4-6 weeks of treatment. Thus, reassurance and multimodal approach is often necessary.

DISCLOSURE

No disclosures.

REFERENCES

1. Hupp JR, Near RM. Facial Neuropathy. In: Hupp JR, Ellis E, Tucker MR, editors. Contemporary oral and maxillofacial surgery. 6th edition. St. Louis: Elsevier Mosby; 2014. p. 618–25.
2. International Association for the Study of Pain, IASP Taxonomy. Pain terms, 2017, Neuropathic Pain. https://www.iasp-pain.org/resources/terminology/.
3. Kraft RM. Trigeminal Neuralgia. Am Fam Physician 2008;77:1291–6.
4. Olesen J. Trigeminal Neuralgia. In: International Classification of Headache Disorders. 2018. Available at: https://ichd-3.org/13-painful-cranial-neuropathies-and-other-facial-pains/13-1-trigeminal-neuralgia/13-1-1-classical-trigeminal-neuralgia/. Accessed November 20, 2023.
5. Chole R, Ranjitkumar P, et al. Drug Treatment of Trigeminal Neuralgia: A Systematic Review of the Literature. J Oral Maxillofac Surg 2007;65:40–5.
6. Zakrzewska JM, Jorns TP. Evidence-Based Approach to the Medical Management of Trigeminal Neuralgia. Br J Neurosurg 2009;21:253–61.
7. Wiffen PJ, McQuay HJ, et al. Carbamazepine for Acute and Chronic Pain. Cochrane Database Syst Rev 2005;3:CD005451.
8. Merren MD. Gabapentin for Treatment of Pain and Tremor: A Large Case Series. South Med J 1998;91:739–44.
9. Zakrzewka JM, Chaudhry Z, et al. Lamotrigine (Lamictal) in Refractory Trigeminaml Neuralgia: Results from a Double-Blind Placebo Controlled Crossover Trial. Pain 1997;73:223–30.
10. Fromm GH, Terrence CF, et al. Baclofen in the Treatment of Trigeminal Neuralgia: Double-Blind Study and Long-Term Follow up. Ann Neurol 1984;15:240–4.
11. Gilron I, Booher SL, et al. Topiramate in Trigeminal Neuralgia a Randomized, placebo-controlled Multiple Crossover Pilot Study. Clin Neuropharmacol 2001; 24:109–12.
12. Carasso RL, Yehuda S, et al. Clomipramine and Amitriptyline in the Treatment of Severe Pain. Int J Neurosci 1979;9:191–4.

13. Piovesan EJ, Teive HG, et al. An Open Study of Botulinum-A Toxin Treatment of Trigeminal Neuralgia. Neuroology 2005;65:1306–8.
14. Epstein JB, Marcoe JH. Topical Application of Capsaicin for Treatment of Oral Neuropathic Pain and Trigeminal Neuralgia. Oral Surg Oral Med Oral Pathol 1994;77:135–40.
15. Shah RJ, Padalia D. Glossopharyngeal neuralgia. [Updated 2022 Feb 17]. In: StatPearls [Internet]. Treasure Island (FL): StatPearls Publishing; 2022. Available at: https://www.ncbi.nlm.nih.gov/books/NBK541041/.
16. Graff-Radford SB, Newman A, et al. Treatment Options for Glossopharyngeal Neuralgia. Therapy 2005;2:733–7.
17. Gobel H. 13.1.2.5 Idiopathic painful trigeminal neuropathy. ICHD-3. Available at: https://ichd-3.org/13-painful-cranial-neuropathies-and-other-facial-pains/13-1-trigeminal-neuralgia/13-1-2-painful-trigeminal-neuropathy. Accessed March 13, 2023.
18. Mallick-Searl T, Snodgrass B, et al. Postherpetic Neuralgia: Epidemiology, Pathophysiology, and Pain Management Pharmacology. J Multidiscip Healthc 2016;9:447–54.
19. Kuma B, Kaltia J, et al. Central Poststroke Pain: A Review of Pathophysiology and Treatment. Pain Med 2009;108:1645–55.
20. Zagaria MA. Central Poststroke Pain Syndrome. US Pharm 2016;41:21–3.
21. Kilt H, Finnerup N, et al. Central Post-Stroke Pain: Clinical Characteristics, pathophysiology, and management. Lancet Neurol 2009;8:857–65.
22. Taylor SS, Noor N, et al. Complex Regional Pain Syndrome: A Comprehensive Review. Pain Ther 2021;10:875–92.
23. Treister AK, Hatch MN, et al. Demystifying Post-Stroke Pain: From Etiology to Treatment. Pharm Manag PM R 2017;9:63–75.
24. Mackey S, Feinberg S. Pharmacological Therapies for Complex Regional Pain Syndrome. Curr Pain Headache Rep 2007;11:38–43.
25. Aggarwal A, Panat S. Burning Mouth Syndrome: A Diagnostic and Therapeutic Dilemma. J Clin Exp Dent 2012;4:180–5.
26. Aravindhan R, Vidyalakshmi S, et al. Burning Mouth Syndrome: A Review on its Diagnostic and Therapeutic Approach. J Pham Bioallied Sci 2014;6:S21–5.

Treatment of Oral Dysplasia

Earl Clarkson, DDS[a], Reza Hadioonzadeh, DDS[c],
Scott M. Peters, DDS[b],*

KEYWORDS

- Dysplasia • Leukoplakia • Erythroplakia • Proliferative verrucous leukoplakia
- Lichen planus • Oral submucosal fibrosis • Actinic cheilitis
- Squamous cell carcinoma

KEY POINTS

- The reader will be able to define dysplasia and understand how it is diagnosed.
- The reader will be able to identify the different types of oral premalignant lesions.
- The reader will be able to explain how oral premalignant lesions are treated.

INTRODUCTION

There are over 300,000 cases of oral squamous cell carcinoma (SCC) diagnosed worldwide each year, including more than 30,000 cases in the United States and more than 3000 cases in Canada. Oral SCC is the most common cancer of the head and neck. Despite advances in surgical technology, the 5-year survival rate has remained at 50% for many years. Most clinicians attribute this plateau in survival rate to the fact that most cases of SCC are diagnosed and treated in advanced stages. However, in patients who are treated in early stages, the 5-year survival rate increases to as high as 80%. In addition, these patients tend to report improved quality of life when compared to those who are treated at advanced stages of disease. This highlights the importance of screening, diagnosis, and treatment of premalignant and early stage malignant lesions.[1]

The term epithelial dysplasia refers to a precancerous lesion with an increased risk for transformation to malignancy, specifically squamous cell carcinoma. Dysplasia is a diagnosis which is rendered through microscopic analysis of diseased tissue. Within the oral cavity, dysplastic lesions may have many different clinical presentations.[2] This article will first define the term dysplasia and explain how a diagnosis of dysplasia is rendered. Then, it will review the different clinical forms dysplasia may take within

---

[a] Oral and Maxillofacial Surgery, Woodhull Medical Center, Brooklyn, NY, USA; [b] Oral and Maxillofacial Surgery, Woodhull Medical Center, Brooklyn, NY, USA; [c] Oral and Maxillofacial Pathology, Geisinger Medical Center, Wilkes-Barre, PA, USA
* Corresponding author. Geisinger Medical Center, 675 Baltimore Drive, Wilkes-Barre, PA 18702.
E-mail address: Smpeters1@geisinger.edu

Dent Clin N Am 68 (2024) 133–149
https://doi.org/10.1016/j.cden.2023.07.008

the oral cavity. Finally, it will discuss both current treatment recommendations for dysplastic lesions and emerging therapeutic options.

DISCUSSION

Before the term dysplasia can be defined and discussed, it is important to briefly review the histology of oral mucosa. On histologic examination, oral mucosa appears as connective tissue covered by stratified squamous epithelium. Some portions of the oral mucosa (hard palate, gingiva, dorsal tongue) also contain a layer of surface keratin, while others (soft palate, buccal mucosa, labial mucosa) are non-keratinized (**Fig. 1**). Epithelial cells originate from the basal (bottom-most) layer of the surface epithelium and migrate upward (closer to the surface) as they mature. Epithelial dysplasia is a microscopic finding within the surface epithelium of tissue. It refers to changes in the epithelial cells including nuclear hyperchromasia, enlargement, and pleomorphism, increased mitotic activity, loss of orderly stratification, cellular dyskeratosis, and bulging of rete ridges (**Fig. 2**).[3] In the oral cavity, a 3-tier grading system for dysplasia is used. Mild epithelial dysplasia refers to changes limited to the basal and parabasal layers of the epithelium (**Fig. 3**). When these changes involve the lower one-half of the epithelium, the term moderate epithelial dysplasia is used (**Fig. 4**). Extension into the upper half of the epithelium results in a diagnosis of severe epithelial dysplasia (**Fig. 5**). Changes involving the full thickness of the epithelium are referred to as carcinoma in situ (**Fig. 6**). Dysplasia is distinguished from SCC in that the latter shows the invasion of atypical epithelial cells into the underlying connective tissue while the former does not (**Fig. 7**).[4]

The term potentially malignant disorder may be used to describe lesions of the oral mucosa which are associated with a greater than normal risk of developing malignancy. When biopsied and examined microscopically, these lesions may show features of dysplasia. Some of the potentially malignant disorders which will be discussed in this article include leukoplakia and proliferative verrucous leukoplakia, erythroplakia, actinic cheilitis, and oral submucosal fibrosis. The relationship between oral lichen planus and squamous cell carcinoma will also be reviewed.

A leukoplakia is defined as a white patch or plaque that is adherent to the oral mucosa (cannot be removed with a gloved finger, gauze, or dental instrument) and cannot be diagnosed as another specific disease (**Fig. 8**). This definition is, in essence, a

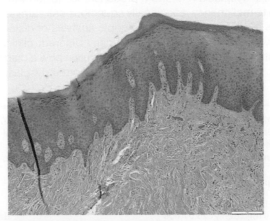

Fig. 1. Histologic appearance of benign oral mucosa.

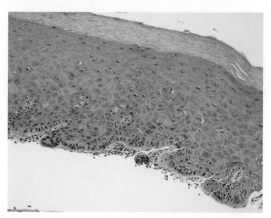

Fig. 2. Histologic features of epithelial dysplasia, including the bulging of rete ridges, loss of orderly stratification of epithelial cells, and increased mitotic activity.

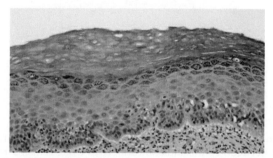

Fig. 3. In mild epithelial dysplasia, the cytologic atypia is limited to the basal one-third of the epithelium.

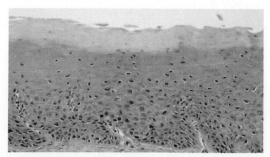

Fig. 4. Histologic appearance of moderate epithelial dysplasia, showing cytologic atypia involving the basal one-half of the epithelium.

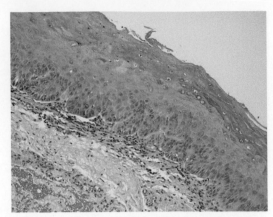

Fig. 5. Severe epithelial dysplasia. The cellular atypia extends into the upper third of the epithelium.

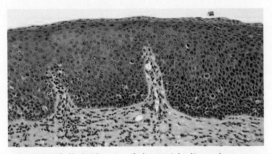

Fig. 6. Carcinoma in situ. The full thickness of the epithelium demonstrates dysplasia. However, the boundary between epithelium and connective tissue remains intact.

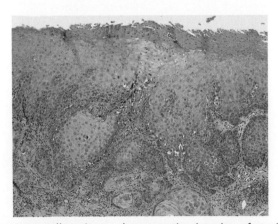

Fig. 7. Invasive squamous cell carcinoma demonstrating invasion of atypical epithelial cells into the underlying connective tissue.

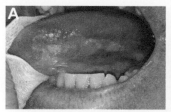
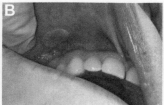
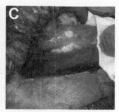

Fig. 8. (A–C) Clinical examples of leukoplakias. Although these lesions vary in location, size, and thickness, all represent non-removable white lesions which cannot be given a specific and definitive diagnosis without biopsy.

diagnosis of exclusion. The term leukoplakia is not a single or specific diagnosis, rather it is a clinical descriptor for any white lesion of uncertain etiology.[2] As a general rule, any oral leukoplakia that has not resolved after 2 weeks should be biopsied to establish a definitive diagnosis. Broadly speaking, when a leukoplakia is examined microscopically, the findings will fall into one of the 3 diagnostic categories. The largest percentage of oral leukoplakias demonstrate benign findings on histology. They show epithelial hyperplasia and/or hyperkeratosis and can be thought of as the oral equivalent to a callous of the skin (**Fig. 9**). Approximately 5% to 25% of oral leukoplakias show dysplasia on biopsy (**Fig. 10**). The smallest percentage of leukoplakic lesions will demonstrate invasive cancer (squamous cell carcinoma) (**Fig. 11**).[3] The clinical challenge is that there is no reliable way to predict which leukoplakic lesions will be benign and which will be premalignant or cancerous based on appearance alone. Therefore, the treatment recommendation for any non-resolving leukoplakia is biopsy to establish a definitive diagnosis. Thinner, homogenous leukoplakias will often (but not always) show earlier dysplastic features (mild dysplasia) on biopsy (**Fig. 12**). Clinical features such as the thickening of the lesion, granular or irregular surface texture, or a mixed red and white appearance ("speckled" leukoplakia or erythroleukoplakia) are all clinical features which may be associated with higher degrees of dysplasia or outright malignancy (**Fig. 13**).

Proliferative verrucous leukoplakia (PVL) is a unique form of leukoplakia with a high rate of transformation to malignancy. It is most commonly seen in elderly females, often without any history of tobacco use. The gingiva is involved most frequently, although any oral mucosal site may be affected. Lesions of PVL progress through

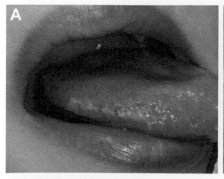
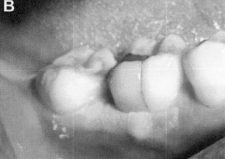

Fig. 9. (A, B) Clinical examples of leukoplakias diagnosed as epithelial hyperplasia with overlying hyperkeratosis on biopsy.

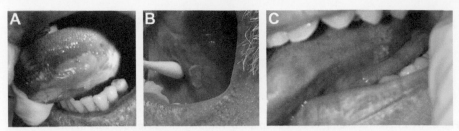

Fig. 10. (*A*) Leukoplakia diagnosed as mild epithelial dysplasia on biopsy. (*B*) Leukoplakia diagnosed as moderate epithelial dysplasia on biopsy. (*C*) Leukoplakia diagnosed as severe epithelial dysplasia on biopsy

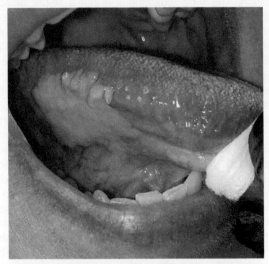

Fig. 11. Leukoplakic lesion which demonstrated squamous cell carcinoma on biopsy.

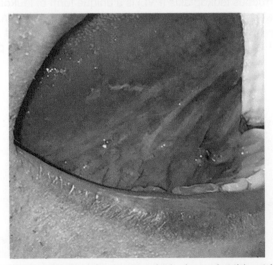

Fig. 12. Thin, homogenous leukoplakic lesion which showed mild epithelial dysplasia on biopsy.

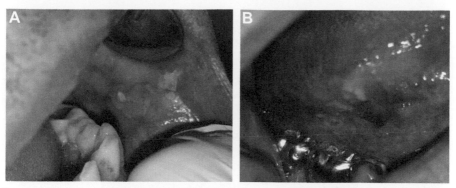

Fig. 13. (A) A thick leukoplakic lesion which demonstrated moderate to focally severe dysplasia on biopsy. (B) An erythroleukoplakia (speckled leukoplakia) which showed carcinoma in situ on microscopic examination.

four clinical stages. In the earliest stage, the lesions appear as flat, white, focally thickened patches (**Fig. 14**). In some instances, they may clinically resemble oral lichen planus. As the lesions progress to the next clinical stage, they will increase both in number and in thickness (**Fig. 15**). After this stage, the lesions will begin to develop an exophytic or verrucous growth profile (**Fig. 16**). Oftentimes, it is at this stage that the lesions first begin to demonstrate dysplasia on histologic examination. In the final clinical stage, there is transformation to malignancy, most often verrucous carcinoma or squamous cell carcinoma (**Fig. 17**).[2] The management of PVL can be challenging for several reasons. Due to the innocuous clinical appearance of early lesions, the diagnosis of PVL may often be overlooked at this stage. If early stage lesions are biopsied, they may not show microscopic features of dysplasia, leading to failure to appropriately diagnose the condition (**Fig. 18**). The authors' recommendation is that any gingival lesion demonstrating thick and/or verrucous epithelial hyperplasia and hyperkeratosis should be viewed as suspicious for PVL in the appropriate clinical context (a clinical presentation of multiple white gingival lesions).

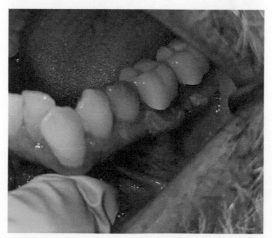

Fig. 14. Early stage proliferative verrucous leukoplakia presenting as thin white patches on the gingiva.

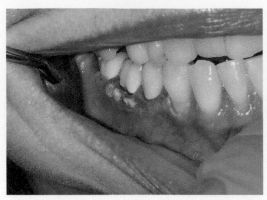

Fig. 15. As the lesions of proliferative verrucous leukoplakia progress, they start to become thicker clinically.

The definition of an erythroplakia is similar to that of a leukoplakia. It is a red patch or plaque that cannot be wiped off and cannot be diagnosed as another specific disease. While the majority of leukoplakias yield benign findings on pathology, most erythroplakias demonstrate dysplasia or invasive carcinoma on microscopic examination (**Fig. 19**). Therefore, the relative risk of malignancy of an idiopathic erythroplakia is much higher when compared to its leukoplakic counterpart. Similar to a leukoplakia, the current recommendation for the initial management of an erythroplakia is a biopsy of any lesion which has failed to resolve after 2 weeks.[5]

Actinic cheilitis, also known as solar cheilitis, refers to precancerous lesions of the labial (lip) mucosa which are the direct result of sun damage. A similar term, actinic

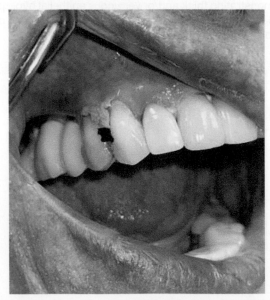

Fig. 16. A later stage lesion of proliferative verrucous leukoplakia which now demonstrates an exophytic growth profile.

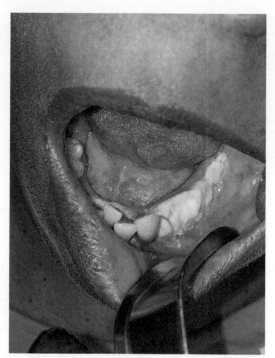

Fig. 17. Proliferative verrucous leukoplakia which has transformed into verrucous carcinoma.

keratosis, is used to describe premalignant lesions of the skin. The lower labial mucosa is much more frequently affected than the upper lip, due to the direct effect of ultraviolet radiation on this location.[6] Historically, actinic cheilitis has been seen more often in patients with a history of outdoor occupational exposures, such as farmers and sailors. Early lesions of actinic cheilitis will appear as discrete, often subtle

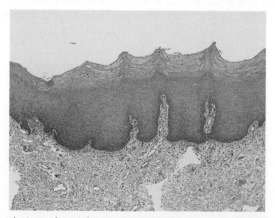

Fig. 18. Biopsy of a lesion of proliferative verrucous leukoplakia which was diagnosed as verrucous epithelial hyperplasia and hyperkeratosis (*thick*). Although no dysplasia was seen at this time, this lesion progressed to the clinical lesion illustrated in **Fig. 17**.

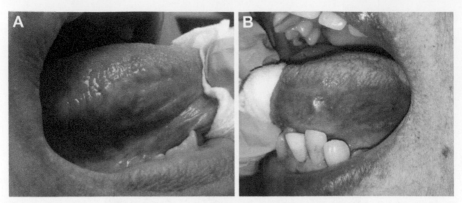

Fig. 19. (*A*) Clinical example of an erythroplakia diagnosed as severe epithelial dysplasia. (*B*) Erythroplakic lesion diagnosed as squamous cell carcinoma.

leukoplakic patches of the lip (**Fig. 20**). As these lesions progress, they will become larger in size and the boundaries between lesion and the vermillion border of the lip will begin to blur (**Fig. 21**). In later stages of actinic cheilitis, the labial mucosa will appear crusted, cracked, or ulcerated (**Fig. 22**). Actinic cheilitis is by definition a premalignant lesion, and therefore a biopsy will demonstrate dysplasia on microscopic examination. In addition, the underlying connective tissue (dermis) will often exhibit changes secondary to sun damage (solar elastosis) (**Fig. 23**).[7] Actinic cheilitis may be treated by surgical excision of the lesion, however this may not always be feasible or preferred due to lesion size and cosmetic concerns at the site. Unlike the treatment of intraoral dysplasias, there are approved non-surgical therapies for the management of actinic cheilitis. Anti-neoplastic agents, such as Imiquimoid or Fluorouracil, may be applied to the lesion to promote resolution. Similarly, some studies have advocated for therapies such as liquid nitrogen, laser ablation, chemical peels, or phototherapy in lieu of surgical removal.

Oral submucosal fibrosis is a premalignant condition which is strongly associated with the use of betel quid. Betel quid is a substance which consists of a betel leaf wrapped around an areca nut, slaked lime, tobacco, and a mixture of various sweeteners and spices. Betel quid is frequently used in South and Southeastern Asia, and

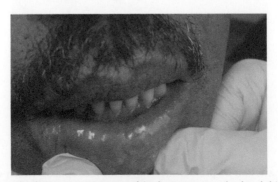

Fig. 20. Early actinic cheilitis presenting as a thin, homogenous leukoplakia of the lower lip. Microscopic examination revealed mild epithelial dysplasia.

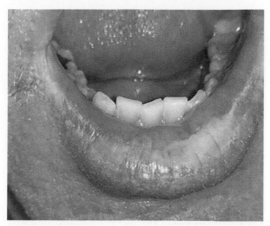

Fig. 21. As actinic cheilitis progresses clinically, the boundary between lesion and vermillion border will blur.

oral submucosal fibrosis is seen most often in these populations. Patients with oral submucosal fibrosis develop a generalized pallor and fibrosis of the affected mucosa.[8] They will have resultant limited jaw opening (trismus) and may complain of oral mucosal burning. In addition, the epithelium in this field of fibrosed tissue is at a higher risk to undergo dysplastic or malignant changes.[9] Patients with oral submucosal fibrosis should be screened regularly for oral cancer, as the relative risk for SCC in this population group is almost twenty times that of a patient without oral submuocsal fibrosis. Due to severe trismus, however, it may be challenging to detect and diagnose precancerous lesions.

Oral lichen planus (OLP) is a chronic mucocutaneous disorder with a somewhat controversial association with oral SCC. The etiology of OLP is still unknown, but it is often classified as an autoimmune condition. It is seen most frequently between the ages of forty to 60 years of age. A slight female predilection has been reported. Lichen planus will most often present as bilateral and/or multifocal lesions which may involve any aspect of the oral mucosa. The buccal mucosa and gingiva tend to be affected with the highest frequency.[10] Oral lichen planus will take many clinical

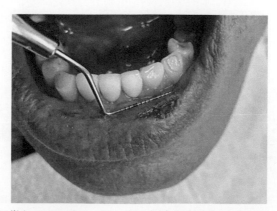

Fig. 22. Actinic cheilitis presenting with a cracked and ulcerated appearance. This lesion showed severe dysplasia on biopsy.

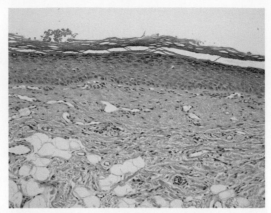

Fig. 23. Histologic examination of actinic cheilitis will demonstrate dysplasia of the epithelium and solar elastosis of the superficial connective tissue.

forms. The reticular variant of lichen planus is seen most commonly and presents as a series of white, lace-like lesions known as Wickham Striae (**Fig. 24**). In erosive or ulcerative lichen planus, the mucosa appears erythematous and may bleed easily. Tan-grey ulcerations may also be identified (**Fig. 25**). Wickham Striae may be encountered in erosive lichen planus, however they are often subtler when compared to their reticular counterpart. Plaque-form lichen planus describes thick leukoplakic patches of lichen planus (**Fig. 26**). This form is often limited to the dorsal aspect of the tongue. Other clinical subtypes of lichen planus, such as the papular and bullous forms, have also been documented, but are seen with less frequency (**Fig. 27**).[11] Although an in-depth discussion regarding lichen planus treatment is beyond the scope of this article, OLP is included here because it is now considered a premalignant condition. A small percentage (approximately 1%–2%) of patients with lichen planus may develop oral squamous cell carcinoma. This is seen most frequently in patients with erosive forms of lichen planus. The exact reason as to why patients develop SCC is unclear. Some have argued that the lichenoid lesions themselves may undergo malignant

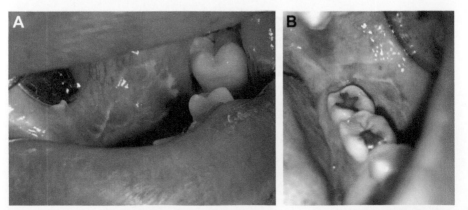

Fig. 24. (*A, B*) Clinical examples of reticular lichen planus presenting with white, lace-like lesions.

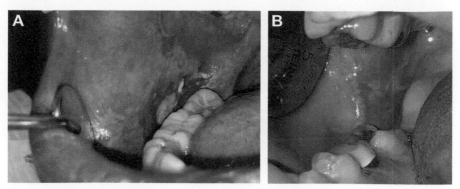

Fig. 25. (*A, B*) Clinical examples of erosive lichen planus. The lesions demonstrate varying areas of erythema and ulceration. Wickham striae can be seen, however they represent a less prominent component of these lesions.

transformation, however evidence of this event is poorly documented.[12] Another possibility is that because lichen planus is a chronic inflammatory disease, there is an increased risk of cytologic atypia due to a constant inflammatory stimulus, leading to malignant transformation.[13] However, this is not documented in other chronic inflammatory mucosal diseases such as mucosal pemphigoid or pemphigus vulgaris. A more cynical explanation is that lesions that were diagnosed as lichen planus may have been misclassified. As previously discussed, early lesions of PVL may closely resemble the clinical appearance of OLP (**Fig. 28**). PVL has a very high rate of transformation to malignancy. Similarly, sometimes lesions may appear lichenoid clinically or microscopically however they demonstrate histologic evidence of dysplasia. Historically, these lesions were referred to as "lichenoid dysplasia" however it is unlikely that they actually represent examples of lichen planus (**Fig. 29**).

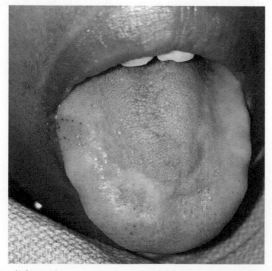

Fig. 26. Plaque-form lichen planus presenting as thick hyperkeratotic patches of the dorsal tongue.

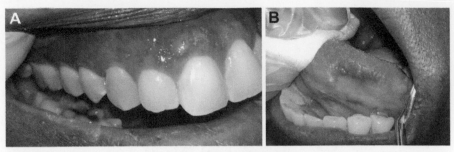

Fig. 27. (*A*) Papular lichen planus. (*B*) Bullous lichen planus.

Now that the different clinical forms of oral dysplasia have been described, treatment strategies will be discussed. The general recommendation for any oral dysplastic lesion is complete surgical excision. Although the relative risk of malignant transformation of mild dysplasia is less than moderate or severe dysplasia, there is no way to reliably predict the biologic activity of dysplastic lesions.[2] In addition, mild dysplasia of the upper aerodigestive tract may undergo a phenomenon known as drop-down or drop-off carcinoma, meaning it can progress directly to malignancy without first showing features of higher grade dysplasia. Under certain circumstances, the clinician may elect to observe mild dysplasia although this is often not recommended as these lesions have shown malignant transformation rates of 0.13% to 36% with overall transformation rate of 7% in oral leukoplakias.[14–16]

The most important advantage of conventional scalpel excision is the ability to obtain a reliable tissue sample for histopathologic examination. However larger lesions that heal via secondary intension may lead to restriction in function due to the generation of fibrous tissue. In these cases, mucosal grafts or split-thickness skin grafts may be considered as an adjunct to surgical excision for improved healing and post-operative function. An alternate treatment is use of CO_2 laser. The CO_2 beam is well absorbed by tissue with high water content, which leads to the vaporization of cellular contents and cell death. When using a CO_2 laser, it is essential to excise

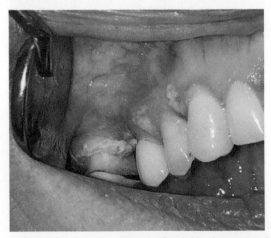

Fig. 28. Early lesions of proliferative verrucous leukoplakia demonstrating a faintly lichenoid appearance.

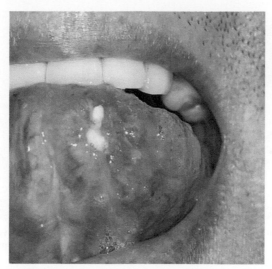

Fig. 29. This lesion appears lichenoid clinically, with a central zone of erythema and a white, radiating, somewhat lace-like border. However, biopsy of this lesion demonstrated severe epithelial dysplasia.

the lesion rather than ablate it in order to allow for reliable histopathologic examination and inspection of the specimen for clear margins.[17] With ablation, a tissue sample is not obtained and it is assumed that appropriate depth has been reached based on the clinical examination of the surgical site. In addition, CO_2 vaporization may not remove the entire lesion in thick keratinized tissue as this type of tissue is more resistant to vaporization. Incomplete excision of lesions may lead to rapid epithelialization by remnant dysplastic cells and recurrence at the site.[18] A major advantage of laser treatment is related to post-operative healing and analgesia due to minimal damage to nearby bone and teeth, hemostatic and anesthetic surgical bed due to sealed blood vessels and nerve ending. In addition, the reduced number of myoepithelial cells has been documented at the periphery which in turn leads to reduced contracture of the surgical wound.[19–21]

There are an increasing number of clinical trials for the non-surgical management of these lesions. Chemopreventive therapies using medications such as Imiquimoid, Nivolumab, and Retinoids have shown promising results in small patient cohorts. If these medications are deemed to be efficacious in the treatment of oral dysplasia, then they could be used for the management of patients who are not surgical candidates or in those who have multiple premalignant lesions (PVL) where surgical treatments would lead to significant morbidity.[22]

In summary, surgical excision of a dysplastic lesion via scalpel remains gold standard treatment in order to properly assess margins upon microscopic examination (**Fig. 30**). Although lesions can be removed via laser ablation, this technique makes the interpretation of clinical margins difficult and should be performed in special cases only. These may include larger lesions in geriatric patients in which the risk of surgical intervention outweighs the benefit or patients who are not candidates for complete excision due to other comorbidities. In these instances, the site should be kept under strict surveillance and should be periodically re-biopsied if necessary to assess for recurrence and progression of disease. After removal of the lesion, patients should

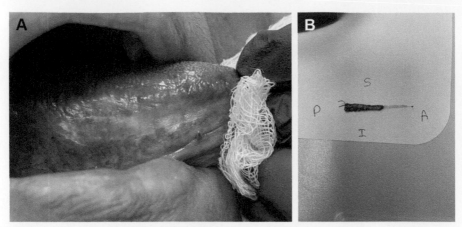

Fig. 30. (*A*) Leukoplakic lesion of the lateral tongue. (*B*) Excisional biopsy specimen of this lesion, with sutures indicating specimen orientation. The histology demonstrated mild to moderate epithelial dysplasia.

be placed on continued, long-term follow-up. More long-term studies are required to examine effectiveness of chemotherapies on oral dysplastic lesions.

CLINICS CARE POINTS

- Oral epithelial dysplasia is synonymous with premalignancy. It is diagnosed on the basis of histology.

- There are a variety of clinical oral lesions which may demonstrate dysplasia on microscopic examination. These include oral leukoplakias, erythroplakias, proliferative verrucous leukoplakia, actinic cheilitis, and oral submucosal fibrosis. Tissue biopsy of these lesions is required in order to establish a definitive diagnosis.

- Oral lichen planus is classified as a premalignant condition, although the exact association between lichen planus and oral cancer is unclear.

- Epithelial dysplasia in the oral cavity is graded using a three-tier system (mild, moderate, severe).

- A complete removal of any oral dysplastic lesion is recommended. This is usually performed via surgical excision.

DISCLOSURE

The authors have nothing to disclose.

REFERENCES

1. Epstein JB, Zhang L, Rosin M. Advances in the diagnosis of oral premalignant and malignant lesions. Journal (Canadian Dental Association). 2002;68(10):617-621. Accessed March 18, 2023. https://pubmed.ncbi.nlm.nih.gov/12410942/.
2. Silverman S. Oral lichen planus: A potentially premalignant lesion. J Oral Maxillofac Surg 2000;58(11):1286–8.
3. Villa A, Woo SB. Leukoplakia—a diagnostic and management algorithm. J Oral Maxillofac Surg 2017;75(4):723–34.

4. Woo SB. Oral epithelial dysplasia and premalignancy. Head and Neck Pathology 2019;13(3):423–39.
5. Saini R, Lee N, Liu K, et al. Prospects in the application of photodynamic therapy in oral cancer and premalignant lesions. Cancers 2016;8(9):83.
6. Zide Michael F. Actinic keratosis: from the skin to the lip. J Oral Maxillofac Surg 2008;66(6):1162–76.
7. Cavalcante A, Anbinder AL, Carvhalo YR. Actinic cheilitis: clinical and histological features. J Oral Maxillofac Surg 2008;66(3):498–503.
8. Pal US, Maurya H, Ganguly R, et al. Complications of platysma myocutaneous flap in patients with oral submucosal fibrosis: A systematic review. J Oral Biol Craniofacial Res 2022;12(4):421–6.
9. Yang SW, Tsai CN, Lee YS, et al. Treatment outcome of dysplastic oral leukoplakia with carbon dioxide laser—emphasis on the factors affecting recurrence. J Oral Maxillofac Surg 2011;69(6):e78–87.
10. Cortés-Ramírez DA, Gainza-Cirauqui ML, Echebarria-Goikouria MA, et al. Oral lichenoid disease as a premalignant condition: the controversies and the unknown. Med Oral, Patol Oral Cirugía Bucal 2009;14(3):E118–22.
11. Moosavi MS, Tavakol F. Literature review of cancer stem cells in oral lichen planus: a premalignant lesion. Stem Cell Invest 2021;8(25):25.
12. González-Moles MÁ, Warnakulasuriya S, González-Ruiz I, et al. Dysplasia in oral lichen planus: relevance, controversies and challenges. A position paper. Med Oral, Patol Oral Cirugía Bucal 2021;26(4):e541–8.
13. Shirani S, Kargahi N, Razavi SM, et al. Epithelial dysplasia in oral cavity. Iran J Med Sci 2014;39(5):406–17. https://www.ncbi.nlm.nih.gov/pmc/articles/PMC4164887/.
14. Bouquot Jerry E. Common oral lesions found during a mass screening examination. J Am Dent Assoc 1986;112(1):50.
15. Lumerman H, Freedman P, Kerpel S. Oral epithelial dysplasia and the development of invasive squamous cell carcinoma. Oral Surg Oral Med Oral Pathol Oral Radiol Endod 1995;79(3):321–9.
16. Waldron CA, Shafer WG. Leukoplakia Revisited.A clinicopathologic study 3256 oral leukoplakias. Cancer 1975;36(4):1386–92.
17. Meltzer C. Surgical management of oral and mucosal dysplasias: The case for laser excision. J Oral Maxillofac Surg 2007;65(2):293–5.
18. Kademani D, Dierks E. Surgical management of oral and mucosal dysplasias: the case for surgical excision. J Oral Maxillofac Surg 2007;65(2):287–92.
19. Fisher SE, Frame JW, Browne RM, et al. A comparative histological study of wound healing following CO_2 laser and conventional surgical excision of canine buccal mucosa. Arch Oral Biol 1983;28(4):287–91.
20. Gabbiani G, Ryan GB, Majne G. Presence of modified fibroblasts in granulation tissue and their possible role in wound contraction. Experientia 1971;27(5):549–50.
21. Montandon D, D'andiran G, Gabbiani G. The mechanism of wound contraction and epithelialization: clinical and experimental studies. Clin Plast Surg 1977;4(3):325–46.
22. Azevedo LH, Galletta VC, de Paula Eduardo C, et al. Treatment of oral verrucous carcinoma with carbon dioxide laser. J Oral Maxillofac Surg 2007;65(11):2361–6.

Controversies in Dental Traumatology

Orrett E. Ogle, DDS*

KEYWORDS

- Dental trauma • Tooth luxation • Tooth avulsion • Replantation of avulsed teeth
- Alveolar fracture

KEY POINTS

- Avulsed primary teeth should never be replanted.
- Traumatic dental injuries require long-term follow-up.
- Alveolar bone fractures, subluxation, luxation, avulsion, and certain root fractures will require splinting.
- Tooth avulsion has an unpredictable prognosis, and endosseous implant may be an alternative in older patients.

INTRODUCTION

Trauma to the dental structures may occur with or independent of other facial injures (**Table 1**). This article is limited only to injuries of the dentition. Dental injury occurs as the result of a sudden physical impact to the teeth, gums, or alveolar process. The injury may occur as a result of falls, contact sports, interpersonal violence, or bicycle and motor vehicle accidents. There are several types of injuries that fall under the category of dental trauma.

EPIDEMIOLOGY

Dental trauma is the most common cause of trauma in the head and neck region,[1] with most of them occurring in children and teenagers. Approximately 10% of children between the ages of 2 and 18 years have sustained significant tooth trauma, accounting for 18% of all somatic injuries in the age group 0 to 6 years.[2] In a report by Andersson, oral injuries account for as much as 17% of all bodily injuries in children aged 0 to 6 years.[3]

Although dental trauma is a common occurrence worldwide, its prevalence and incidence is not well documented and varies within countries. A lot of the reported figures are estimates. Most studies are based on small samples, with very few studies of

Oral and Maxillofacial Surgery, Woodhull Hospital, Brooklyn, NY 11206, USA
* 4974 Golf Valley Court, Douglasville, GA 30135.
E-mail address: oeogle@aol.com

Dent Clin N Am 68 (2024) 151–165
https://doi.org/10.1016/j.cden.2023.07.011
0011-8532/24/© 2023 Elsevier Inc. All rights reserved.

Table 1
Guidelines for fixation time and type of splint to be used

Type of Injury	Fixation Time	Type of Splint
Subluxation	2 wk	Flexible splint
Extrusive luxation	2 wk	Flexible splint
Lateral luxation	4 wk	Flexible splint
Intrusive luxation	4 wk	Flexible splint
Root fracture	4 wk	Flexible splint
Root fracture (cervical 1/3)	4 mo	Flexible splint
Avulsion	2 wk	Flexible splint
Avulsion. Dry time >60 min	4 wk	Flexible splint
Alveolar fracture	4 wk	No recommendation regarding rigidity of the splint.

Adapted from IADT recommendations for splinting time and type for various types of injuries. (International Dental Association of Dental Traumatology. Available at: URL: 'http://www.iadt-dentaltrauma.org/1-9%20%20iadt%20guidelines%20combined%20-%20lr%20-%2011-5-2013.pdf) Accessed Feb 2023.

nationally representative samples. The results from the few studies that have been reported gives the incidence rates of traumatic dental injuries ranging from 1% to 3% per year in the general population.[3] In the primary dentition, the greatest incidence of trauma to the teeth occurs at ages 2 to 3 years, which is most likely because motor coordination is not fully developed at this age. For the permanent dentition, age 9 to 12 years is considered the peak age for occurrence. Incidence rates are higher among men than among women, with some studies reporting twice as many injuries among men.[4]

In the United States, the prevalence of traumatic dental injuries (TDIs) is 2.9% among 6- to 8-year-old children and 11.1% among children who are 9 to 11 years old. TDIs are also reported to be more prevalent among men than women.[4,5] An older US survey reported a much higher prevalence of traumatic dental injuries varying between 16.7% and 18.4% in 6- to 20-year old and 27.1% and 28.1% in 21 to 50-year-old age groups.[6]

In both the primacy and permanent dentition the maxillary incisors are the teeth mostly involved. Mandibular incisors are rarely injured in the primary dentition.[7]

TYPES OF DENTAL TRAUMA

Dental trauma can be divided into 8 fractures and 6 luxation entities. Combination injuries in which both luxation and fracture occur are not uncommon. There are therefore 48 combinations that must be seen as 48 distinct healing situations. The complexity is further increased by the fact that trauma to the primary and the permanent teeth must be treated as separate entities; this results in 96 distinct trauma events.[8] A traumatized tooth may therefore suffer 1 of 96 distinct trauma conditions.

Classification

- Crown fracture:
  Enamel infraction
  Enamel fracture only
  Enamel-dentine fracture
  Enamel-dentine-pulp fracture

- Crown and root fracture
- Isolated root fracture
- Retained root fracture
- Alveolar fracture
- Concussion
- Subluxation (loosening)
- Medial/lateral luxation
- Intrusive luxation (dislocation into alveolar bone)
- Extrusive luxation (partial avulsion)
- Complete avulsion

The IADT (International Association of Dental Traumatology) has established treatment guidelines for TDIs but because of the multitude of possible trauma scenarios and the broad variety of possible treatment options much of the dental trauma treatment worldwide is far from being universal or ideal.[8]

PRIMARY DENTITION

In general, there is limited evidence to support many of the treatment options in the primary dentition. It has been suggested that observation is often the most appropriate option in the emergency situation unless there is risk of aspiration, ingestion, or interference with the occlusion.[9]

In significant numbers, parents of children sustaining TDIs take their children to hospital emergency departments (EDs). Isolated dental trauma results in thousands of ED visits every year. Several studies have shown that emergency room physicians and pediatricians have limited knowledge and understanding of the critical management of dental trauma.[10] The controversy is whether the hospital ED is a good choice for the management of TDIs. Unless a hospital ED has dental providers (generally dental interns or oral surgery residents), treatment of dental trauma will be less definitive than care rendered in a dedicated dental facility. The dental facility and the practitioners in the facility are also an important factor. Lots of dental trauma, however, occur after hours and, in reality, the hospital ED is the only option because no dentists are readily available. Overcrowded emergency rooms may delay treatment and adversely affect the dental outcome. The other controversy is which dental specialist is best suited to render emergency care to the child—oral surgeon, pedodontist, endodontist, or general dentist? Understandably, this would depend on the nature of the injury. Clearly, a fractured crown in a child would be treated by a pedodontist, whereas an alveolar fracture would be best treated by an oral and maxillofacial surgeon. In most of the cases the primary urgent care is frequently provided by the oral and maxillofacial surgeon because they are on hospital staff and on-call schedules. Subsequently, the patient may be referred to a pedodontist, general dentist, or an endodontist for secondary level care. Later care may further involve the orthodontist and prosthodontists. In rural areas there may only be a small number of pediatric dentists or endodontists, and general dentist may be the only option. Lack of specialist will affect outcome.

The traumatic incident will create a lot of anxiety in the child, which may present a management problem to the treating dentist. The maturity of the child and the ability to deal with the treating situation is an important factor that will influence treatment decisions and outcome. At a young age, the child may resist all attempts at any, and all interventions and extraction/s may become the easiest but not necessarily the best option. Injections are often the one thing most children are universally afraid of. Attempting to use local anesthesia to treat the dental injury may make the clinical situation worse. The controversy is should the child be sedated or physically restrained?

According to the American Academy of Pediatric Dentistry physical restraint is acceptable if the patient requires immediate diagnosis and/or treatment and cannot cooperate because of lack of maturity or mental or physical disability.[11] The TDI would meet the criteria for physical restraint. Another likely indication for the use of restraint would be when sedation/general anesthesia may be contraindicated because the child has a full stomach, is allergic to one of the drugs, or has a history of adverse reactions to general anesthesia. Use of restraints does not require special training. Sedation would decrease the anxiety, help to keep the child calm and comfortable during treatment, and prevent the psychological trauma from physical restraint. However, sedation poses a greater risk, requires special training, and will need equipment such as oxygen source, drugs, and emergency equipment among other items.

Dental Issues

The IADT has developed treatment guidelines based on a comprehensive review of the dental literature and recommendations from experienced researchers and clinicians from various specialties and the general dentistry community.[12,13] These guidelines for the management of every type of TDI have become the standard of care and they have universally become accepted as such.

Crown fractures and luxations are the most commonly occurring of all dental injuries.[14] Despite the fact that most of the injuries to the primary anterior dentition are luxations, the diagnosis and management of luxation injuries in the primary dentition is a topic of controversy.[15]

Tooth luxation occurs when trauma disrupts the ligaments and bone and the tooth is dislocated within the socket but maintains some attachment. Luxation injuries can be classified as intrusion, lateral luxations, and extrusion.

Intrusion

An intrusive luxation is the displacement of a tooth into the alveolar bone. It has been reported to be the injury with the highest prevalence of developmental disturbances of permanent teeth because of the traumatized damage to the enamel epithelium of the permanent successors.[16] One source cites that 65% of intruded primary teeth caused developmental disturbances in the permanent successor.[17] The management of intrusive luxations in the primary dentition is not universally agreed on, and there are various options that differ from the IADT guidelines in which management is dictated by the orientation of the primary tooth apex relative to the developing permanent tooth germ. The guidelines further indicate extraction of the intruded primary tooth if there is clinical and/or radiographic evidence of displacement into the developing permanent tooth germ. Some investigators have argued that regardless of the type of intrusion injury, the permanent successor will usually be within 3 mm of the apex of the primary tooth and that this space seen on radiographs may consist of connective tissue only, thus extraction should be the treatment of choice for all intrusive injuries to avoid damage to the developing permanent tooth.[18] Other investigators argue that the degree of intrusion should dictate management and extraction should not be universal. Reeruption or repositioning may be options. Based on observations from a 2018 retrospective study, it was suggested that if the primary tooth intrusion clearly has not compromised the permanent tooth germ then conservative measures (observation) may be acceptable, unless there are issues with patient cooperation and follow-up.[19] If one adopts a conservative option of leaving an intruded primary tooth to observe for reeruption, the clinician must follow-up for signs of periapical infection or pulp necrosis.[15]

Intrusive luxations usually crush the bone at its apex, which is often associated with comminuted bone fractures; this produces intramedullary inflammation, which could be deleterious to the underlying tooth bud. The goal of treating intrusive luxation is to prevent damage to the tooth germ of the permanent tooth.

LATERAL AND EXTRUSIVE LUXATIONS

There are some controversial/alternative management options for the management of lateral and extrusive luxation injuries in the primary dentition. Most of the controversial/ alternative treatment options are concerned with the technique to manage occlusal interference that results from lateral or extrusive luxation. The evidence in the literature is unclear about the definite approach for lateral luxation injuries in primary teeth in terms of prognostic outcomes according to different treatment methods.[15] The IADT recommend that cases involving extrusive luxation greater than 3 mm in the primary dentition should be extracted.[20]

Avulsed teeth should never be reimplanted in the primary dentition, even if they will have a few years before exfoliation. Splint placement and removal would be strenuous for a young child. Also, there is the possibility of causing further harm to the permanent tooth and may interfere with its eruption.

PERMANENT DENTITION

Typically, the first permanent teeth erupts in the lower anterior when a child is between 6 and 7 year old. They are followed by the 2 upper central incisors. Between the ages of 6 and 12 years there is the "mixed dentition," in which children will have both primary and permanent teeth. During the mixed dentition period and for a few years after, the permanent teeth can be divided into 2 groups according to the stage of root development. The stages of root development are defined as immature (open apex) versus mature (closed apex) permanent teeth. IADT guidelines that offer treatment of specific TDIs are different for the 2 stages.

Although luxation injuries are the most common TDIs in the primary dentition, crown fractures are the most common in the permanent teeth.[21] Most of the isolated crown fractures of a permanent tooth occur more commonly in children and young adults, with most of the injuries occurring before age 19 years.[21] Adult dental injuries, however, are often more complex than just a fractured crown because they frequently involve greater forces associated with facial trauma due to motor vehicle accidents, sports-related injuries, and interpersonal violence. The IADT guidelines that are aimed at providing information for the immediate and urgent care of TDIs are well accepted; but with complex dental injuries, with or without facial injuries, the health care provider must use clinical judgment in managing the conditions present in the given traumatic situation. The goal in both the initial and longer term care is to preserve teeth and adjacent structures.

The treatment of crown fractures in permanent teeth is based on the severity of the fracture using either the Ellis classification of teeth fractures or the classification by Andreasen that is closely related to the desired treatment. These treatment modalities are well accepted by the dental community but the recommended treatment procedures used for dental traumas are not evidence-based. One controversy involves the required follow-up time for traumatized teeth with or without crown fractures. Treatment can be followed by multiple and extremely varied posttreatment responses, ranging from no lasting effects and immediate pulp death to a long-term slow pulp necrosis or absorption. Pulp necrosis is a frequent complication, with some cases not manifesting until years after the injury occurred. The risk of pulp necrosis in permanent teeth increases, with the extent of the injury with lateral luxation and intrusion posing the greatest risk.[22] Andreasen and Pedersen reported that pulp necrosis in mild injuries such as concussion could appear within 3 months, whereas in cases of luxation injuries such as lateral luxation and intrusion it may typically not be manifested for 2 years.[22] However, most cases of pulp necrosis occur within the first year after trauma. Teeth with invasive cervical resorptions were diagnosed after more than 4 to 5 years following the injury.[23] Complications such as inflammatory root resorption and ankylotic root resorption usually are radiographically evident within the first 2 to 3 years after avulsion.[24] Crown fractures occurring with luxation injuries significantly increases the risk of pulp necrosis. Follow-up periods should therefore be based on the type of traumatic dental injury and the severity of the injury. Current recommendations for follow-up time range from 4 weeks to 5 years, depending on the trauma characteristics.[25] This recommended follow-up period is not consistently followed nor fully accepted. Some investigators suggest that the recommended follow-up time should be revised to reflect the need for more frequent and overall prolonged follow-up to catch late-developing complications. One late complication is the development of pulp canal obliteration and possible pulp necrosis following traumatic dental injuries; this is a frequent finding after luxation injuries of young permanent teeth caused by accelerated hard tissue formation within the pulp cavity leading to a reduction in the size of the coronal pulp chamber and eventual gradual narrowing of the entire root canal. Crown discoloration to a yellowish hue is a common finding in this condition and is caused by the excessive deposition of dentin, which affects the light-transmitting properties of the tooth, resulting in a gradual opacity of the crown.[26] The discoloration may take a while to develop, and even when not associated with pulp necrosis, it may require endodontic intervention to help restore esthetics by internal bleaching. Although the current available endodontic arsenal with microscopes offers successful techniques, the treatment may still pose a real challenge. However, there is no supportive evidence to indicate early prophylactic endodontic intervention, and time is the only determining factor. Because the response to pulp sensibility tests and tooth discoloration are not reliable for diagnosing pulp canal obliteration, the frequency of this condition is found to increase with longer follow-up periods.

The dental pulp will be involved in dental trauma. Two types of pulp injuries may occur: pulp exposure to oral bacteria via exposed dentinal tubules or direct exposure of the pulp wound surface in complicated crown fractures and[2] rupture or detachment of the neurovascular supply to the pulp, which may occur at the apical foramen in luxation injuries or at the level of the root fracture site in cases of root fractures. Pulp necrosis without infection would occur when the trauma causes a sudden, complete severance of the apical blood supply, leading to an avascular necrosis of the pulp.

Direct bacterial invasion can also lead to pulp necrosis even with a good blood supply. Bacterial infection of the pulp can occur very easily in the oral cavity because of its high and varied bacterial content. Oral bacteria and their toxins may invade the pulp through exposed dentinal tubules or can go directly into the exposed pulp tissue. In cases of enamel-dentin fractures the quality of the bacteria-tight seal is thought to be an important factor in the success of pulp survival. To decrease the chances of pulp necrosis due to bacterial invasion in an enamel-dentin crown fracture, the importance of sealing exposed dentinal tubules after the trauma is emphasized. However, there is no evidence that this treatment is necessary to protect the pulp.[27] Contradictions exists in the treatment of vital pulpal exposure in crown fractures involving the pulp. With pulp exposure, vital pulpal treatments with pulp capping are usually the treatment of choice for immature permanent teeth, but some believe it can be performed for both immature and mature permanent teeth. This concept of direct pulp capping in mature permanent teeth is considered controversial by many clinicians.

Fractures of a healthy tooth with vital noninfectious pulp can be treated similar to an accidental mechanical exposure in restorative dentistry. If aseptic conditions are maintained and the tissue thoroughly irrigated to decrease the bacterial inoculum, the underlying pulp usually does not become infected. Pulpal healing and repair have been reported at a high rate in both experimental and clinical follow-up studies in cases where the tissue was injured by accidental trauma. In a report by Al-Hiyasat and colleagues[28] the repair of mechanical exposure by pulp capping produced a 92% success rate. (Other studies have reported lower success rates however). The success rate for traumatized tooth was not available. The use of dental materials such as calcium hydroxide, bonded composite resins, and mineral trioxide aggregate have been proved to facilitate both the formation of reparative dentin and the maintenance of vital pulp. Some endodontists disagree with this treatment method, however, claiming that the predictability of pulp capping procedures is inferior to the proven long-term success rate that endodontic therapy (pulpectomy and root filling) have had. Another opposing reason is that if pulp capping fails, the patient may have a very painful condition. The subsequent endodontic treatment may furthermore become complex and more difficult to carry out than at the initial exposure, because the reparative phenomena, developing in the pulp during the healing phase, may result in a narrowing of the pulpal space[29]

Avulsed Teeth

Avulsed teeth should be replanted in the socket as soon as possible. There is a high success rate if the tooth is reimplanted within 20 minutes. Fully developed teeth with an extraoral dry time of 1 hour or less or teeth stored in a biological medium should be successful if IADT guidelines are followed. A major complication of reimplanted avulsed teeth is root resorption. Treatment modalities have been proposed to delay or prevent root resorption and thus increase the long-term success rate of avulsed teeth. It has been suggested that Emdogain can be used for treating avulsed teeth before replantation to prevent or delay root resorption by regenerating a healthy periodontium.[30] The mechanism of action of Emdogain is based on its ability to produce new periodontal ligament from the socket side cell population. To date, clinical evidence regarding the success rate of avulsed teeth treated with Emdogain before replantation is lacking. Similarly, some advocate placing an antibiotic on the root surface before replantation. There is no clear evidence that this is effective.

Tooth avulsion is a severe dental injury that has an unpredictable prognosis. Reports on replanted avulsed teeth gave survival rates between 50.0% and 83.3%.[31]

Tooth avulsion in young patients in whom continuous growth of the facial skeleton is expected, replantation, fixation, and suturing should always be the treatment of choice whenever feasible.

Because of unpredictable prognosis and low long-term survival rates for replanted avulsed tooth, dental implants, which offers more reliable treatment outcome, is suggested in the older individual. It should be noted that this is not the recommendation of the IADT or of the American Association of Endodontists (AAE). In older adults, avulsion of a mature tooth without damage to the supporting bone and soft tissues can be compared with a tooth extraction and an implant placed within 24 hours after the TDI. This has to meet the following conditions, however: intact socket walls and a facial bone wall thickness of at least 1 mm and bone apical and palatal to the socket to provide primary implant stability and healthy soft tissue.[32] Early implant placement can be done in most cases provided that the existing bone can ensure ideal early implant stability. Early implant stability is the most critical factor in achieving osseointegration. Six to eight weeks of healing will lead to complete soft tissue closure. However, simultaneous contour augmentation of the facial bone wall is most often necessary to provide long-term support of the facial soft tissues.[33]

Alveolar bone fractures, subluxation, luxation, avulsion, and certain root fractures will require splinting. In the case of luxation injuries, the IADT stresses that outcome depends more on the duration of the splinting than on the method of splinting although flexible splinting is always recommended. Despite the IADT recommendations, an evidence-based appraisal of luxated, avulsed, and root-fractured teeth found that splinting duration was generally not a significant variable when related to healing outcomes.[34]

Many types of splints have been used to stabilize luxated teeth with clinicians generally using what they are familiar with or in some cases what is available. Although the IADT has issued recommendations for the types of splints to be used for specific injuries, the recommended guidelines are not always followed. The types of splints in current use are as follows:

- Composite and wire splints
- Composite and nylon fishing line splints
- Orthodontic wire and bracket
- Titanium trauma splints
- Wire ligature splints
- Composite
- Acrylic splints
- Arch bar
- Fiber splints (polyethylene or Kevlar fiber mesh)

Composite and wire splints are the most commonly used and are flexible splints when the wire has a diameter of no greater than 0.3 to 0.4 mm.[35] An alternative to wire is nylon fishing line.

Orthodontic bracket splints allow teeth that have been intruded or not correctly repositioned to have the alignment and occlusal relationships modified at a later date. This is also a flexible splint.

The *titanium trauma splint* is a flexible splint made of 0.2-mm thick titanium. The disadvantage of this splint type is its high cost.

Wire ligature splints are mainly used by oral surgeons. They are generally rigid and impinge on the gingival tissues, with resulting inflammation. The technique can be modified, however, to place the arch wire away from the gingiva and closer to the incisal edge.

Composite resin applied to the surfaces of teeth is a rigid splint and accordingly is not recommended in the IADT guidelines. It is easy to apply but difficult to remove.

Acrylic splints are typically used in hospital EDs by oral surgeons because that is what is generally available. It is inexpensive and easy to place. Similar to composite resin, this splint does not meet the IADT guidelines. This splint is also difficult to remove.

Arch bar splints used by oral surgeons will create large compression zones in the periodontal ligament due to tightening of the steel wires at the cementoenamel junction and establish invasion pathways for bacteria along the subgingivally placed wires. This splint is rigid and does not meet the IADT guidelines.

Duration

Specific splinting durations have been established by the IADT guidelines for the different injury types. Although the duration of splinting for luxation injuries are universally accepted, there is controversy regarding replanted avulsed teeth however. A systematic analysis of splinting duration and periodontal outcomes for replanted avulsed teeth by Hinckfuss and Messer[36] found that periodontal outcomes were unaffected by splinting duration when comparing short-term splinting (14 days) and long-term splinting (longer than 14 days). According to this review it makes no difference in splinting for 2 weeks as opposed to a longer period of time. Further, Andreasen and colleagues[24] in a study of 400 avulsed and replanted teeth found that there were no significant differences between teeth splinted from 0 to 20 days and those splinted for 21 to 40 days. According to this study therefore, it is inconsequential whether avulsed teeth are splinted for either 2 or 4 weeks. To further the controversy, an animal study showed that replanted teeth splinted for 30 days developed a higher incidence of resorption than teeth splinted for only 1 week.[37]

As opposed to the IADT guidelines, the AAE[25] recommendations make no distinction between avulsed teeth with extraoral drying time greater than 60 minutes and those less than 60 minutes. In either of these avulsion categories the AAE recommend splinting for 2 weeks only. Kahler and colleagues[38] noted that both animal and human studies have demonstrated that strong gingival attachment to support a tooth in the socket is attained after just 1 week, suggesting that the shorter duration of 2 weeks is indicated for both types of avulsion.

ALVEOLAR FRACTURES

Alveolar fractures occur primarily in dentate arches but can also occur in edentulous arches. The anterior maxilla and mandible are the most common sites due to their location, but they occur most often in the thinner maxilla. The fracture may involve a single tooth, or it may involve a segment containing multiple teeth with labial or palatal/lingual displacement of the dentoalveolar segment, resulting in loss of the arch form and occlusal interference.

In contrast to the IADT-recommended fixation for luxation injuries, the fixation for alveolar fractures should be rigid in order to allow proper bone healing. The IADT guidelines do not offer a recommendation for the rigidity of splint for alveolar fractures. Fixation methods in current use are arch bars, figure-eight and loop wiring, orthodontic bands, and acrylic or metallic cap splints. The type of splint used depends on the type of alveolar fracture and the number of teeth presented in the segment.

The recent protocols recommend fixation for 4 to 6 weeks.[37]

Some investigators have questioned if it is really possible to obtain an accurate anatomic reduction and reestablishment of pretrauma occlusion with just digital repositioning of the fractured segment. One suggestion to improve the accuracy of the reduction is to get alginate impressions and do model surgery on a plaster model to recreate the normal anatomic relationship of the fractured segment and allow fabrication of an accurate splint.[39] Another point of contention is if large alveolar fractures should be internally fixed with miniplates. Open reduction of alveolar fractures is mostly indicated for alveolar fractures in the posterior maxilla. This would be definitely indicated if open reduction and internal fixation of an associated fracture is being performed. Another indication for open reduction with or without internal fixation would be an alveolar fracture, which cannot be reduced using a closed technique.

ANTIBIOTICS AND ANALGESICS
Antibiotics

There is no evidence in the literature to support the use of systemic antibiotics in the management of crown fractures, root fractures, or luxation injuries.

No positive effect on pulpal healing in cases of luxation injury or root fracture has been reported with the use of systemic of antibiotics. Despite the lack of supporting evidence, in cases of luxation injuries that are accompanied by significant soft tissue damage or require sutures, the use of systemic antibiotic is at the discretion of the clinician and is possibly not a bad idea. In pediatric dental trauma, the child's medical history may warrant antibiotic coverage. A recommendation is that intraoral wounds that seem to have been contaminated by extrinsic bacteria, debris (eg, dirt, soil, gravel), or foreign body have an increased risk of infection and should be managed by systemic antibiotics.[40] Amoxicillin is the drug of choice but the use of amoxicillin-clavulanic acid has been suggested for highly contaminated wounds because it covers a broader spectrum than amoxicillin. There is no evidence to support this however. The use of clavulanic acid in the pediatric population has been associated with gastrointestinal disturbances (diarrhea), and its use is questionable.

At present there is no clear consensus that systemic antibiotics should be administered at replantation of an avulsed permanent tooth. There is no high-quality evidence to support the use of systemic antibiotics at replantation of avulsed permanent teeth. A meta-analyses showed no significant associations between the administration of systemic antibiotics on the one hand and tooth survival, periodontal healing, and pulpal revascularization on the other hand.[41]

Although the value of systemic administration of antibiotics for avulsed teeth is questionable, some experts postulate that because the periodontal ligament of an avulsed tooth becomes contaminated by bacteria from the oral cavity, the storage medium, or the environment in which the avulsion occurred, the use of systemic antibiotics after replantation is justified to prevent infection-related reactions and decrease the occurrence of inflammatory root resorption.[42] Systemic antibiotics have been recommended as adjunctive therapy for avulsed permanent incisors with an open or closed apex. Again, amoxicillin or penicillin is the drug of choice due to effectiveness against oral flora and low incidence of adverse.[43]

Another belief is that subsequent to replantation, cleansing of the root surface for contamination followed by systemic antibiotics is essential for pulp and periodontal healing. These treatment concepts have been derived from experimental animal studies and have not been verified in human clinical studies. The effect of topical antibiotics placed on the root surface before replantation with respect to pulp revascularization remains controversial. Animal studies have shown great potential but human studies have failed to demonstrate improved pulp revascularization when teeth are soaked in topical antibiotics.[44]

Tetanus Vaccine

A tetanus booster may be required if environmental contamination of the oral injury has occurred, depending on how dirty the wound is and how long it has been since the last vaccine. If in an avulsive injury, for example, the tooth fell on a dirty surface such as soil a tetanus vaccine would be indicated. According to the UK Public Health "Green Book" on vaccination, tetanus immunoglobulin is indicated if the socket or tooth has been contaminated through contact with soil or foreign bodies or the injury is associated with fracture of the jaw bone. Vaccination against future tetanus infection is advised if the immunization status is unknown, incomplete, or the patient is immunocompromised.[45]

It is very unlikely that children younger than 12 years will require tetanus vaccine. Based on a review of the literature regarding tetanus, the investigators concluded that tetanus toxoid is recommended in adults only if it has been more than 10 years since their last immunization.[46] A more recent paper published in the journal *Clinical Infectious Diseases*[47] suggested that tetanus booster vaccines are not necessary for adults who have completed their childhood vaccination series. (This advice aligns with the current World Health Organization recommendations). In the study they found that antibody responses to tetanus declined with an estimated half-life of 14 years.

Using mathematical models combining antibody magnitude and duration the researchers predict that 95% of the population will remain protected against tetanus and diphtheria for 30 years or more without requiring further booster vaccination.

PAIN MANAGEMENT

There is no doubt that trauma to the dentition and supporting tissues will be associated with pain and discomfort. However, there is no fixed protocol how to manage the pain. The degree of pain depends on the nature and severity of the injury but it can vary and does not always correlate with the extent of the injuries. In general, the acute pain will resolve after the initial dental treatment and will continue to decrease with healing of the involved tissues.

The pain management will basically be pharmaceutical. It will require assessment of the level of pain and selection of the appropriate analgesic to relieve the assessment score. Age-specific pharmacologic pain management must also be considered. Adequate pain management will promote early healing and reduce patient's stress responses. The level of pain will be highly correlated with the level of inflammation, which activates the pain producing mediators. For this reason, nonsteroidal antiinflammatory drugs (NSAIDs) are the most rational first-line agents.[48] A multimodal pain management technique using 2 or more drugs with different mechanisms of action will give the best result. Combinations of analgesic drugs can produce better pain relief in cases in which a single drug has not been very effective. The purpose of combining 2 or more drugs with different mechanisms of action is to achieve a synergistic interaction. Combining acetaminophen with NSAIDs that have different mechanisms or location of action can produce adequate control of pain from traumatic dental injuries. Acetaminophen works in the central nervous system, whereas the site of action for the NSAID is peripheral, where the inflammation is present. Effective pain relief is achieved by attacking the pain at 2 different sites—centrally and peripherally.[48] Although steroids are not analgesics, on rare occasions they may be useful in controlling pain.

In the early stage following the traumatic incidence cold therapy can be used to help control soft tissue pain. The cold will reduce blood flow to the traumatized areas, which will tend to reduce the inflammation that causes pain. It may also temporarily reduce nerve activity, which can further relieve pain. Salt water rinses can help reduce inflammation by reverse osmosis. Edema fluid comes out of the cells because the salt concentration in the saline solution is of a higher concentration than that in the cells.[48] Pain control should be evaluated either by phone or in the dental office.

Pain management for children with traumatic dental injuries have no clear evidence-based guidelines and in a lot of cases children are not given any analgesic of any kind. One study demonstrated that ibuprofen was significantly more effective than acetaminophen in treating traumatic injuries in children.[49] That is because ibuprofen has the added benefit of fighting inflammation, which acetaminophen does not. Ibuprofen is the most widely studied and used NSAID in children for the management of acute pain and is the only NSAID approved for use in children as young as 6 months. Ibuprofen, however, can sometimes irritate the stomach. Naproxen is safe to use in children aged 12 years and older, and aspirin is contraindicated in children younger than 16 years. As with adult patients it is generally safe to take acetaminophen and ibuprofen together, as long as proper dosing is followed.

SUMMARY

The management of traumatic dental injuries is more a shade of gray than it is black and white; this is because nearly all treatment procedures used for dental traumas are not evidence-based. Because it is unethical to perform randomized studies on trauma victims, analysis of the long-term outcome of healing and its relationship to treatment cannot be determined. Some of the treatment concepts have been derived from experimental studies in animals but their relevance has not been verified in large human clinical studies. Other sources of evidence have been systematic reviews of relevant clinical literature. The IADT has established treatment guidelines for TDIs that are based on a comprehensive review of the dental literature and recommendations from experienced researchers and clinicians from various specialties. Even though most of the guidelines are evidence based, it is not beyond belief that personal opinions, anecdotal evidence, and unproven treatments may have been incorporated into the guidelines. Wide scale studies have not found definitive evidence to contraindicate their current guidelines; however, some controversies have been found that do contradict some of the IADT guidelines.

This chapter has highlighted some of the gray areas related to the treatment and outcome of traumatic dental injuries. Significant controversies in the management of luxation and avulsive injuries have been brought out. Adjunctive treatment such as antibiotic usage, tetanus vaccination, and pain management was addressed. What is evident is that further research and consensus statements are needed to narrow the gray areas.

CLINICS CARE POINTS

- Primary tooth should be extracted if there is clinical and/or radiographic evidence of displacement into the developing permanent tooth germ.

- Extrusive luxation greater than 3 mm in the primary dentition should be extracted. Avulsed teeth should never be reimplanted in the primary dentition.

- Tooth avulsion in young patients in whom continuous growth of the facial skeleton is expected, replantation, fixation, and suturing should always be the treatment of choice whenever feasible.

- Avulsed permanet teeth should be reimplanted within 60 minutes.

DISCLOSURE

The author has nothing to disclose.

REFERENCES

1. Bohm L.A. and Roby B.B., Pediatric facial fractures. In: Lesperance M.M., *Cummings pediatric otolaryngology*, 2nd edition, 2021, Elsevier, 105–117, Chapter 7.
2. Kliegman RM. Dental trauma. In: Nelson textbook of pediatrics. 21st edition. Elsevier Inc; 2020. p. 1922–8. PART XVII, Chapter 340.
3. Andersson L. Epidemiology of traumatic dental injuries. Pediatr Dent 2013;35(2): 102–5.
4. Baskaradoss JK, Bhagavatula P. Measurement and distribution of malocclusion, trauma, and congenital anomalies. In: Mascarenhas AK, Okunseri C, editors. Dye BABurt and eklund's dentistry, dental practice, and the community. 7th edition. St Louis, MO: W.B. Saunders; 2021. p. 208–17.
5. Dye BA, Tan S, Smith VM.et al Trends in Oral Health Status: United States, 1988–1994 and 1999–2004. Vital and health statistics. Series 11, TABLES 18, 33, 34. Available at https://stacks.cdc.gov/view/cdc/6834 Accessed Jan. 2023.

6. Kaste LM, Gift HC, Bhat M, et al. Prevalence of incisor trauma in persons 6 to 50 years of age: United States, 1988-1991. J Dent Res 1996;75(2_suppl):696–705.

7. Day PF, Flores MT, O'Connell AC, et al. International Association of Dental Traumatology guidelines for the management of traumatic dental injuries: 3. Injuries in the primary dentition. Dent Traumatol 2020;36(4):343–59.

8. The Dental Trauma Guide - Evidence based dental trauma treatment. Available at : https://dentaltraumaguide.org/evidence-based-dental-trauma-treatment/. Accessed Feb 2023.

9. Cunha RF, Pugliesi DM, Percinoto C. Treatment of traumatized primary teeth: a conservative approach. Dent Traumatol 2007;23(6):360–3.

10. Alrashdi M, Limaki ME, Alrashidi A. Oral Health Knowledge Gaps and Their Impact on the Role of Pediatricians: A Multicentric Study. Int J Environ Res Public Health 2021;18(19):10237.

11. Use of Protective Stabilization for Pediatric Dental Patients. Available at https://www.aapd.org/media/Policies_Guidelines/BP_Protective.pdf. Accessed Feb; 2023.

12. Guidelines for the management of traumatic dental injuries. III. Primary teeth. Available at https://onlinelibrary.wiley.com/doi/full/10.1111/j.1600-9657.2007.00627.x. Accessed February 2023.

13. International Association of Dental Traumatology guidelines for the management of traumatic dental injuries: Available at https://onlinelibrary.wiley.com/doi/full/10.1034/j.1600-9657.2001.170401.x Accessed Feb 2023.

14. Kramer PF, Onetto J, Flores MT, et al. Traumatic Dental Injuries in the primary dentition: a 15-year bibliometric analysis of Dental Traumatology. Dent Traumatol 2016;32(5):341–6.

15. Lai YYL. Traumatic dental injuries in children: the controversies of managing primary tooth luxation injuries. J Pak Dent Assoc 2019;28(2):85–91.

16. von Arx T. Developmental disturbances of permanent teeth following trauma to the primary dentition. Aust Dent J 1993;38(1):1–10.

17. Andreasen JO, Andreasen FM. Intrusive Luxation. In: Andreasen JO, Andreasen FM, Andersson L, editors. Textbook and color atlas of traumatic injuries of the teeth. 4th edition. Oxford, UK: Wiley-Blackwell; 2018.

18. Smith R, Rapp R. A cephalometric study of the developmental relationship between primary and permanent maxillary central incisor teeth. ASDC (Am Soc Dent Child) J Dent Child 1980;47(1):36–41.

19. Soares TR, Silva LP, Luiz RR, et al. Profile of intrusive luxation and healing complications in deciduous and permanent teeth - a retrospective study. Act OdontolScand 2018;76(8):567–71.

20. Malmgren B, Andreasen JO, Flores MT, et al. International Association of Dental Traumatology guidelines for the management of traumatic dental injuries: 3. Injuries in the primary dentition. Dent Traumatol 2012;28(3):174–82.

21. DENTAL TRAUMA GUIDELINES. International Association of Dental Traumatology 2012 REVISION. Available at: https://www.iadt-dentaltrauma.org/1-%20%20iadt%20guidelines%20combined%20-%20lr%20-%2011-5-2013.pdf. Accessed February 2023.

22. Andreasen FM, Pedersen BV. Prognosis of luxated permanent teeth — the development of pulp necrosis. Dent Traumatol 1985;1(6):207–20.

23. Lin S, Pilosof N, Munir Karawani M, et al. Occurrence and timing of complications following traumatic dental injuries: A retrospective study in a dental trauma department. J Clin Exp Dent 2016;8(4):429–36.

24. Andreasen JO, Borum MK, Jacobsen HL, et al. Replantation of 400 avulsed permanent incisors. 4. Factors related to periodontal ligament healing. Endod Dent Traumatol 1995;11(2):76–89.

25. The recommended guidelines of the American Association of Endodontists for the treatment of traumatic dental injuries. AAE Publication; 2014. Available at: https://www.aae.org/specialty/clinical-resources/treatment-planning/traumatic-dental-injuries/. Accessed February 2023.

26. Bastos JV, de Souza Côrtes ML. Pulp canal obliteration after traumatic injuries in permanent teeth – scientific fact or fiction? Braz Oral Res 2018;32(suppl 1):159–68.

27. Andreasen JO, Lauridsen E, Andreasen FM. Contradictions in the treatment of traumatic dental injuries and ways to proceed in dental trauma research. Dent Traumatol 2010;26(1):16–22.

28. Al-Hiyasat AS, Barrieshi-Nusair KM, Al-Omari MA. The radiographic outcomes of direct pulp-capping procedures performed by dental students: a retrospective study. J Am Dent Assoc 2006;137(12):1699–705.

29. Bergenholtz G, Spångberg L. Controversies in Endodontics. Crit Rev Oral Biol Med 2004;15(2):99–114.

30. Caglar E, Tanboga I, Süsal S. Treatment of avulsed teeth with Emdogain–a case report. Dent Traumatol 2005;21(1):51–3.

31. Müller DD, Bissinger R, Reymus M, et al. Survival and complication analyses of avulsed and replanted permanent teeth. Sci Rep 2020;10:2841. Available at. https://www.nature.com/articles/s41598-020-59843-1. Accessed March, 2023.

32. Morton D, Chen S, Martin W, et al. Consensus statements and recommended clinical procedures regarding optimizing esthetic outcomes in implant dentistry. Int J Oral Maxillofac Implants 2014;29(Suppl):216–20.

33. Jensen SS. Timing of implant placement after traumatic dental injury. Dent Traumatol 2019;35(6):376–9.

34. Kahler B, Heithersay GS. An evidence-based appraisal of splinting luxated, avulsed and root fractured teeth. Dent Traumatol 2008;24(1):2–10.

35. Oikarinen K. Comparison of the flexibility of various splinting methods for tooth fixation. Int J Oral Maxillofac Surg 1988;17(4):249–52.

36. Hinckfuss SE, Messer LB. Splinting duration and periodontal outcomes for replanted avulsed teeth: a systematic review. Dent Traumatol 2009;25(2):150–7.

37. Berman LH, Blanco L, Cohen S. Alveolar fractures. In: Berman LH, Blanco L, Cohen S, editors. A clinical guide to dental traumatology. St. Louis, MO: CV Mosby; 2007. p. 147.

38. Kahler B, Hu JY, Marriot-Smith CS, et al. Splinting of teeth following trauma: a review and a new splinting recommendation. Aust Dent J 2016;61(S1):59–73.

39. Gutmacher Z, Peled E, Norman D, et al. Alveolar bone fracture: pathognomonic sign for clinical diagnosis. Open Dent J 2017;11:8–14.

40. Goel D, Goel GK, Chaudhary S, et al. Antibiotic prescriptions in pediatric dentistry: A review. J Family Med Prim Care 2020;9(2):473–80.

41. Bourgeois J, Carvalho JC, De Bruyne M, et al. Antibiotics at replantation of avulsed permanent teeth? A systematic review. J Evid Based Dent Pract 2022; 22(2):101706.

42. Hammarstrom L, Blomlof L, Feiglin B, et al. Replantation of teeth and antibiotic treatment. Endod Dent Traumatol 1986;2(2):51–7.

43. Fouad AF, Abbott PV, Tsilingaridis G, et al. International Association of Dental Traumatology guidelines for the management of traumatic dental injuries: 2. Avulsion of permanent teeth. Dent Traumatol 2020;36(4):331–42.

44. Tsilingaridis G, Malmgren B, Skutberg C, et al. The effect of topical treatment with doxycycline compared to saline on 66 avulsed permanent teeth–a retrospective case-control study. Dent Traumatol 2015;31(3):171–6.
45. Tetanus: the green book, chapter 30. Tetanus immunisation information for public health professionals, including updates. Available at : https://www.gov.uk/government/publications/tetanus-the-green-book-chapter-30. Accessed Mar. 2023.
46. Rhee P, Nunley MK, Demetriades D, et al. Tetanus and Trauma: A Review and Recommendations. J Trauma 2005;58(5):1082–8.
47. Hammarlund E, Thomas A, Poore EA, et al. Durability of Vaccine-Induced Immunity Against Tetanus and Diphtheria Toxins: A Cross-sectional Analysis. Clin Infect Dis 2016;62(9):1111–8.
48. Ogle OE. New Approaches to Pain Management. Dent Clin North Am 2020;64(2): 315–24.
49. Clark E, Plint AC, Correll R, et al. A randomized, controlled trial of acetaminophen, ibuprofen, and codeine for acute pain relief in children with musculoskeletal trauma. Pediatrics 2007;119(3):460–7.

Diagnosis and Treatment of Periimplant Mucositis and Periimplantitis
An Overview and Related Controversial Issues

Michael H. Chan, DDS[a,b,*], Joseph Kang, DDS[b]

KEYWORDS

- Perimucositis • Periimplantitis • Nonsurgical treatment • Surgical treatment
- Resective surgery • Implantoplasty • Regenerative surgery

KEY POINTS

- Periimplant disease progresses more rapidly than periodontitis, and therefore, practitioners need to recognize and treat periimplant disease early and aggressively.
- Good patient selection and avoidance of certain risk factors can minimize the incidence of periimplantitis.
- Nonsurgical therapy always precedes surgical therapy.
- There is no clear consensus on the choice of instrumentation and/or adjuncts materials for implant surface debridement is superior in the long term.
- Standardization of research parameters in periimplant disease and outcome assessment in future studies may provide a foundation for consensus on the treatment modalities.

INTRODUCTION

Branemark certainly revolutionized how teeth replacement has gone on a global scale. Whether a person is missing one tooth or an entire arch, dental implants can provide support to prosthesis with long-term success and patient satisfaction. Despite its worldwide acclaim, diseased implants can be problematic to both patients and clinicians.

Periimplant diseases are inflammatory conditions that affect the tissues surrounding dental implants, in particular hard and soft components. Periimplant mucositis is characterized by inflammation of the soft tissues, without loss of supporting bone,[1]

[a] Oral & Maxillofacial Surgery, Department of Veterans Affairs, New York Harbor Healthcare System (Brooklyn Campus), 800 Poly Place (Bk-160), Brooklyn, NY 11209, USA; [b] Oral & Maxillofacial Surgery, Department of Oral and Maxillofacial Surgery, The Brooklyn Hospital Center, 121 DeKalb Avenue (Box-187), Brooklyn, NY 11201, USA
* Corresponding author. 800 Poly Place (BK- 160), Brooklyn, NY 11209.
E-mail address: chanoms@yahoo.com

Dent Clin N Am 68 (2024) 167–202
https://doi.org/10.1016/j.cden.2023.08.001
0011-8532/24/© 2023 Elsevier Inc. All rights reserved.

whereas periimplantitis includes the aforementioned clinical signs with associated bone loss.[2,3] The prevalence of perimucositis and periimplant has been presented to be 19% to 65% and 1% to 47%, respectively.[4] The latest meta-analysis reported the mean prevalence for periimplantitis at patient level (12.53%) and at implant level (19.53%).[5] The growing number of periimplantitis cases have researchers fervently trying to find adequate solutions to this enigmatic global problem.

PATHWAY TO PERIIMPLANTITIS

The differences between dental implant and natural teeth are on 2 anatomic levels. Implants have less vascular supply, and their connective tissue fibers configuration make them more vulnerable. These collagenous fibers are situated only in the soft tissue collar and are arranged in parallel fashion (**Fig. 1**).[6,7] The pathogen invasion is much more rapid in implants than natural teeth because of the lack of cementum and Sharpey fibers found in implants. These fibers provide a strong connective tissue attachment between periosteum and bone and, in turn, prevent direct progression of infection.[6] Additionally, the vulnerability of the "periimplant mucosal seal" is one of the main reasons for the insidious onset and the aggressive accelerated bone loss pattern observed in periimplantitis.[8]

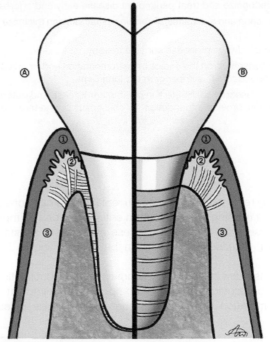

Fig. 1. Periodontal and periimplant fibers. 1 = sulcus epithelium, 2 = junctional epithelium, and 3 = connective tissue. A = Cross-section of natural tooth: all 3 layers form a coronal seal around the tooth with collagenous fibers (junctional epithelium layer). These fibers extend into the periodontal ligament (PDL) inserting onto the root surface in perpendicular arrangement, creating a stronger seal. B = Cross-section of dental implant: also, all 3 layers form a periimplant mucosal seal; however, these fibers are only arranged in parallel configuration in the junctional epithelium. Unlike natural teeth, there are no fibers adhering to the implant surface, making it more suspectable to breakdown. (Image courtesy of Maya Nunez.)

Farhan and colleagues have extracted gram-negative anaerobic bacteria, spirochetes and *Tannerella forsythia*, to be associated with periimplantitis.[9] Although Sahamann and colleagues concluded that identification of specific microorganism was not consistently isolated nor reproducible within all studies compared, however, gram-positive aerobes, gram-negative anerobes, and fusiform were the commonest microbiome that make up for periimplantitis.[10]

Although identifying periopathogens is important, the discovery of microbiome dysbiosis has prompted scientists to investigate how some of these "native" microorganisms change into "bad" pathogens during the diseased state. Moreover, studies investigate how these tenacious pathogens build an ecosystem with great stability around the periodontium, which is capable of causing severe local destruction.[11]

RISK FACTORS

There is an established consensus for these risk factors to contribute to the development of periimplantitis. Such risks include patients with a history of severe periodontitis, poor plaque control, and noncompliance after surgery. Interestingly, there is inconclusive evidence in regard to smoking and diabetes as risk factors for periimplantitis. In addition, studies show that there is limited evidence linking periimplantitis to residual cement and implant location interfering with cleaning. Lastly, the consensus group states there is inconclusive evidence on the necessity of keratinized mucosa and occlusal overload as a risk factor.[3]

Unlike the consensus's group findings, some studies support these risk factors for perIimplantitis development and are described later.

Diabetes

In general, diabetics with hyperglycemia are known to have impaired wound healing secondary to deranged cellular recruitment and bone metabolism, leading to increased bone resorption surrounding dental implants. The effects of hyperglycemia can be a risk factor for developing these complications: (1) delayed osseointegration, (2) long-term development of periimplantitis, and (3) poor long-term survival. However, diabetics with euglycemia have good successful outcome when compared with healthy individuals.[12]

Smoking

A systemic review and meta-analysis by Chranovic and colleagues in 2015 highlighted 3 main detrimental effects that smokers have on dental implants when compared with nonsmokers: (1) increased failure rate, (2) increased postop infection, and (3) increased bone loss around implant. The cause and effect of cigarette smoke on the periimplant environment has been theorized to negatively affect vascular supply and maintenance of bone turnover for deposition. These failure rates were reported for smokers to be 6.35% and for nonsmokers at 3.18%.[13]

Genetic Factors

The osteoprogetergin (OPG)/RANKL/RANK system helps regulate bone metabolism. In particular, an OPG/RANKL binding will favor prevention of bone resorption, whereas, an RANKL/RANK connection will favor activation and differentiation of preosteoclast into osteoclast for bone resorption. A recent meta-analysis has discovered a mutated OPG gene (rs2073618) could significantly increase the development of periimplantitis. As such, these patients with periimplantitis were found to have low levels of OPG in their gingival sulcus. The investigators concluded that this genetic variant may be a useful biomarker for identifying individuals at risk of periimplantitis.[14]

History of Periodontal Disease

A systemic review and meta-analysis demonstrated there is 2 times the risk for patients with a history of adult periodontitis to develop periimplantitis than those without.[15] The risk is decreased if periodontal disease is eradicated before implant therapy.[16]

Occlusal Overload

Similar to clenching and bruxism, excessive or poorly balanced occlusion can cause occlusal overload, leading to increased marginal bone loss around implant. One systemic reviewed concluded that there is such an association based on 4 out of 7 studies. However, these results were not consistently reproducible in either animal or human model. The investigators suggested future studies are needed to investigate the following question and to standardize studies and eliminate bias: (1) threshold for overload in a quantifiable number, (2) using digital technology to access these findings to better understand load distribution.[17]

Residual Cement on Restoration

Of the 74 implants investigated in this retrospective study, every patient (n = 39) with a history of periodontal disease with residual cement on restoration developed periimplantitis as opposed only 3 patients (n = 34) without a history of periimplantitis. These data suggested those who have a history of periodontal disease with residual cement would have a strong correlation for developing periimplantitis. The investigator further recommends screw-retain restoration for this population to reduce the incident.[18]

Clenching/Bruxism

Clenching and bruxism have been listed as a contraindication for implant placement due to the heavy forces generated on these prostheses and related supporting structures causing prosthetic and biological complications. Prosthetic complications include fracture/loosening of related prosthetic components. Crestal bone loss is associated with excessive stress at the implant coronal portion contributing to periimplantitis. Most of these failures were seen with fixed restorations.[19]

A systemic review and meta-analysis has found a statistical significance related to these complications with bruxers. The cause and effect of this relationship is still controversial. Some of the studies did not demonstrate these results with bruxers even with short implants. Poorly occlusal design resulted in occlusal overload, and not the act of bruxium may be the contributory factor.[19]

As a remedy, the investigator proposed the following: (1) an implant with a larger surface area for osseointegration in correct prosthetically driven position (eg, longer and wider), (2) occlusal scheme (centric only and avoid lateral excursion), (3) metal occlusal surface and reduction of size of prosthetic restoration, (4) reduction of cantilever length, (5) nightguard, and (6) enrollment in implant maintenance therapy program.[19]

Malpositioned Implant

Poorly positioned implant is one of the contributing factors for unsuccessful implant therapy. When these are placed out of the alveolar housing (eg,; buccal), esthetic compromise and gingival recession could lead to periimplantitis. One study reported that as the implant is placed buccally by 1 mm, there will be 0.22 mm of crestal bone loss on the same surface observed at 4 months.[20]

Keratinized Tissue

Keratinized gingival tissue around implants may have a beneficial and protective role in periimplant health and maintenance; 2 mm is the common cut off for adequate KT, although the optimal width of KT may depend on other factors (eg, mucosal thickness, supracrestal tissue height, periimplant bone thickness, pocket depth, prosthetic design).[21]

Through systematic review and meta-analysis, Ramanuskaite and colleagues investigated the influence of KT on overall periimplant health in both cross-sectional and longitudinal studies.[22] Data extrapolated from their studies showed that dental implants with reduced KT width (eg, < 2 mm or ≤ 0 mm) had a higher incidence of periimplantitis, exhibited higher bleeding on probing (BOP), plaque scores, marginal bone loss, and mucosal recession compared with those with adequate KT (eg, ≥ 2 mm or > 0 mm). However, there was no difference in pocket depth between the 2 groups.[22] Furthermore, the lack of KT (eg, ≤ 2 mm) led to patient discomfort when brushing, which detrimentally affects oral hygiene habits and can lead to signs and symptoms of periimplant inflammation.[23]

However, the necessity of KT for periimplant health is still controversial. Heitz-Mayfield suggested KT is not significant to implant health if the patient is able to maintain proper hygiene.[1] Furthermore, through retrospective analysis, Ravidà and colleagues investigated the impact of periimplant KT width (>2 mm vs < 2 mm) on surgical clinical outcomes when treating periimplantitis for both resective and regeneration surgery.[24] They found regenerative surgery yielded a higher success rate for the (<2 mm KT group) at 23.5% versus (>2 mm KT group) with 7.7%. However, the overall surgical success rates were very similar between the 2 groups: 7.7% for (<2 mm KT group) and 10.3% for (>2 mm KT group), both with low percentages. In addition, (< 2 mm KT group) had most of these implants with greater than 50% of bone explanted due to failure (n = 7/11). Their investigation concluded that it is the amount of preoperative bone loss that will provide a better predictor of surgical success rather than the amount of KT present. The other conclusion drawn from this study is that having greater than 2 mm of KT may influence the degree of how severe the disease progression will be (eg, BOP, SOP, PD) and how these clinical parameters can influence bone loss or marginal bone level.[24]

Titanium Particles

A recent systematic and meta-analysis showed periimplantitis is associated with residual titanium particles released from implant surfaces that can cause an intense inflammatory reaction.[25] Lymphocytes, macrophages, and controversially neutrophils were identified, with plasma cells to be predominantly found at the base of the implant pocket at the connective tissue layer. This layer that surrounds the implant is sometimes referred as the "periimplant seal," which represents the last line of defense. The investigators found approximately 90% of the tissue biopsied to have titanium particles under histologic examination. These particles are thought to have originated either from surgery or through an induced corrosion process (electrochemical). Because bacteria have an affinity for corrosives surfaces, they further congregate and increase in numbers. As a result, they will cause more titanium particles to leach out through their enzymatic process. Furthermore, this continuous inflammatory process, in particular with macrophages going unchecked, will release inflammatory mediators; this in turn will cause further bone destruction. Under this environment, there is an increased amount of vascularization seen in the connective tissue layer, causing hyperemia. Lastly, there are reports of similar cell types found among periimplantitis, chronic periodontitis, and aggressive periodontitis.[25]

CLASSIFICATION

A consensus was reached between the American Academy of Periodontics and the European Federation of Periodontology on defining periimplant diseases and reclassified in 2017. They were categorized into (1) periimplant health, (2) periimplant mucositis, and (3) periimplantitis (**Table 1**).[26]

CLINICAL AND RADIOGRAPHIC PRESENTATION

Although periimplant health denotes the absence of disease surrounding the restored fixture, periimplant mucositis and periimplantitis are 2 common complications associated with dental implants. They are characterized by inflammation (eg, hyperemia, swelling, or pain) and infection around the implant.

Periimplant mucositis features[2]:

1. Bleeding on *mild* probing (BOP) or suppuration on probing (SOP) with signs of gingival inflammation
2. Pocket depth (PD) increased from baseline
3. Without signs of bone loss beyond initial osseointegration allowance (up to 2 mm)

Periimplantitis features[2]:

1. BOP (± SOP) on *easy* probing with signs of inflammation
2. Progressive bone loss around the implant greater than initial osteointegration physiologic allowance (>2 mm) from baseline
3. Increased PD after placement of restorations
4. If there is no comparative imaging, BOP with probing depth greater than 6 mm, and radiographic evidence of bone loss greater than 3 mm

Bone loss from remodeling after a successful osseointegrated implant has been documented between 0.5 mm and 2 mm in the first year,[2] whereas up to 4 mm of perimucosal tissue is considered healthy.[28] Unlike traditional periodontal probing on natural teeth, probing depths can exist variably in healthy perimucosal implant complex.[3] For example, probing measurements of 1 mm or 5 mm without pathologic BOP/SOP can represent normalcy; this may be influenced by the depth of implant platform and type of restoration as well as periodontal tissue type. Be aware that aggressive probing could induce bleeding, which can lead to a false-positive finding. Diseased periodontal tissue will have increased severity of bleeding with *gentle* probing (± SOP).[2] This finding accompanied with increase in pocket depth and absence of radiographic bone loss is suggestive of periimplant mucositis. Further insult from the bacterial biofilm accompanied with radiographic bone loss will lead to a diagnosis of periimplantitis.[27]

BONE DEFECT MORPHOLOGY

By definition, periimplantitis is associated with bone loss. Typical bone loss can be categorized into vertical, horizontal, or combination. Furthermore, the number of existing walls will dictate the radiographic and morphologic defect in periimplantitis. Morphology of the bone defect may affect the type of treatment rendered that is most appropriate for that pattern of bone loss.

Although not adopted universally, the classification of bone defect morphology surrounding periimplantitis was initiated by Schwarz and colleagues[29] and was later modified by Monje and colleagues[30]

Table 1
Periimplant health and complications

	Clinical Signs of Inflammation BOP	PD	SOP	Radiographic Bone Loss
Periimplant health	–	Varies, but generally ≤ 5 mm	–	< 2 mm (after initial bone remodeling)
Periimplant mucositis	+	Increased compared with baseline	+ or –	< 2 mm (after initial bone remodeling)
Periimplantitis (with baseline measurements)	+	Increased compared to baseline	+ or –	Increased compared with baseline
Periimplantitis (without baseline measurements)	+	≥ 6 mm	+ or –	≥ 3 mm

Abbreviations: BOP, bleeding on probing; PD, pocket depth; SOP, suppuration on probing.

Adapted from Characteristics of peri-implant health, peri-implant mucositis, and peri-implant health. Information from 2017 World Workshop: Peri-implant health, peri-implant mucositis, and peri-implantitis: Care definitions and diagnostic considerations.[2,26,27]

1. Class I = intraosseous defect
   a. Class Ia = buccal dehiscence
   b. Class Ib = 2- to 3-wall defect
   c. Class Ic = circumferential defect
2. Class II = supracrestal/horizontal defect
3. Class III = combined defect (with additional horizontal bone component)
   a. Class IIIa = buccal dehiscence + horizontal bone loss
   b. Class IIIb = 2- to 3-wall defect + horizontal bone loss
   c. Class IIIc = circumferential defect + horizontal bone loss

Each implant was subclassified to defect severity based on the defect depth from the implant neck and ratio of bone loss/total implant length.

1. Grade S (Slight) = 3 to 4 mm or less than 25% of the implant length
2. Grade M (Moderate) = 4 to 5 mm or greater than or equal to 25% to 50% of the implant length
3. Grade A (Advanced) = greater than 6 mm or greater than 50% of the implant length

After review of 158 implant, Monje and colleagues found the most common was class Ib defect (2- to 3-wall defect) in 55% of the implants. The next most common was shown to be 16.5% for class Ia (buccal dehiscence) and 13.9% for class IIIb (2- to 3-wall defect + horizontal defect).[30]

PROGNOSTIC FACTORS

Baseline clinical examination and radiographic imaging should be performed at the onset before diagnosis and treatment are rendered. Six-point probing per implant site has been advocated along with dental radiographs showing implant platform and crestal bone height. Digital parallel radiographs can be used for comparisons.

Many clinical and radiographic parameters are used to gauge treatment outcomes. Commonly referenced are bleeding extent (site) and bleeding severity (degree of bleeding), BOP, PD, SOP, plaque index (PI), clinical attachment loss (CAL), soft tissue level (STL), marginal bone level (MBL), and radiographic fill.

Recently, it has been proposed BOP extent and severity has the most influence on predicting future bone loss.[31] Although this has been suggested as a prognostic indicator, the cause and effect to determine periimplantitis is not known.[2]

GOALS OF TREATMENT

General treatment goals for both periimplant mucositis and periimplantitis share similar objectives:

1. To eliminate inflammation
2. Prevent bone loss
3. To restore periimplant tissue health

Ultimately treatment success of perimucositis is judged by arresting BOP/SOP and prevent pocket depth worsening, whereas periimplantitis includes the aforementioned in addition to bone level stabilization.

TREATMENT OPTIONS

Identifying the cause would help mitigate future recurrences. These causes include systemic causes (eg, smokers, or poor glycemic control), biological causes (eg, poor hygiene status), and/or technical causes (eg, prosthetic wear, poor implant positioning, residual cement suspension, and prosthesis interference for hygiene access). After performing baseline clinical examinations and radiographs, nonsurgical and surgical options are available. Both would entail the removal of plaque/biofilm from the periimplant complex surfaces either by mechanical, chemical, physical means or by a combination of the aforementioned.

Nonsurgical therapy is the mainstay of initial treatment.[32] Mechanical intervention such as curettes, rotary brushes, ultrasonic devices, or air-abrasive devices are currently used. Antiseptics, antibiotics, and other detoxifying agents are labeled as chemical means. Laser and photodynamic therapy (PDT) are categorized as physical intervention. Surgical treatment, generally at 6 months, is usually sought after a failed nonsurgical attempt, which is documented to occur more than 50% of the time.[2] Surgical therapy can be instituted as soon as 4 weeks for worsening situations. However, if a patient cannot undergo surgical procedure, retreatment using nonsurgical therapy has been supported.[32]

Perhaps the low success rate of nonsurgical periimplantitis is due to limited access to implant surface, which makes proper debridement and decontamination difficult. Surgical approaches include open flap debridement, resective surgery with or without implantoplasty, and regenerative procedures; these options can improve outcome of periimplantitis treatment.[33] Open flap debridement gains direct access to the implant surface for unimpeded debridement. Many different types of instruments and chemical adjuncts can be used and are discussed in the next section. The gingival tissue is then readapted to the original position to maintain the tissue height. Resective surgery is indicated for suprabony defects and pocket reduction; an apical positioned flap facilitates patient's home hygiene. An implantoplasty consists of removing the roughened surface and implant threads down to a polished finish to deter future bacterial adhesion. Regenerative surgery uses various grafting materials with or without a barrier membrane around an infrabony defect site.[34]

NONSURIGCAL THERAPY

Mechanical, chemical, and physical modalities of nonsurgical therapy are discussed in the following section.

MECHANICAL DEBRIDEMENT

Mechanical debridement is the cornerstone to nonsurgical and surgical treatment of periimplant disease. Removal of the plaque, calculus, and debris via implant surface debridement is critical to reduce the bacterial load causing inflammation and periimplant disease. Available instrumentation includes curettes, ultrasonic devices, rotary brushes, and air-abrasive system (**Table 2**).

CURETTES

Curettes are often the first instruments considered for mechanical debridement of implants perhaps from the similarities drawn from treatment of natural dentition. Stainless steel surface instruments have been shown to cause irreversible damage on implant surfaces in an in vitro study. This damaged surface provides a nidus for bacterial attachment, leading to future biofilm development.[41] In addition, the particles released from the implant surface can induce an inflammatory response.[42] However, long-term effects of these metal instruments on implant surfaces are unknown at this time.[43]

Table 2
Mechanical debridement using different instrumentation and chemical and physical adjuncts used for treatment of periimplant disease[33,35–40]

Mechanical		
Curette	1. Titanium 2. Carbon fiber 3. Polytetrafluoroethylene (PTFE) 4. Plastic	
Ultrasonic	1. Titanium 2. Carbon fiber 3. Polyetheretherketone (PEEK)-coated tip	
Rotary brush	1. Titanium 2. Chitosan	
Air-abrasive system	1. Amino acid glycine powder 2. Erythritol-based powder	
Chemotherapeutic		
Local	Antibiotic	Minocycline microspheres (*Arestin*) Minocycline ointment (*Periocline*) Doxycycline hyclate gel (*Atridox*) Metronidazole gel (*Elyzol*) Lincomycin gel Erythromycin gel Tetracycline fibers (*Actisite*)
	Antiseptic	Citric acid Hydrogen peroxide Chlorhexidine Sodium hypochlorite
	Other	Saline
Systemic	Antibiotic	Amoxicillin Metronidazole Azithromycin Tetracycline Doxycycline Clindamycin
	Other	Probiotic (*Lactobacillus*)
Physical		
Laser	1. Er:YAG 2. Er,Cr:YSGG 3. Carbon dioxide (CO2) 4. Diode laser 5. Nd:YAG	
Photodynamic therapy	Diode laser	—

Currently, many curettes exist on the market that are implant surface compatible: titanium, carbon fiber, polytetrafluoroethylene (PTFE)-coated, and plastic. Materials softer than titanium, such as plastic, PTFE-coated, or other nonmetallic ultrasonic tips, do not cause damage to implant surfaces,[42] but an in vitro study examining efficacy of these nonmetallic materials suggest they may not properly remove bacterial biofilm from implant with rough surfaces.[33,44] Many studies use curettes as the control treatment, and therefore, there are no head-to-head studies comparing different material curettes with each other. Nonetheless, regardless of material, such as PTFE,[45] titanium,[46] and plastic,[47] mechanical debridement showed improvements in BOP and PD from baseline at 6 months and up to 12 months.

ULTRASONIC DEVICES

Ultrasonic devices are commonly used for oral hygiene prophylaxis and implant bio-film removal. Similar to stainless steel curettes, these stainless steel ultrasonic tips must be avoided. Three types of ultrasonic tips have shown not to cause damage to implant surfaces, which include titanium, carbon fiber, and polyetheretherketone (PEEK)-coated tips.

In an in vitro study, ultrasonic debridement showed a wide range of efficacy to remove biofilm (represented as red ink). Furthermore, stainless and PEEK-coated tips both showed inferior cleaning capabilities when compared with titanium brushes and air-abrasive units. The order of effectiveness for surface ink removal was demonstrated in the following ascending order: ultrasonic tips with PEEK (43.3%–49.4%), stainless steel (53.5%–57.4%), air-polishing systems (87.1%–88.7%), and titanium brushes (88.0%–90.0%).[48]

Conversely, Keim and colleagues' results showed ultrasonic debridement was effective (11.4%–19.7% residual ink remaining).[41] Ultrasonic with titanium tip debridement showed to be the most effective when compared with titanium brush or beta-tricalcium phosphate air-abrasive system.[49] In clinical studies, Blasi and colleagues found ultrasonic with plastic tip to show better outcomes than air-polishing device with glycine powder in treatment of mucositis.[50] Comparing carbon fiber ultrasonic tip with carbon fiber curette, Karring and colleagues found no difference in BOP, PD, and plaque index after 6 months.[51]

ROTARY BRUSHES

Rotary brushes are attached to implant handpieces for mechanical debridement of implant surface. Titanium and chitosan-based brush materials are the most common. When compared with steel curettes, titanium brushes made from titanium bristles have improved biofilm removal.[52] In another in vitro study, Park and colleagues found titanium brushes did not significantly modify the implant's microsurface when examined under scanning electron microscopy, confocal laser microscopy, and contact profilometry.[53] Chitosan is a polysaccharide produced from the chitin of crustaceans and insects that is nontoxic and bioabsorbable with antibacterial and antiinflammatory properties.[46] Chitosan brushes have shown improved clinical signs of inflammation (eg, reduction in PD and BOP) when compared with titanium curettes in the early healing phase at week 2 and 4 but no difference at 6 months.[46]

AIR-ABRASIVE SYSTEM

Air-abrasive systems use kinetic energy from compressed air, water, and different powdered materials for air-powder ablation against bacterial biofilm on implant surfaces.[54] Examples of powders include glycine and erythritol. Glycine, a water-soluble amino acid, has been shown to remove subgingival biofilm and promote bone healing.[55] Erythritol is a low-abrasive sugar material that possesses antibacterial properties, which improves gingival and bone tissue healing.[56] Studies compare air-abrasive systems with other nonsurgical instrumentation (eg, ultrasonic, curettes, lasers, and so on) but not to each other (glycine vs erythritol). More importantly, the air-powder abrasion is effective at removing biofilm from implant without causing damage to its surfaces.[54]

In a recent systematic review and meta-analysis investigating the nonsurgical treatment of periimplantitis using air-abrasive devices, it has shown to have improved clinical and radiographic outcome particularly with decreased BOP when compared with mechanical debridement techniques (curettes and ultrasonics). However, an increased mucosal recession was also noted. Both of these parameters (BOP and mucosal recession) were observed for up to 6 months with statistical differences.[43] The investigators were inconclusive to endorse one instrumentation over another for surface decontamination because they all had similar outcomes within a short time period.[43] It is noteworthy that a rare complication occurred with one case report of air emphysema developed with the use of air-abrasive system.[57]

PHYSICAL DECONTAMINATION
Lasers

Laser therapy can cause bacterial cell death and has the potential to induce new bone formation while being compatible and nondestructive to the implant's surface.[58,59] Multiple laser systems exist, including yttrium-aluminum-garnet (Er:YAG) erbium, chromium-doped yttrium, scandium, gallium and garnet (Er,Cr:YSGG), carbon dioxide (CO_2), diode, and neodymium-doped:yttrium-aluminum-garnet (Nd:YAG) (see **Table 2**).

Er:YAG Laser

Er:YAG laser (2940 nm) is the most used laser for nonsurgical treatment of periimplantitis.[60] The laser wavelength is absorbed by water molecules and generates microblasting to cut soft and hard tissue.[61] Er:YAG laser is effective at removing calculus without causing surface changes when used with irrigation.[62] Abduljabbar and colleagues investigated whether a single use of Er:YAG as an adjunct to mechanical debridement with plastic instruments would provide clinical benefit versus only mechanical debridement. They found Er:YAG adjunct provided significant differences in mean plaque score, BOP, and PD, but only at 3 months follow-up. At 6 months, there was no difference between the 2 groups.[63] Similarly, Renvert and colleagues compared the effectiveness of Er:YAG versus air abrasion and found that both groups have improvements at 1-month follow-up but no difference at 6 months.[64] Moreover, a study by John and colleagues found that Er:YAG was effective as monotherapy compared with mechanical debridement with local antiseptic therapy (eg, chlorhexidine [CHX]) over a 34-month follow-up period but was unable to attain full disease resolution.[65]

Er,Cr:YSGG Laser

Er,Cr:YSGG (2780 nm) is similar to Er:YAG in that the laser wavelength is absorbed by water with similar thermal properties and is therefore used in similar fashion to eliminate bacteria in small spaces such as in periimplantitis.[58] In a randomized controlled trial (RCT), investigators compared laser-assisted mechanical debridement using Er,Cr:YSGG and diode lasers and found only decrease in PD at 6 months in the Er,Cr:YSGG, whereas no difference between diode laser and control (only mechanical debridement).[66]

Carbon Dioxide Laser

Carbon dioxide laser has bactericidal effects and may improve osteoblast attachment to titanium surfaces after irradiation without significant surface alteration seen on scanning electron microscope, as demonstrated in an in vitro study.[67] Two studies have shown clinical improvement (eg, reduction in PD, BOP, and increase in bone level) by using CO_2 laser for surface detoxification.[36] However, if the laser settings are used improperly, localized osteonecrosis can occur.[36]

Diode Laser

Diode laser exerts antibacterial effects by increasing localized temperature on implant surfaces; therefore, irrigation is necessary to prevent damage on implant surfaces.[68] Studies reviewed combined diode laser and mechanical debridement, either nonsurgical or surgical, and found mixed results for the effectiveness of diode lasers. Investigators found clinical improvements (eg, reduction in BOP, PD) when used as surgical therapy, whereas others report no added clinical benefit during surgical therapy.[36]

Nd:YAG Laser

Nd:YAG is useful for coagulation but can melt titanium implant surfaces due to its high temperature and is therefore contraindicated in periimplantitis.[36] However, an RCT study by Abduljabbar and colleagues[63] showed that Nd: YAG along with mechanical debridement performed in nonsurgical surgical debridement had good clinical outcome (eg, PD reduction) in 3 months but not at 6 months.[63,69]

Review of all Lasers

Mostafa's systemic review examined various lasers used for treatment of periimplantitis and acknowledged some studies have shown its short-term effectiveness for implant surface decontamination to improve some clinical parameters. However, she cannot conclude which laser system is superior because of the heterogenicity and recommended further large-scale controlled studies to ascertain these findings.[36]

Photodynamic Therapy

PDT exerts antibacterial effects via release of free oxygen. When a low-power diode laser is used to activate photosensitive dyes inserted into the periimplant sulcus, toxic oxygen species (eg, singlet oxygen, free radical) are released and cause microbial destruction.[35] PDT has not been shown to damage the implant surface.[70] Comparing PDT as adjunct with mechanical debridement alone (either nonsurgical or surgical), some studies resulted in minimal to no difference in clinical measurements.[71,72] On the other hand, Karimi and colleagues has shown implants that have undergone PDT with nonsurgical mechanical debridement yielded significant improvements in both PD and CAL compared with implants that underwent only mechanical debridement (without PDT) at 3 months follow-up.[73] Others found improvements in only BOP at 12 months.[74]

Overall, PDT shows benefits in some clinical improvements, especially in the short-term. However, more evidence is needed to recommend PDT as the standard of treatment.

ADJUNCTIVE THERAPY

Chemotherapeutics are antibiotic and antiseptic treatments used to decontaminate implant surfaces by targeting microorganisms that form and maintain biofilm, which cause periimplant disease.

There is a wide range of chemotherapeutics agents studied in the literature including local and systemic agents for treatment of periimplantitis (see **Table 2**).

LOCAL CHEMOTHERAPEUTICS
Local Antibiotics

Local administration of antibiotics can be given alone or in combination with nonsurgical or surgical treatment of periimplantitis. Antibiotics delivered into the periimplant space include minocycline microspheres (*Arestin*), minocycline ointment (*Periocline*), doxycycline gel (*Atridox*), metronidazole gel (*Elyzol*), lincomycin gel, erythromycin gel, and tetracycline fibers (*Actisite*), among others.[40] Toledano and colleagues investigated the efficacy of local delivery of antibiotics as the sole treatment (eg, without mechanical debridement or other periimplant treatments), and the meta-analysis showed an additional PD reduction by 0.3 mm and 85% increase in odds of BOP reduction with local antibiotics compared with control groups without local antibiotics.[40]

When combined with mechanical debridement, significant improvements in clinical outcomes are seen with local delivery of antibiotics in combination with mechanical debridement.[61] In a review, one study investigated 8.5% doxycycline hyclate and mechanical debridement compared with mechanical debridement and found improvements in attachment levels, BOP and PD, in the doxycycline group.[75] Furthermore, in another study, mechanical debridement with either submucosal minocycline microspheres or 0.1 mL 1% CHX gel showed minocycline microspheres improved PD and BOP, whereas CHX gel only resulted in BOP reduction at 12 months.[76] Another study looked at surgical debridement with either 10 mg minocycline ointment (0.5 g) or placebo to show improvements only in gingival index and not in other clinical parameters (eg, PD, BOP, PI) or microbiological outcomes at 6 months.[77]

In 2 studies investigating PDT compared with chlorhexidine gel or minocycline microspheres, it also did not find statistically significant differences in clinical outcomes between the 2 groups, other than BOP reduction.[78,79] Ultimately, in their review, Passarelli and colleagues concluded there were no clinical differences (eg, BOP, PD, PI) between minocycline microspheres and 0.1 mL 1% CHX gel.[75]

LOCAL ANTISEPTIC
Citric Acid

Citric acid is acidic (pH = 1) and therefore has antibacterial effectiveness on biofilms of tooth roots and dental implants. Forty percent citric acid for 1 minute is commonly used to treat implants, although one in vitro study found that rubbing 10% citric acid for 4 minutes was the most optimal length of time to achieve significant removal of biofilm.[80] In a clinical study with titanium rings to represent titanium implants, citric acid did not display significant bactericidal effects as compared with other antimicrobial agents (eg, hydrogen peroxide, chlorhexidine, sodium hypochlorite, or Listerine).[39] Because of its acidic nature, higher concentration citric acid (40%) may cause implant and periimplant tissue damage when used for more than 30 to 60 seconds.[81] Both Investigators recommend limited within 1-minute application with 40% citric acid for decontamination of implant surface.

Hydrogen Peroxide

Hydrogen peroxide exerts its antibacterial effects by generating cytotoxic hydroxyl radical and disrupt bacterial cell membranes, causing cell death.[82] Hydrogen peroxide can be used on implant surfaces as an adjunct with mechanical debridement, effectively removing biofilm on implant surfaces. The strength ranges from 3% to 10% and is physically rubbed on implant surfaces for 1 minute. Of note, 10% hydrogen peroxide can cause gingival irritation and should be used with caution.[81]

Chlorhexidine

CHX is an antiseptic commonly used for disinfection in the oral cavity. CHX works by attaching to the bacterial cell wall, disrupting its integrity, and therefore causing bacterial death.[83] In their systematic review and meta-analysis, Ye and colleagues found when CHX was used as an adjunct in nonsurgical treatment with mechanical debridement, there was significant reduction in PD in perimucositis during a follow-up period ranging from 12 weeks to 8 months. However, for periimplantitis, investigators did not find similar results in PD; this may be due to the increased depth of pockets in periimplantitis versus periimplant mucositis. When reviewed in more detail, they gathered mixed results for CHX mouthwash, but improved clinical outcomes testing the CHX gel and CHX chips. They concluded the efficacy of CHX as adjunctive treatment of periimplant disease is not yet clear.[84]

Sodium Hypochlorite

Sodium hypochlorite (1%) is a disinfectant used in dentistry, owing its powerful cytotoxicity characteristic to its undissociated hypochlorous acid.[85] In an RCT, 68 implants with periimplant mucositis were treated with either sodium hypochlorite gel or a placebo gel before mechanical debridement and was repeated 5 times. No statistically significant differences were found between the 2 groups after 6 months follow-up.[86]

OTHER
Saline

Saline is an isotonic solution that is commonly used for irrigation fluid after debridement. In 4 RCTs, investigators used either surgical gauze or cotton pellets soaked in sterile saline with curettes as controls to test against other adjuncts (eg, chlorhexidine cetylpyridinium chloride, and diode laser).[87–90] All 4 studies found significant improvements in BOP and PD from baseline when investigating mechanical debridement with saline gauze or pellets. It seems likely that most of the clinical improvement is from the act of mechanical debridement under surgical access rather than the chemotherapeutics of sterile saline in gauze/cotton pellet. Nonetheless, it is possible the gauze or cotton pellet may contribute to improving mechanical debridement with the curette by acting as an abrasive material against the implant surface.

SYSTEMIC CHEMOTHERAPEUTICS
Systemic Antibiotics

Systemic antibiotics are commonly prescribed to treat oral manifestations of disease such as odontogenic infections, periodontal disease, and periimplant disease. Biofilm, similar to those around implants causing periimplant disease, prevent antibiotics and host immune cells from access to the microorganisms that contribute to the damaging effects such as surrounding inflammation of tissues.[91] A growing public health concern for overuse of antibiotics is the rapid development of antibacterial resistance of microbial species.[92] Therefore, use of systemic antibiotics to treat periimplant disease has come under closer scrutiny. Some examples of systemic antibiotics include amoxicillin, metronidazole, azithromycin, tetracycline, doxycycline, and clindamycin.

Antibiotics were given along with mechanical debridement compared with mechanical debridement alone (with or without placebo). Toledano and colleagues reviewed literature looking at amoxicillin alone, metronidazole alone, amoxicillin with metronidazole, or other combinations (eg, clindamycin + amoxicillin + azithromycin + tetracycline) in combination with mechanical debridement that did not improve BOP and PD but resulted in improvements in other areas (eg, CAL, SOP, recession, bacterial count). However, they concluded that the minimal benefits in clinical outcomes should be weighed against the risk of antibiotic resistance.[40] In contrast, Wang and colleagues gathered improvements in BOP and PD for up to 12 months from azithromycin with mechanical debridement and amoxicillin and metronidazole with mechanical debridement.[93] Furthermore, Zhao and colleagues found that amoxicillin and metronidazole with ultrasonic debridement and clarithromycin with PDT showed significant improvements in BOP, CAL, and PD.[61] Overall, the consensus on systemic use of antibiotics is not well supported in the literature currently.

Probiotics

Probiotics (such as *Lactobacillus* bacteria) have shown antibacterial effects against subgingival periodontal bacterial species seen in periimplant disease, in an in vitro study.[92] Probiotics have been considered as an adjunct to periimplant disease maintenance due to their overall health benefits and antimicrobial effect on harmful oral bacteria.[94] Gao and colleagues investigated effects of probiotics on PD, BOP, and PI on periimplant mucositis and periimplantitis. Their systematic review of 6 studies showed no significant differences on the effectiveness of *Lactobacillus* in conjunction to nonsurgical treatment of periimplant disease compared with control (mechanical debridement).[37] More studies are required to see if there is a true beneficial effect of probiotics as an adjunctive treatment of periimplant disease.

LASER THERAPY/AIR-ABRASIVE SYSTEM/ULTRASONIC DEVICE AND ADJUNCTIVE CHEMICAL AND PHYSICAL AGENTS VERSUS MECHANICAL DEBRIDEMENT FOR NONSURGICAL TREATMENT OF PERIIMPLANT MUCOSITIS

A recent systemic review concluded that using either mechanical or physical means (eg, air polishing devices with glycemic powder, chitosan brush, ultrasonic device with various tips [carbon fiber tip or plastic-coated tip], titanium curettes, plastic curettes, adjunctive diode laser) and adjunctive antiseptic could not demonstrate which instrumentation was better in removing plaque around the implant than traditional home oral care.[95] In addition, Ramanauskaite and colleagues, through their systemic review and meta-analysis, concluded mechanical debridement alone with home oral hygiene is the best treatment option for periimplant mucositis. In addition, none of the other debridement devices or adjunctive chemicals had any advantageous effects over professional mechanical debridement combined with good home hygiene[96]; this is considered as the standard of care[47] and is also supported by the others.[1,97]

LASER THERAPY/AIR-ABRASIVE SYSTEM/ULTRASONIC DEVICE VERSUS MECHANICAL DEBRIDEMENT ± CHEMICAL AGENTS FOR TREATMENT OF NONSURGICAL PERIIMPLANTITIS

Regarding laser therapy versus mechanical debridement (hand curettes ± CHX), a recent systematic review demonstrated both groups had good clinical outcomes. Nd:YAG and Er,Cr:YSGG had PD reduction with statistical difference in 3 to 6 months but only Er,Cr:YSGG held up in 6 months. When comparing among all lasers, 1 with Nd:YAG and 2 with Er:YAG demonstrated significant BOP reduction with statistical difference over the mechanical debridement group in 3 to 6 months. This time only Er:YAG persisted for 6 months. Mean PD reduction of 0.8 to 1.5 mm and BOP reduction of 11% to 48% were recorded within all laser groups tested.[69] In addition, SOP and MBL were not recorded between both test and control groups.[63,98,99]

In the same systemic review, comparing air-abrasion or ultrasonic device versus mechanical debridement (curettes and/or ultrasonic) with or without local antiseptics, all groups tested had PD and BOP reduction in 6 months. The mean PD reduction was recorded at less than 1.3 mm and 7% to 70% of BOP within all studies. Four air-abrasive system studies demonstrated better PD reduction but no statistical difference in 3- to 6-month period against mechanical debridement. Although all treatments rendered had BOP reduction, only 1 air-abrasion device study combined with local

CHX application showed statistically significant BOP reduction against the control group.[100] In reference to SOP and MBL, there was no statistical significance between the test and control groups. The investigator concluded the evidence within this review is limited due to the small sample size and heterogenicity to draw any meaningful conclusions.[69]

The aforementioned findings also concur with Ramanauskaite and colleagues' review in that air-abrasive system with glycemic powder and Er:YAG laser demonstrated higher BOP reduction against mechanical debridement group in the short-term. However, it was not true for PD reduction. In addition, adjunctive application of either local antiseptics, antibiotics, or probiotics was not helpful in reducing PD or BOP. Furthermore, ultrasonic devices failed to show superiority in terms of PD or BOP reduction against mechanical debridement $\pm$ CHX.[47]

This is also in line with Atieh and colleagues' review demonstrating increase in BOP reduction with statistical difference in 6 months with air-abrasive devices when compared with mechanical debridement. PD values were also in line with the aforementioned reviews such that it was not statistically significant against the control group up to 6 months.[41] However, the investigators commented that further controlled studies are needed to ascertain these results.[43]

Surgical Treatment

Several surgical approaches can treat periimplantitis and are discussed later (**Table 3**).

1. Open flap debridement
2. Resective surgery
3. Adjunctive implantoplasty

Table 3
Surgical techniques and materials for treatment of periimplantitis[33,101–103]

Surgical Technique	Description	Materials Used
Open Flap Debridement	Surgical procedure involving the lifting of a flap of soft tissue to expose the implant surface, followed by removal of the bacterial biofilm and debris by mechanical, physical, and/or chemical means	Mechanical: ultrasonic scaler, curettes, titanium brushes, air-abrasive system Physical: laser, PDT Antibiotics: tetracycline fibers, minocycline microspheres Antiseptic: citric acid, CHX
Resective surgery	Surgical procedure involving the pocket reduction, with possible osteoplasty and apical repositioned flap	Scalpel, rotary instruments, chisels
Implantoplasty	Surgical procedure involving the removal of rough or contaminated implant surface and thread to a smooth finish	Titanium brushes, diamond burs, Arkansas stones, polishing burs
Regenerative surgery	Surgical procedure involving the placement grafting material used for bone regeneration and reosseointegration	Bone grafts: autogenous, allograft, xenograft, alloplast, porous titanium granules Bioactive materials: EMD, PRF Membrane: resorbable and nonresorbable, PRF

Abbreviations: EMD, enamel matrix derivates; PRF, platelet-rich fibrin

4. Resective surgery with or without adjunctive implantoplasty
5. Regenerative surgery

The treatment outcome of surgical success is commonly judged, after 6 months, by these parameters.[104]

1. PD ≤ 5 mm
2. No BOP or SOP
3. No additional bone loss

Open Flap Debridement

Open flap debridement requires a full-thickness reflection of the gingiva, allowing direct access to the implant surface for decontamination. PD reduction, decreased BOP, and stabilization of bone loss have been noted with this technique.[101] Success rate of 53% has been reported[105] (**Table 4**). However, significant postoperative peri-implant soft tissue recession of 1.8 to 1.9 mm were documented after 1 to 5 years.[102]

OPEN FLAP DEBRIDEMENT WITH OR WITHOUT ADJUNCTIVE ANTIBIOTICS

Two RCTs showed no difference between the 2 groups treated with or without systemic antibiotics in these clinical parameters (eg, PD, BOP, SOP, or RBL) in 1-year period[101] and over 3-year period.[108] In fact, Hallstrom and colleagues were perplexed with the discovery of a higher bacterial repopulation for the antibiotic group than the control group after 1 year of treatment. Furthermore, the success rates for the test group and control group were 46.7% and 25%, respectively (case definition = PD ≤ 5 mm, absent BOP/SOP, no bone loss ≤ 5 mm)[101] (see **Table 4**).

Resective Surgery

The goal of this technique is to reduce redundant hyperplastic tissue surrounding the implant with an apical repositioned flap and bony recontouring for negative architecture. Also, this technique is indicated for horizontal bone defect not amenable for bone grafting. According to Schwarz,[105] resective surgery has a success rate ranging from 33% to 75% over a 2- to 5-year period (see **Table 4**).

Adjunctive Implantoplasty

Several studies have investigated the effectiveness of implantoplasty in treating periim-plantitis. A recent systematic review and meta-analysis evaluated the outcome of implantoplasty. A total of 8 articles qualified for systematic review and 7 of them were included in the quantitative analysis. Significant probing depth reduction with implanto-plasty was noted (mean difference = −3.37 mm) through meta-analysis. Kaplan-Meier analysis was used to calculate the probability of implant success to be 94.7% at 2 years

Table 4 Success rate of surgical treatment of periimplantitis[101–107]	
Surgical Treatment	**Success Rate (%)**
Open flap debridement	25–53
Resective surgery	33–75
Implantoplasty	94.7
Regenerative surgery	11.1–42[a]

[a] 10 y.

(see **Table 4**). This analysis showed that implantoplasty resulted in statistically significant improvement in clinical parameters such as PD, BOP, and SOP compared with baseline despite 10.7% to 33% of residual bleeding were noted.[103]

The investigators noted implantoplasty should be used with caution for patients with narrow diameter implants (eg, 3.5 mm) because it may reduce implant wall thickness and fracture resistance.[109] In addition, controversies still surround the type of materials best used for surface decontamination for implantotplasty. Materials such as hydrogen peroxide, tetracycline, ethylenediaminetetraacetic acid (EDTA), and chlorohexidine have been tried.[103] Overall, the investigators recommended implantoplasty for treatment of periimplantits despite the small sample size reviewed.[103]

Resective Surgery with or Without Adjunctive Implantoplasty

Overall, implants treated with resective surgery and adjunctive implantoplatsy had significant PD reduction when compared with sites without (**Fig. 2**). Soft tissue level changes were compatible for both groups. Of note, 2 RCTs showed increased mucosal recession despite improvement in all other parameters (eg, BOP, PD, SOP, and MLB) using adjunctive implantoplasty when compared with control group.[110,111]

Regenerative Surgery

The goal of regenerative surgery is to promote bone regeneration of infrabony defects around implants by proper decontamination and placement of biological bone graft material outlined in **Table 5**. Controversies exist regarding the superiority of material and the necessity for use of collagen membrane for regeneration. This section reviews the following outcome for bony regeneration against other materials and techniques such as other adjunctive and alternative means, for specific bone defect morphology, on different implant surfaces, and against open flap debridement technique (**Fig. 3**).

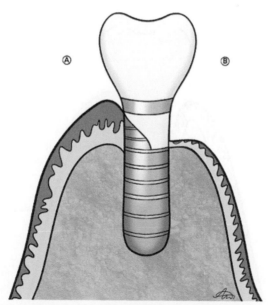

Fig. 2. Periimplantitis bone loss and implantoplasty. A = Horizontal bone loss with hyperplastic tissue around dental implant. B = Resective surgery with implantoplasty and apical repositioned gingiva. (Image courtesy of Maya Nunez.)[105]

Table 5
Materials available for regenerative surgery

	Material
Bone Graft Materials	1. Autogenous 2. Allograft 3. Xenograft 4. Alloplastic 5. Titanium granules
Biological Active Materials	1. Enamel matrix derivates (EMD) 2. Bone morphogenic protein (BMP) 3. Platelet-rich fibrin (PRF)
Membrane	1. Resorbable 2. Nonresorbable 3. Platelet-rich fibrin (PRF)

Indications for regenerative surgery proposed by the 15th European workshop[104]:

1. At least 3 mm of infrabony defect
2. 3- to 4-wall defect
3. With surrounding KT present

BONE GRAFT MATERIALS USED FOR REGENERATIVE SURGERY
Autogenous Bone Versus Xenograft

The findings of a randomized controlled clinical trial by Aghazadeh and colleagues indicated significantly better clinical and radiographic outcomes with the use of xenograft over autogenous bone both with collagen membrane coverage.[106] The study was

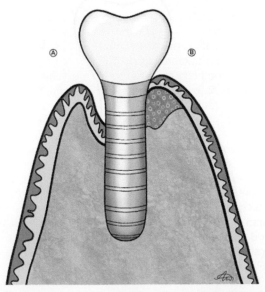

Fig. 3. Periimplantitis defect and regeneration. A = Infrabony defect around dental implant. B = Regenerative surgery showing bone graft material placement in infrabony defect site. (Image courtesy of Maya Nunez.)[105]

conducted at a single center and involved 45 participants who were randomly assigned to placement of autogenous bone or bone-derived xenograft. At 12 months, the actual radiographic mean bone gain was only 1.1 mm ± 0.3 and 0.2 mm ± 0.3 for both xenograft and autogenous bone, respectively. The success rate (case definition: ≤ 5 mm pocket depth, no further bone loss, no BOP/SOP) for xenograft is 20.5% and 11.1% for the autogenous group (see **Table 4**). In conclusion, this study showed that xenograft had more radiographic bone gain and higher clinical success rate than autogenous bone.[106]

Another study conducted by Aghazadeh and colleagues compared the outcomes of regenerative surgical treatment of periimplant defects using autogenous bone versus bovine-derived xenograft over a span of 5 years.[112] By the fifth year, both groups exhibited a reduction in BOP and PD. The bovine-derived group showed a greater mean reduction in PD (2.8 mm) compared with the autogenous group (1.7 mm). Regarding the change in bone level at the implant site, the autogenous group experienced a mean decrease of −0.7 mm, whereas the bovine-derived group demonstrated a mean increase of 1.6 mm. Case definition of success is defined as no bone loss, no SOP, PD less than or equal to 5 mm, and maximum of one implant surface showing BOP. This success was achieved in 36% of implants treated with autogenous bone regeneration and 78.3% of implants treated with xenograft regeneration. In conclusion, these 2 studies by Aghazadeh and colleagues showed that xenograft had better radiographic bone gain and higher success rates.[106,112]

Titanium Particles Versus Xenograft

When compared with xenograft, the use of titanium particles resulted in significantly higher radiographic fill of bone defects. A prospective clinical study by Guler and colleagues compared the effects of porous titanium granules and the use of xenograft in the treatment of periimplant defects.[113] Twenty-two patients were included in the study with clinical measurements and 3-dimensional imaging recorded at baseline and in 6 months. The porous titanium granule group showed a statistically significant increase in radiographic values over the xenograft group. The mean bone fill increase was 1.74 mm (± 0.65 mm) for porous titanium granules and 1.05 mm (± 0.54 mm) for the xenograft group. Again, this reiterates that vertical bone fill is difficult to achieve. However, only these clinical outcomes (eg, PD and CAL) were observed to be the most improved, favoring the titanium group in the immediate postop phase, but this was not sustained with statistical differences at the 6-month period.[113]

REGENERATIVE SURGERY VERSUS OPEN FLAP DEBRIDEMENT

An RCT by Jepsen and colleagues reported on regenerative surgery using porous titanium granules compared with open flap debridement alone for nonsubmerged implants with 3- to 4-wall defects.[114] The study included 63 patients and followed a protocol of open flap debridement using titanium brushes, hydrogen peroxide and regenerative protocol that filled 33 defects with porous titanium particles. At 12 months, the regenerative group showed a higher radiographic defect fill with mean of 3.6 mm compared with open flap debridement by only 1.0 mm. In comparison with open flap debridement alone, the regenerative group exhibited a reductions in probing depth (2.8 mm vs 2.6 mm) and BOP (89.4%–33.3% vs 85.8%–40.4%). However, surgical success (case definition = PD ≤ 4 mm, no BOP at 6 sites, and no bone loss from baseline) was only observed in 30% with the titanium granule group and 23% with the control group. Lastly, the investigators pointed out the histomorphology studies could not be performed with proof, and these results are purely radiographically enhanced.[114]

A systematic review and meta-analysis by Tomasi and colleagues evaluated the efficacy of regenerative therapy for periimplantitis bone defects.[115] The benefit of regenerative surgery over open flap debridement was evaluated only in 3 out of 16 studies with a total of 116 implants. The meta-analysis identified a larger improvement in marginal bone level (weighted mean difference = 1.7 mm) and bone defect fill (weighted mean difference = 57%) for regenerative surgery over open flap debridement. This bone gain was only radiographic interpretation without histologic evidence. The study, however, found no differences in clinical measurements, specifically PD and BOP. At the end of 12 months, 30% of the implant sites still had BOP for both groups. The investigators acknowledged this review had small sample size, and the control group did not consistently represent same materials used, with outcome measures variable among groups compared.[115]

A randomized clinical study conducted by Renvert and colleagues compared the outcomes of regenerative surgery and open flap debridement in the treatment of periimplantitis for 3-wall defect (270-degree defect).[116] The study included 66 patients, of which 32 patients had open flap debridement alone and 34 had open flap debridement with regenerative surgery using xenograft and a collagen membrane. The results showed that both treatments led to significant improvements in clinical parameters such as PD reduction and CAL gain. However, the regenerative surgery group had significantly better results in terms of bone fill 2.7 mm (± 1.3 mm) compared with the open flap debridement group 1.4 mm (± 1.2 mm). Surgical success (case definition = defect bone fill radiographically ≥ 0 mm, no BOP/SOP, PD ≤ 5 mm) was 35% for test group and 30% for the control group. Again, this confirms the challenges in regenerative surgery.[116]

BIOLOGICALLY ACTIVE MATERIALS USED FOR REGENERATIVE SURGERY

There are several animal and human studies on the use of biologically active materials such as enamel matrix derivates (EMD), bone morphogenic protein (rhBMP-2), platelet-rich fibrin (PRF), and platelet-derived growth factors during regenerative treatment of periimplantitis.

Enamel Matrix Derivates

A randomized controlled trial by Isehed and colleagues investigated the effects of enamel matrix derivates on periimplant bone defect over a 5-year period.[117] The study included 25 patients randomized to surgical treatment with and without EMD. At the 5-year follow-up, 11 out of 13 (85%) of implants in the EMD group survived, and 9 out of 12 (75%) of the patients without EMD group survived. The clinical treatment outcomes (PD and BOP reduction) were comparable between the 2 groups. Data revealed baseline median bone level decreased from 5.6 mm at baseline to 4.1 mm at 5 years for the EMD group and 4.2 mm at baseline to 3.3 mm at 5 years for the nonEMD group. The median bone gain for both groups was approximately 1 mm after 5 years, again demonstrating vertical bone augmentation is difficult to achieve; however, it did satisfy the definition of no further bone loss.[117]

A 3-year prospective cohort study by Mercado and colleagues evaluated the use of enamel matrix derivative and doxycycline in regeneration of bone defects associated with periimplantitis.[118] There were 30 patients in the study, and protocol included surgical access and debridement, decontamination of implant surface with 24% EDTA, xenograft bone, enamel matrix derivative, and doxycycline powder as well as connective tissue grafts where KT is lacking. At 36 months, the mean PD and bone loss reduction was 3.5 mm (± 0.60 mm) and 2.6 mm (± 0.73 mm) from a baseline of 8.9 mm

(± 1.9 mm) and 6.92 mm (± 1.26 mm), respectively. The investigators reported only 56.6% of implants were treated successfully (case definition = PD ≤ 5 mm, no BOP/ SOP, bone loss limited to within 10%, and no gingival recession of >0.5 mm and >1.5 mm for anterior and posterior regions, respectively). They concluded that regenerative treatment using combination of enamel matrix derivative, doxycycline, EDTA, and xenograft showed promising results.[118]

Bone Morphogenic Protein

There are a limited number of conflicting human and animal studies using BMP for treatment of periimplantitis. A study completed by Hanisch and colleagues used rhesus monkeys as an animal model and reconstructed a periimplantitis defect using rhBMP-2 in an absorbable collagen sponge carrier.[119] The results showed there was a vertical bone gain of 2.6 mm (± 1.2 mm) versus 0.8 mm (± 0.8 mm) for the control group. The investigators of this study concluded that there was significant evidence that the rhBMP-2 has potential for bone formation for advanced periimplantitis. A study by Esporrin and colleagues used beagle dogs as an animal model and reconstructed a periimplantitis defect using xenograft and 10% collagen soak loaded with rhBMP-2 covered with a natural collagen membrane versus xenograft and 10% collagen but soaked with saline and membrane.[120] After a period of 8 weeks of healing, histometric bone gain was 1.01 mm (± 0.29 mm) for the rhBPM-2 group and 0.92 mm (± 0.6 mm) for the control without being statistically significant.

MEMBRANE USED FOR REGENERATIVE SURGERY
Membrane Versus No Membrane

There is conflicting data in the literature regarding the use of barrier membranes to improve the outcomes of regenerative treatment. A longitudinal trial was conducted by Khoury and colleagues[121] This study included 25 patients and 41 periimplant defects that were treated with open flap debridement with autogenous bone graft alone, with nonresorbable membrane, and/or with a resorbable membrane. A case series by Roos and colleagues included 12 patients with periimplantitis.[34] After 1 year, resorbable membranes and submerged implants demonstrated clinical and radiographic improvement with a PD decrease of 4.2 mm and defect fill 2.3 mm. At 3 years postsurgery, the 3 surgical treatment protocols did not affect the treatment outcome, and the author mentions that routine application of membranes should be approached with caution. However, the case series by Schwarz and colleagues found the use of collagen barrier membrane to be beneficial.[122] Daugela and colleagues concluded through their meta-analysis that the use of a membrane is not a useful adjunct for regenerative periimplant surgery.[123]

Platelet-Rich Fibrin

PRF is a fibrin matrix containing autogenous leukocytes and growth factors. PRF has been advocated during regenerative surgery for its use as a resorbable membrane and to promote healing. PRF during regenerative surgery for periimplantitis has shown to have the benefit of less bleeding, milder pain, and greater bone density at 2 and 4 months postop.[124]

ALTERNATIVE AND ADJUNCTIVE MEANS FOR REGENERATIVE SURGERY

The use of various alternative (eg, all lasers tested) and adjunctive (eg, CHX, phosphorus or citric acid) means for decontamination of implant surface for regenerative surgery did not provide long-term superiority against the control group (eg, saline) regardless of surface type.[125] These findings applied to implant surfaces that are left to heal in a nonsubmerged environment. The investigators claimed failure was directly from recontamination of the implant under constant exposure to the oral environment.[125]

OUTCOME OF REGENERATIVE SURGERY FOR SPECIFIC BONE DEFECT MORPHOLOGY

The bone defect morphology and the effect on regeneration remains controversial in the literature and can be influenced by the defect configuration. Schwartz and colleagues examined 3 different types of bone defect configurations by using xenograft and collagen membrane with an open flap technique. Twenty-seven patients selected had infrabony defects, which were described as follows: class Ib (buccal dehiscence and 180° of bone loss), class Ic (buccal dehiscence and 360° of bone loss), and class Ie (360° of bone loss, with a crater like defect).[126] The primary outcome for this study was to investigate these clinical parameters (eg, PI, BOP, PD, mucosal recession, and clinical attachments). Of these 5 parameters, class Ie group had the most decrease in PD and CAL reduction in 12 months. The mean PD and mean CAL were 2.7 mm (± 0.7 mm) and 2.4 mm (± 1.0 mm) when compared with class Ib 1.6 mm (± 0.9 mm) and 1.2 mm (± 0.9 mm) and class Ic 1.6 mm (± 0.7 mm) and 1.1 mm (± 0.9 mm), respectively, without statistical differences. Although the investigators pointed out that different defect configurations, in particular a craterlike defect (eg, class Ie), may produce better clinical results, it was interesting that radiographic bone fill was not included as an outcome assessment for these regenerative clinical trials. Moreover, they concluded surgical remedies are not amenable for the other 2 classes of defects.[90]

Roccuzzo and colleagues investigated clinical parameters for a 1-year study using xenograft with 10% collagen to repair an infrabony defect using Schwarz bone defect classification.[126] When comparing these results, class Ie had mean PD reduction slightly better at 3.10 mm ± 2.69 mm, whereas class Ib and class Ic exhibited a PD reduction at 2.6 mm ± 1.50 mm and 3.45 mm ± 1.74 mm, respectively, in 12 months. In addition, 3 out of 13 implants (23%) were lost in class Ie, and 1 implant was lost in class Ib (4.5%). It would have been helpful and interesting to include radiographic measurements to assess the outcome of these bone grafting procedures. Surgical success (case definition = PD ≤ 5 mm and no BOP/SOP) was reported at 49.3% (37/75). Lastly, the investigators pointed out more studies will need to be conducted to ascertain if these bony defects can be reconstructed and maintained in the long-term.[126]

OUTCOME OF REGENERATIVE SURGERY FOR DIFFERENT IMPLANT SURFACE TYPES

Studies have found that implants with a rougher titanium plasma-sprayed (TPS) surface had lower success than implants with moderately roughened, sandblasted, large grit, acid-etched (SLA) surface. A study by Roccuzzo and colleagues investigated the outcomes of surgical open flap debridement and regenerative periimplantitis treatment of defects around either SLA or TPS implants. At 7 years, the treatment success (case definition: PD ≤ 5 mm, absent BOP/SOP, and no further bone loss) with SLA was 58.3% compared with TPS implants at 14.3%.[127] Furthermore, by the same group, the 10-year results showed SLA implants had continual decline at 42% but an uptick with TPS fixtures at 29%.[107] These results may suggest implant surface may have an influence on long-term success outcome. Although a vague description of "modified" implant surface was described by Berglundh and colleagues, they have reported that "nonmodified" implant surface had better BOP and PD results when compared with "modified" surface through an 11-year period.[128] Incidentally, this was also in line with Carcuac and colleagues' RCT studies of 1 and 3 years.[108,129]

OUTCOME SUCCESS FOR REGENERATIVE SURGERY SHORT- AND LONG-TERM

Regenerative procedures have been documented to have good short-term outcome (≤1 year). Unfortunately, these results do not sustain in the long run.[115] La Monaca and colleagues demonstrated a precipitous drop from 91% to 59% success rate between 1- and 5-year period, respectively.[130] Furthermore, as previously noted, a 10-year study using regenerative technique (deproteinized bovine bone mineral with 10% collagen) for SLA implants and TPS implants had low success rate of 42% and 29%, respectively[107] (see **Table 4**).

SUMMARY

- General goals of treatment of both periimplant mucositis and periimplantitis share similar objectives:
  1. To eliminate inflammation
  2. Prevent bone loss
  3. To restore periimplant tissue health
- Early recognition and intervention are recommended to prevent disease progression.
- Be aware when comparing treatment outcomes between periimplantitis success versus periimplantitis effectiveness. They both have different sets of criteria.
- Absence of inflammation especially without signs of BOP/SOP is considered as disease resolution.

RISK FACTORS FOR PERIIMPLANTITIS

- Poor oral hygiene, lack of maintenance therapy, and history of periodontitis are risk factors for periimplantitis.[3]
- The risk of periimplantitis is decreased if proper preop periodontal therapy is provided for patients with history of periodontitis.[16]
- Diabetes, smoking, occlusal overload, and necessity of KT are still controversial issues without definitive conclusion.[3]
- Limited evidence linking periimplantitis to residual cement and malpositioned implant.[3]
- Clenching/bruxism are risk factors for periimplantitis, but the cause and effect are still controversial.[19]
- Gene mutation OPG (rs2073618) could potentially be a biomarker to determine those at risk for periimplantitis. Further investigation is needed.[14]
- Residual titanium implant particle is associated to cause inflammation in the gingival sulcus and implant interface.[25]

Nonsurgical Periimplant Mucositis Therapy

- Most agree traditional debridement and reinforced oral hygiene is the standard of care for periimplant mucositis.[1,2]
- There is no superiority in which alternative device (eg, air-abrasive with glycemic powder and Chitosan brush) or physical/adjunctive agent (eg, diode laser, PDT, local antiseptic, systemic antibiotics, and probiotics) is better than professional mechanical debridement[47] or good oral hygiene[95]; these are based on 1-year studies.[47,95]

- Nonsurgical periimplant mucositis treatment *effectiveness* (using combined mechanical debridement and hygiene instructions)[2]:
  1. Reduced BOP extent (15%–40%) from baseline
  2. Pocket depth improvement (0.5–1.0 mm) from baseline

Nonsurgical Periimplantitis Therapy

- Nonsurgical therapy for periimplantitis always takes precedent before surgical therapy. It has been suggested that bacterial load reduction is a prelude for increased success and potentially provides a favorable environment for surgical therapy.[32]
- Air-abrasion system and Er:YAG laser have shown to have better BOP reduction but not PD when compared with mechanical debridement ± CHX in the short-term (<12 months).[47]
- Titanium curettes are also effective for nonsurgical therapy.[47]
- The addition of antiseptic, antibiotics, or probiotics was not useful for reducing BOP and PD in the short-term.[47]
- All the aforementioned instrumentations and materials tested had similar effects on soft tissue levels for both test and control groups.[47]
- Laser therapy (eg, Er,Cr:YAGG, Er:YAG, and Nd:YAG) has good short-term effect (</6 months with BOP reduction when compared with mechanical debridement).[69]
- Nonsurgical periimplantitis treatment *effectiveness* (just mechanical debridement)[2]:
  1. Reduced BOP extent (20%–50%) from baseline
  2. Pocket depth improvement (≤1 mm) from baseline
- Despite these efforts, greater than 50% of those treated nonsurgically will still have persistent disease (eg, persistent BOP, increased PD, and radiographic bone loss), which will necessitate surgical intervention.[2,32]

Surgical Periimplantitis Therapy

- Surgical success is commonly judged, after 6 months, by these parameters[104]:
  1. PD ≤ 5 mm
  2. No BOP or SOP
  3. No additional bone loss

Open Flap Debridement

- Open flap debridement has a 53% success rate over a 1- to 5-year period when enrolled in the supportive implant therapy program.[105]
- 3% to 14% implant failure rate was reported within 5 years of surgery.[105]
- 1.8 to 1.9 mm soft tissue recession has been associated with open flap debridement over 1- to 5-year period.[102]
- No difference was reported between open flap debridement–treated implants with or without adjunctive antibiotics in over 1- to 3-year period.[101,108]
- Success rate for open flap debridement with antibiotics group and open flap debridement alone were 46.7% and 25%, respectively.[101]

Resective Surgery

- Resective surgery has a success rate of 33% to 75% over a 2- to 5-year period when enrolled in the supportive implant therapy program.[105]
- Mucosal recession can be an unpleasant outcome.[110,111]

Implantoplasty

- A recent systematic review and meta-analysis calculated the probability of implantoplasty success to be 94.7% at 2 years.[103]
- No adjunctive materials (eg, hydrogen peroxide, tetracycline, EDTA, and chlorohexidine) were found to be superior for surface treatment of implantoplasty.[103]
- Controversies still surround the type of materials best used for surface decontamination for implantotplasty.[103]
- Avoid implantoplasty for narrow size implants for potential weakening and fracture prone (eg, 3.5 mm).[109]

Resective Surgery with Implantoplasty

- Resective surgery with implantoplasty demonstrated overall improved clinical parameters (eg,: BOP, PD, SOP, MBL) especially with significant with pocket reduction.[110,111]

Regenerative Surgery

- Concept for regeneration surgery:
  1. For infrabony defect
  2. Debridement of implant surface ± adjunctive chemicals
  3. Bone graft material ± membrane
- Regenerative surgery has been documented to have good short-term outcome (≤1 year). Unfortunately, these results do not sustain in the long run.[115]
- Success rate for regenerative surgery has been documented between 11.1% and 42% (1 and 10 years, respectively).[106,107]
- All types of bone grafting materials can be used for regenerative technique without one type being superior.[131]
- Although some successful surgical outcomes were reported, recurrence did develop, and some cases worsened; 3% to 25% implant failure rate was reported within 5 years of surgery.[105]
- There is not enough data to determine which surgical technique is superior due to a lack of a large volume of studies available.[105]
- A negative treatment outcome has been found with poor prognosis in cases with bone loss greater than 7 mm, PD greater than 8 mm, SOP, modified implant surface (implant with treated surfaces), and smoking.[105]

Regenerative Surgery Versus Open Flap Debridement

- Success rate of 30% to 35%for the regenerative group and 23% to 30% for open flap debridement group were observed in 2 clinical trials after 12 months. Overall improvement in clinical parameters was noted.[114,116]
- There were too few studies with adequate sample size in systemic review and meta-analysis to draw any meaningful conclusions to evaluate the efficiency of regeneration therapy for periimplantitis.[115]

Regenerative Surgery with or Without Membrane

- 58.6% who used nonresorbable membrane developed an infection (eg, fistula).[131]
- Others have supported the use of resorbable membrane.[34,122]
- Meta-analyzed paper concluded it is not useful for regenerative surgery.[123]

Alternative and Adjunctive Means for Regenerative Surgery

- The use of various alternative (eg, all lasers tested) and adjunctive (eg, CHX, phosphorus or citric acid) means for decontamination of implant surface for regenerative surgery did not provide long-term superiority against the control group (eg, saline) regardless of surface type.[125]

Regenerative Surgical Success for Specific Bone Defect Morphology

- The bone defect morphology and the effect on regeneration remains controversial in the literature and can be influenced by the defect configuration.
- Infrabony defect type (eg, class Ie−360 horizontal bone loss) with craterlike defect produces better clinical results (eg, PD and CAL) in 12 months than the other 2 defect types.[90,126] Surgical success (case definition = PD ≤ 5 mm and no BOP/SOP) was reported at 49.3% (37/75).[126]

Regenerative Surgery for Different Implant Surface

- A 10-year longitudinal study demonstrated a rougher implant surface has a lower success rate of 29% compared with that of a moderate rough implant of 42%.[107]

Supportive Periimplant Therapy

- If the patient has signs of disease stabilization, a maintenance program should be outlined and tailored individually; this is usually a 6-month recall, although a more frequent scheduling can be instituted if necessary.
- One of the signs of good oral health is to achieve a low plaque index.[1]
- Patient compliance for supportive periimplant therapy has been suggested to be crucial for long-term success.[16,127,132] The study reported survival rates ranging from 76% to 100% at 5 years and 70% to 99% at 7 years.[133]

SUMMARY

In conclusion, despite all the current research performed thus far, superiority of instrumentation and materials used for treatment of periimplantitis is still lacking for clinicians to follow. Controversial topics such as the need for KT, necessity of membrane, surface topography of defect, and implant surface will need further investigation. What is certain now is the fact that plaque-induced perimucositis is a reversible condition, with early treatment inception and custom maintenance schedule crucial for positive outcome. The investigators who underwent these reviews with rigor concluded larger and more control studies are needed to ascertain which technique and/or adjunctive measure is superior and more effective to treat periimplantitis.

CLINICS CARE POINTS

- Be aware when comparing treatment outcomes between periimplantitis success versus periimpalntitis effectivness. They both have different sets of criteria.
- Peri-implant disease resolution is based on absence of bleeding upon probing, stabilization of bone loss and eradication of inflammation.
- Early intervention is crucial to prevent further deterioration.
- If treated properly, plaque induced peri-implant mucositis is reversible.
- Nonsurgical therapy for peri-implantitis has < 50% success rate.

- Resective surgery with implantoplasty have some positive reported outcome.
- Regenerative therapy with various bone graft material has improved radiographic bone fill but majority of the success rate is still low (< 50%).
- Supportive Peri-implant Therapy (SPT) in post treatment phase is vital and has been suggested to increase long term success.

DISCLOSURE

The authors listed have nothing to disclose.

REFERENCES

1. Heitz-Mayfield LJA, Salvi GE. Peri-implant mucositis. J Clin Periodontol 2018;45: S237–45. Supp I 20.
2. Renvert S, Persson GR, Pirih FQ, et al. Peri-implant health, peri-implant mucositis, and peri-implantitis: Case definitions and diagnostic considerations. J Periodontol 2018;89(Suppl 1):S304–12. PMID: 29926953.
3. Berglundh T, Armitage G, Araujo MG, et al. Peri-implant diseases and conditions: Consensus report of workgroup 4 of the 2017 World Workshop on the Classification of Periodontal and Peri-Implant Diseases and Conditions. J Clin Periodontol 2018;45(Suppl 20):S286–91. PMID: 29926491.
4. Derks J, Tomasi C. Peri-implant health and disease. A systematic review of current epidemiology. J Clin Periodontol 2015 Apr;42(Suppl 16):S158–71. PMID: 25495683.
5. Diaz P, Gonzalo E, Villagra LJG, et al. What is the prevalence of peri-implantitis? A systematic review and meta-analysis. BMC Oral Health 2022 Oct 19; 22(1):449.
6. Ivanovski S, Lee R. Comparison of peri-implant and periodontal marginal soft tissues in health and disease. Periodontol 2000;76(1):116–30.
7. Berglundh T, Lindhe J, Ericsson I, et al. The soft tissue barrier at implants and teeth. Clin Oral Implants Res 1991;2(2):81–90.
8. Derks J, Schaller D, Håkansson J, et al. Peri-implantitis - onset and pattern of progression. J Clin Periodontol 2016;43(4):383–8.
9. Farhan LS. "The Microbial Etiology and Pathogenesis of Peri-Implantitis.". Oral Health and Dental Management 2018;1–11.
10. Sahrmann P, Gilli F, Wiedemeier DB, et al. The Microbiome of Peri-Implantitis: A Systematic Review and Meta-Analysis. Microorganisms 2020;8(5):661.
11. Ng E, Tay JRH, Balan P, et al. Metagenomic sequencing provides new insights into the subgingival bacteriome and aetiopathology of periodontitis. J Periodontal Res 2021;56(2):205–18.
12. Wagner J, Spille JH, Wiltfang J, et al. Systematic review on diabetes mellitus and dental implants: an update. Int J Implant Dent 2022;8(1):1.
13. Chrcanovic BR, Albrektsson T, Wennerberg A. Smoking and dental implants: A systematic review and meta-analysis. J Dent 2015;43(5):487–98.
14. Xu M, Zhang C, Han Y, et al. Association between Osteoprotegerin rs2073618 polymorphism and peri-implantitis susceptibility: a meta-analysis. BMC Oral Health 2022;22(1):598.
15. Ferreira SD, Martins CC, Amaral SA, et al. Periodontitis as a risk factor for peri-implantitis: Systematic review and meta-analysis of observational studies. J Dent 2018;79:1–10.

16. Renvert S, Quirynen M. Risk indicators for peri-implantitis. A narrative review. Clin Oral Impl Res 2015;26(Suppl. 11):15–44.

17. Di Fiore A, Montagner M, Sivolella S, et al. Peri-Implant Bone Loss and Overload: A Systematic Review Focusing on Occlusal Analysis through Digital and Analogic Methods. J Clin Med 2022;11(16):4812.

18. Linkevicius T, Puisys A, Vindasiute E, et al. Does residual cement around implant-supported restorations cause peri-implant disease? A retrospective case analysis. Clin Oral Implants Res 2013;24(11):1179–84.

19. Zhou Y, Gao J, Luo L, et al. Does Bruxism Contribute to Dental Implant Failure? A Systematic Review and Meta-Analysis. Clin Implant Dent Relat Res 2016; 18(2):410–20.

20. Hämmerle CHF, Tarnow D. The etiology of hard- and soft-tissue deficiencies at dental implants: A narrative review. J Periodontol 2018;89(Suppl 1):S291–303.

21. Ravidà A, Arena C, Tattan M, et al. The role of keratinized mucosa width as a risk factor for peri- implant disease: A systematic review, meta-analysis, and trial sequential analysis. Clin Implant Dent Relat Res 2022;24(3):287–300.

22. Ramanauskaite A, Schwarz F, Sader R. Influence of width of keratinized tissue on the prevalence of peri-implant diseases: A systematic review and meta-analysis. Clin Oral Implants Res 2022;33(S23):8–31.

23. Souza AB, Tormena M, Matarazzo F, et al. The influence of peri-implant keratinized mucosa on brushing discomfort and peri-implant tissue health. Clin Oral Implants Res 2016;27(6):650–5.

24. Ravidà A, Saleh I, Siqueira R, et al. Influence of keratinized mucosa on the surgical therapeutical outcomes of peri-implantitis. J Clin Periodontol 2020;47(4): 529–39.

25. Shafizadeh M, Amid R, Mahmoum M, et al. Histopathological characterization of peri-implant diseases: A systematic review and meta-analysis. Arch Oral Biol 2021;132:105288.

26. Caton JG, Armitage G, Berglundh T, et al. A new classification scheme for periodontal and peri-implant diseases and conditions - Introduction and key changes from the 1999 classification. J Clin Periodontol 2018;45(Suppl 20):S1–8.

27. Schwarz F, Derks J, Monje A, et al. Peri-implantitis. J Periodontol 2018;89:Suppl 1267–S 1290. PMID: 29926957.

28. Araujo MG, Lindhe J. Peri-implant health. J Clin Periodontol 2018;45(Suppl 20): S230–6. PMID: 29926494.

29. Schwarz F, Herten M, Sager M, Bieling K, Sculean A, Becker J, et al. Comparison of naturally occurring and ligature-induced peri-implantitis bone defects in humans and dogs. Clin Oral Implants Res 2007;18(2):161–70.

30. Monje A, Pons R, Insua A, et al. Morphology and severity of peri-implantitis bone defects. Clin Implant Dent Relat Res 2019;21:635–43.

31. Berglundh J, Romandini M, Derks J, et al. Clinical findings and history of bone loss at implant sites. Clin Oral Implants Res 2021;32(3):314–23.

32. Wang CW, Renvert S, Wang HL. Nonsurgical Treatment of Periimplantitis. Implant Dent 2019;28(2):155–60.

33. Schwarz F, Schmucker A, Becker J. Efficacy of alternative or adjunctive measures to conventional treatment of peri-implant mucositis and peri-implantitis: a systematic review and meta-analysis. Int J Implant Dent 2015;1(1):22.

34. Roos-Jansaker AM, Renvert H, Lindahl C, et al. Surgical treatment of peri-implantitis using a bone substitute with or without a resorbable membrane: a prospective cohort study. J Clin Periodontol 2007;34:625–32.

35. Romeo U, Nardi GM, Libotte F, et al. The Antimicrobial Photodynamic Therapy in the Treatment of Peri-Implantitis. Int J Dent 2016;2016:7692387.
36. Mostafa D. Different laser approaches in treatment of peri-implantitis: a review. Lasers in Dental Science 2019;3:71–82.
37. Gao J, Yu S, Zhu X, et al. Does Probiotic Lactobacillus Have an Adjunctive Effect in the Nonsurgical Treatment of Peri-Implant Diseases? A Systematic Review and Meta-analysis. J Evid Base Dent Pract 2020;20(1):101398.
38. Boccia G, Di Spirito F, D'Ambrosio F, et al. Local and Systemic Antibiotics in Peri-Implantitis Management: An Umbrella Review. Antibiotics (Basel) 2023; 12(1):114.
39. Gosau M, Hahnel S, Schwarz F, et al. Effect of six different peri-implantitis disinfection methods on in vivo human oral biofilm. Clin Oral Implants Res 2010; 21(8):866–72.
40. Toledano M, Osorio MT, Vallecillo-Rivas M, et al. Efficacy of local antibiotic therapy in the treatment of peri-implantitis: A systematic review and meta-analysis. J Dent 2021;113:103790.
41. Keim D, Nickles K, Dannewitz B, et al. In vitro efficacy of three different implant surface decontamination methods in three different defect configurations. Clin Oral Implants Res 2019;30(6):550–8.
42. Unursaikhan O, Lee JS, Cha JK, et al. Comparative evaluation of roughness of titanium surfaces treated by different hygiene instruments. J Periodontal Implant Sci 2012;42(3):88–94.
43. Atieh MA, Almatrooshi A, Shah M, et al. Airflow for initial nonsurgical treatment of peri-implantitis: A systematic review and meta-analysis. Clin Implant Dent Relat Res 2022;24(2):196–210.
44. Augthun M, Tinschert J, Huber A. In vitro studies on the effect of cleaning methods on different implant surfaces. J Periodontol 1998;69(8):857–64.
45. De Siena F, Corbella S, Taschieri S, et al. Adjunctive glycine powder airpolishing for the treatment of peri-implant mucositis: an observational clinical trial. Int J Dent Hyg 2015;13(3):170–6. Epub 2014 Nov 14. PMID: 25394856.
46. Wohlfahrt JC, Aass AM, Koldsland OC. Treatment of peri-implant mucositis with a chitosan brush—A pilot randomized clinical trial. Int J Dent Hyg 2019;17(2): 170–6.
47. Ramanauskaite A, Fretwurst T, Schwarz F. Efficacy of alternative or adjunctive measures to conventional non-surgical and surgical treatment of peri-implant mucositis and peri-implantitis: a systematic review and meta-analysis. Int J Implant Dent 2021;7(1):112. PMID: 34779939; PMCID: PMC8593130.
48. Luengo F, Sanz-Esporrín J, Noguerol F, et al. In vitro effect of different implant decontamination methods in three intraosseous defect configurations. Clin Oral Implants Res 2022;33(11):1087–97.
49. Munakata M, Suzuki A, Yamaguchi K, et al. Effects of implant surface mechanical instrumentation methods on peri-implantitis: An in vitro study using a circumferential bone defect model. J Dent Sci 2022;17(2):891–6.
50. Blasi A, Iorio-Siciliano V, Pacenza C, et al. Biofilm removal from implants supported restoration using different instruments: a 6-month comparative multicenter clinical study. Clin Oral Implants Res 2016;27(2):e68–73.
51. Karring ES, Stavropoulos A, Ellegaard B, et al. Treatment of peri-implantitis by the Vectors system. A pilot study. Clin Oral Impl Res 2005;16:288–93.
52. John G, Becker J, Schwarz F. Rotating titanium brush for plaque removal from rough titanium surfaces - an in vitro study. Clin Oral Implants Res 2014;25(7): 838–42.

53. Park JB, Jeon Y, Ko Y. Effects of titanium brush on machined and sand-blasted/acid-etched titanium disc using confocal microscopy and contact profilometry. Clin Oral Implants Res 2015;26(2):130–6.
54. Hentenaar DFM, De Waal YCM, Stewart RE, et al. Erythritol air polishing in the surgical treatment of peri-implantitis: A randomized controlled trial. Clin Oral Implants Res 2022;33(2):184–96.
55. Seki K, Ikeda T, Kamimoto A, et al. Efficacy of glycine air-powder abrasion for treatment of peri-implantitis. J Dent Sci 2022;17(2):1053–5.
56. Schwarz F, Ferrari D, Popovski K, et al. Influence of different air-abrasive powders on cell viability at biologically contaminated titanium dental implants surfaces. Journal of biomedical materials research Part B, Applied biomaterials 2009;88B(1):83–91.
57. Lee ST, Subu MG, Kwon TG. Emphysema following air-powder abrasive treatment for peri-implantitis. Maxillofac Plast Reconstr Surg 2018;40(1):12.
58. Mizutani K, Aoki A, Coluzzi D, et al. Lasers in minimally invasive periodontal and peri-implant therapy. Periodontol 2000 2016;71(1):185–212.
59. Ashnagar S, Nowzari H, Nokhbatolfoghahaei H, et al. Laser treatment of peri-implantitis: a literature review. J Laser Med Sci 2014;5(4):153–62.
60. Charalampakis G, Belibasakis GN. Microbiome of peri-implant infections: Lessons from conventional, molecular and metagenomic analyses. Virulence 2015;6(3):183–7.
61. Zhao T, Song J, Ping Y, et al. The Application of Antimicrobial Photodynamic Therapy (aPDT) in the Treatment of Peri-Implantitis. Comput Math Methods Med 2022;2022:3547398, 8.
62. Matsuyama T, Aoki A, Oda S, et al. Effects of the Er:YAG Laser Irradiation on Titanium Implant Materials and Contaminated Implant Abutment Surfaces. J Clin Laser Med Surg 2003;21(1):7–17.
63. Abduljabbar T, Javed F, Kellesarian SV, et al. Effect of Nd:YAG laser-assisted non-surgical mechanical debridement on clinical and radiographic peri-implant inflammatory parameters in patients with peri-implant disease. J Photochem Photobiol, B 2017;168:16–9.
64. Renvert S, Lindahl C, Roos Jansåker AM, et al. Treatment of peri-implantitis using an Er:YAG laser or an air-abrasive device: a randomized clinical trial. J Clin Periodontol 2011;38(1):65–73.
65. John G, Becker J, Schmucker A, et al. Non-surgical treatment of peri-implant mucositis and peri-implantitis at two-piece zirconium implants: A clinical follow-up observation after up to 3 years. J Clin Periodontol 2017;44(7):756.
66. Alpaslan Yayli NZ, Talmac AC, Keskin Tunc S, et al. Erbium, chromium-doped: yttrium, scandium, gallium, garnet and diode lasers in the treatment of peri-implantitis: clinical and biochemical outcomes in a randomized-controlled clinical trial. Laser Med Sci 2022;37(1):665–74.
67. Romanos G, Crespi R, Barone A, et al. Osteoblast attachment on titanium disks after laser irradiation. Int J Oral Maxillofac Implants 2006;21:232–6.
68. Cobb CM, Low SB, Coluzzi DJ. Lasers and the Treatment of Chronic Periodontitis. Dent Clin 2010;54(1):35–53.
69. Cosgarea R, Roccuzzo A, Jepsen K, et al. Efficacy of mechanical/physical approaches for implant surface decontamination in non-surgical submarginal instrumentation of peri-implantitis. A systematic review. J Clin Periodontol 2023. https://doi.org/10.1111/jcpe.13762.

70. Dörtbudak O, Haas R, Bernhart T, et al. Lethal photosensitization for decontamination of implant surfaces in the treatment of peri-implantitis. Clin Oral Implants Res 2001;12(2):104–8.

71. Albaker AM, ArRejaie AS, Alrabiah M, et al. Effect of antimicrobial photodynamic therapy in open flap debridement in the treatment of peri-implantitis: A randomized controlled trial. Photodiagnosis Photodyn Ther 2018;23:71–4.

72. Ohba S, Sato M, Noda S, et al. Assessment of safety and efficacy of antimicrobial photodynamic therapy for peri-implant disease. Photodiagnosis Photodyn Ther 2020;31:101936.

73. Karimi MR, Hasani A, Khosroshahian S. Efficacy of Antimicrobial Photodynamic Therapy as an Adjunctive to Mechanical Debridement in the Treatment of Peri-implant Diseases: A Randomized Controlled Clinical Trial. J Laser Med Sci 2016; 7(3):139–45.

74. Almohareb T, Alhamoudi N, Al Deeb M, et al. Clinical efficacy of photodynamic therapy as an adjunct to mechanical debridement in the treatment of peri-implantitis with abscess. Photodiagnosis Photodyn Ther 2020;30:101750.

75. Passarelli PC, Netti A, Lopez MA, et al. Local/Topical Antibiotics for Peri-Implantitis Treatment: A Systematic Review. Antibiotics (Basel) 2021;10(11): 1298.

76. Renvert S, Lessem J, Dahlén G, et al. Topical minocycline microspheres versus topical chlorhexidine gel as an adjunct to mechanical debridement of incipient peri-implant infections: a randomized clinical trial. J Clin Periodontol 2006;33(5): 362–9.

77. Cha JK, Lee JS, Kim CS. Surgical Therapy of Peri-Implantitis with Local Minocycline: A 6-Month Randomized Controlled Clinical Trial. J Dent Res 2019;98(3): 288–95. Epub 2019 Jan 9. PMID: 30626263.

78. Rakaševic D, Lazić Z, Rakonjac B. Efficiency of photo-dynamic therapy in the treatment of peri-implantitis: a three- month randomized controlled clinical trial,". Srp Arh Celok Lek 2016;144(9):478–84.

79. Schär D, Ramseier CA, Eick S, et al. Anti-infective therapy of peri-implantitis with adjunctive local drug delivery or photodynamic therapy: six-month outcomes of a prospective randomized clinical trial. Clin Oral Implants Res 2013;24(1): 104–10.

80. Cordeiro JM, Pires JM, Souza JGS, et al. Optimizing citric acid protocol to control implant-related infections: An in vitro and in situ study. J Periodontal Res 2021;56(3):558–68.

81. Rokaya D, Srimaneepong V, Wisitrasameewon W, et al. Peri-implantitis Update: Risk Indicators, Diagnosis, and Treatment. European journal of dentistry 2020; 14(4):672–82.

82. Juven BJ, Pierson MD. Antibacterial Effects of Hydrogen Peroxide and Methods for Its Detection and Quantitation. J Food Prot 1996;59(11):1233–41.

83. Poppolo Deus F, Ouanounou A. Chlorhexidine in Dentistry: Pharmacology, Uses, and Adverse Effects. Int Dent J 2022;72(3):269–77.

84. Ye M, Liu W, Cheng S, et al. Efficacy of Adjunctive Chlorhexidine in non-surgical treatment of Peri-Implantitis/Peri-Implant Mucositis: An updated systematic review and meta-analysis. Pakistan J Med Sci 2023;39(2):595–604.

85. Bürgers R, Witecy C, Hahnel S, et al. The effect of various topical peri-implantitis antiseptics on Staphylococcus epidermidis , Candida albicans , and Streptococcus sanguinis. Arch Oral Biol 2012;57(7):940–7.

86. Iorio-Siciliano V, Blasi A, Stratul SI, et al. Anti-infective therapy of peri-implant mucositis with adjunctive delivery of a sodium hypochlorite gel: a 6-month randomized triple-blind controlled clinical trial. Clin Oral Invest 2020;24(6):1971–9.

87. de Waal YC, Raghoebar GM, Huddleston Slater JJ, et al. Implant decontamination during surgical peri-implantitis treatment: a randomized, double-blind, placebo-controlled trial. J Clin Periodontol 2013;40:186–95.

88. de Waal YC, Raghoebar GM, Meijer HJ, et al. Implant decontamination with 2% chlorhexidine during surgical peri- implantitis treatment: a randomized, double-blind, controlled trial. Clin Oral Implants Res 2014. https://doi.org/10.1111/clr.12419.

89. Papadopoulos CA, Vouros I, Menexes G, et al. The utilization of a diode laser in the surgical treatment of peri-implantitis. A randomized clinical trial. Clin Oral Investig 2015. https://doi.org/10.1007/s00784-014-1397-9.

90. Schwarz F, Sahm N, Schwarz K, et al. Impact of defect configuration on the clinical outcome following surgical regenerative therapy of peri-implantitis. J Clin Periodontol 2010;37(5):449–55. Epub 2010 Mar 24. PMID: 20374416.

91. Sharma D, Misba L, Khan AU. Antibiotics versus biofilm: an emerging battleground in microbial communities. Antimicrob Resist Infect Control 2019;8:76.

92. Carey B, Cryan B. Antibiotic Misuse in the Community-A Contributor to Resistance? Ir Med J 2003;96(44):46, 43.

93. Wang Y, Chen CY, Stathopoulou PG, et al. Efficacy of Antibiotics Used as an Adjunct in the Treatment of Peri-implant Mucositis and Peri-implantitis: A Systematic Review and Meta-analysis. Int J Oral Maxillofac Implant 2022;37:235–49.

94. Kõll-Klais P, Mändar R, Leibur E, et al. Oral lactobacilli in chronic periodontitis and periodontal health: species composition and antimicrobial activity. Oral Microbiol Immunol 2005;20(6):354–61.

95. Verket A, Koldsland OC, Bunaes D, et al. Non-surgical therapy of peri-implant mucositis - mechanical/physical approaches: a systematic review. J Clin Periodontol 2023. https://doi.org/10.1111/jcpe.13789.

96. Ramanauskaite A, Becker K, Juodzbalys G, et al. Clinical outcomes following surgical treatment of peri-implantitis at grafted and non-grafted implant sites: a retrospective analysis. Int J Implant Dent 2018;4(1):27–8.

97. Renvert S, Hirooka H, Polyzois I, et al, Working Group 3. Diagnosis and non-surgical treatment of peri-implant diseases and maintenance care of patients with dental implants - Consensus report of working group 3. Int Dent J 2019 Sep;69(Suppl 2):12–7.

98. Schwarz F, Sculean A, Rothamel D, et al. Clinical evaluation of an Er:YAG laser for nonsurgical treatment of peri-implantitis: a pilot study. Clin Oral Implants Res 2005;16(1):44–52.

99. Schwarz F, Bieling K, Bonsmann M, et al. Nonsurgical treatment of moderate and advanced periimplantitis lesions: a controlled clinical study. Clin Oral Investig 2006;10(4):279–88.

100. Sahm N, Becker J, Santel T, et al. Non-surgical treatment of peri-implantitis using an air-abrasive device or mechanical debridement and local application of chlorhexidine: a prospective, randomized, controlled clinical study. J Clin Periodontol 2011;38(9):872–8.

101. Hallström H, Persson GR, Lindgren S, et al. Open flap debridement of peri-implantitis with or without adjunctive systemic antibiotics: A randomized clinical trial. J Clin Periodontol 2017;44(12):1285–93.

102. Heitz-Mayfield LJA, Salvi GE, Mombelli A, et al. Anti-infective surgical therapy of peri-implantitis. A 12-month prospective clinical study. Clin Oral Implants Res 2012;23(2):205–10.
103. Esteves Lima RP, Abreu LG, Belém FV, et al. Is Implantoplasty Efficacious at Treating Peri-Implantitis? A Systematic Review and Meta-Analysis. J Oral Maxillofac Surg 2021;79(11):2270–9.
104. Jepsen S, Schwarz F, Cordaro L, et al. Regeneration of alveolar ridge defects. Consensus report of group 4 of the 15th European Workshop on Periodontology on Bone Regeneration. J Clin Periodontol 2019;46(Suppl 21):277–86.
105. Schwarz F, Jepsen S, Obreja K, et al. Surgical therapy of peri-implantitis. Periodontol 2000 2022;88(1):145–81.
106. Aghazadeh A, Rutger Persson G, et al. A single-centre randomized controlled clinical trial on the adjunct treatment of intra-bony defects with autogenous bone or a xenograft: results after 12 months. J Clin Periodontol 2012;39(7):666–73.
107. Roccuzzo M, Fierravanti L, Pittoni D, et al. Implant survival after surgical treatment of peri-implantitis lesions by means of deproteinized bovine bone mineral with 10% collagen: 10-year results from a prospective study. Clin Oral Impl Res 2020;31:768–76. https://doi.org/10.1111/clr.13628.
108. Carcuac O, Derks J, Abrahamsson I, et al. Surgical treatment of peri-implantitis: 3-year results from a randomized controlled clinical trial. J Clin Periodontol 2017;44(12):1294–303.
109. Camps-Font O, González-Barnadas A, Mir-Mari J, et al. Fracture resistance after implantoplasty in three implant-abutment connection designs. Med Oral Patol Oral Cir Bucal 2020;25(5):e691–9. PMID: 32683385; PMCID: PMC7473443.
110. Romeo E, Ghisolfi M, Murgolo N, et al. Therapy of peri-implantitis with resective surgery. A 3-year clinical trial on rough screw-shaped oral implants. Part I: clinical outcome. Clin Oral Implants Res 2005;16(1):9–18.
111. Romeo E, Lops D, Chiapasco M, et al. Therapy of peri-implantitis with resective surgery. A 3-year clinical trial on rough screw-shaped oral implants. Part II: radiographic outcome. Clin Oral Implants Res 2007;18(2):179–87.
112. Aghazadeh A, Persson GR, Stavropoulos A, et al. Reconstructive treatment of peri-implant defects-Results after three and five years. Clin Oral Implants Res 2022;33(11):1114–24. Epub 2022 Sep 16. PMID: 36062917; PMCID: PMC9826427.
113. Guler B, Uraz A, Yalim N, et al. The comparison of porous titanium granule and xenograft in the surgical treatment of peri-implantitis: a prospective clinical study. Clin Implant Dent Relat Res 2017;19(2):316–27.
114. Jepsen K, Jepsen S, Laine ML, et al. Reconstruction of Peri-implant Osseous Defects: A Multicenter Randomized Trial. J Dent Res 2016;95(1):58–66.
115. Tomasi C, Regidor E, Ortiz-Vigón A, et al. Efficacy of reconstructive surgical therapy at peri-implantitis-related bone defects. A systematic review and meta-analysis. J Clin Periodontol 2019;46(Suppl 21):340–56.
116. Renvert S, Giovannoli JL, Roos-Jansåker AM, et al. Surgical treatment of peri-implantitis with or without a deproteinized bovine bone mineral and a native bilayer collagen membrane: A randomized clinical trial. J Clin Periodontol 2021;48(10):1312–21.
117. Isehed C, Svenson B, Lundberg P, et al. Surgical treatment of periimplantitis using enamel matrix derivate, an RCT: 3 and 5 year follow up. J Clin Periodontol 2018;45(6):744–53.
118. Mercado F, Hamlet S, Ivanovski S. Regenerative surgical therapy for peri-implantitis using deproteinized bovince bone mineral with 10% collagen,

enamel matrix derivative and doxycycline- A prospective 3 year cohort study. Clin Oral Implants Res 2018;29(6):583–91.

119. Hanisch O, Tatakis DN, Boskovic MM, et al. Bone formation and reosseointegration in peri-implantitis defects following surgical implantation of rhBMP-2. Int J Oral Maxillofac Implants 1997;12(5):604–10. PMID: 9337020.

120. Sanz-Esporrin J, Blanco J, Sanz-Casado JV, et al. The adjunctive effect of rhBMP-2 on the regeneration of peri-implant bone defects after experimental peri-implantitis. Clin Oral Implants Res 2019;30(12):1209–19. Epub 2019 Sep 24. PMID: 31514229.

121. Khoury F, Buchmann R. Surgical therapy of peri-implant disease: a 3-year follow-up study of cases treated with 3 different techniques of bone regeneration. J Periodontol 2001;72(11):1498–508.

122. Schwarz F, Sahm N, Bieling K, et al. Surgical regenerative treatment of peri-implantitis lesions using a nanocrystalline hydroxyapatite or a natural bone mineral in combination with a collagen membrane: a four year clinical follow-up report. J Clin Periodonol 2009;36(9):807–14.

123. Daugela P, Cicciù M, Saulacic N. Surgical Regenerative Treatments for Peri-Implantitis: Meta-analysis of Recent Findings in a Systematic Literature Review. J Oral Maxillofac Res 2016;7(3):e15.

124. Sun G, Cao L, Li H. Effects of platelet-rich fibrin combined with guided bone regeneration in the reconstruction of peri-implantitis bone defect. Am J Transl Res 2021;13(7):8397–402. PMID: 34377334; PMCID: PMC8340191.

125. Ki-Tae Koo, Khoury Fouad, Philip Leander Keeve, et al. Implant Surface Decontamination by Surgical Treatment of Periimplantitis: A Literature Review. Implant Dent 2019;28(2):173–6.

126. Roccuzzo M, Gaudioso L, Lungo M, et al. Surgical therapy of single peri-implantitis intrabony defects, by means of deproteinized bovine bone mineral with 10% collagen. J Clin Periodontol 2016;43(3):311–8. Epub 2016 Mar 9. PMID: 26800389.

127. Roccuzzo M, Pittoni D, Roccuzzo A, et al. Surgical treatment of peri-implantitis intrabony lesions by means of deproteinized bovine bone mineral with 10% collagen: 7-year-results. Clin Oral Implants Res 2017;28(12):1577–83. Epub 2017 Jun 18. PMID: 28626970.

128. Berglundh T, Wennström JL, Lindhe J. Long-term outcome of surgical treatment of peri-implantitis. A 2-11-year retrospective study. Clin Oral Implants Res 2018;29(4):404–10. Epub 2018 Mar 25. PMID: 29575025.

129. Carcuac O, Derks J, Charalampakis G, et al. Adjunctive Systemic and Local Antimicrobial Therapy in the Surgical Treatment of Peri-implantitis: A Randomized Controlled Clinical Trial. J Dent Res 2016;95(1):50–7. Epub 2015 Aug 18. PMID: 26285807.

130. La Monaca G, Pranno N, Annibali S, et al. Clinical and radiographic outcomes of a surgical reconstructive approach in the treatment of peri-implantitis lesions: A 5-year prospective case series. Clin Oral Implants Res 2018;29(10):1025–37. Epub 2018 Sep 28. PMID: 30267445.

131. Khoury F, Keeve PL, Ramanauskaite A, et al. Surgical treatment of peri-implantitis - Consensus report of working group 4. Int Dent J 2019;69(Suppl 2):18–22.

132. Heitz-Mayfield LJA, Salvi GE, Mombelli A, et al. Supportive peri-implant therapy following anti-infective surgical peri-implantitis treatment: 5-year survival and success. Clin Oral Implants Res 2018;29(1):1–6.

133. Roccuzzo M, Layton DM, Roccuzzo A, et al. Clinical outcomes of peri-implantitis treatment and supportive care: A systematic review. Clin Oral Implants Res 2018;29(Suppl 16):331–50. PMID: 30328195.

Immediate Restoration of an Endosseous Implant

Ian Mark, DMD[a],*, Harry Dym, DDS[b], Yijiao Fan, DDS[c,1]

KEYWORDS

- Immediate restoration • Immediate load • Dental implants • Full-arch rehabilitation

KEY POINTS

- Immediate loading of endosseous implants is most successful when performed for full-arch rehabilitation.
- Single implants can be immediately provisionalized, but should not have any occlusal forces.
- Excessive torque and undue surgical trauma should be avoided during implant placement.
- Increasing the surface area of the load and reducing the force applied greatly enhance the bone-implant interface, increasing the likelihood of success.

INTRODUCTION

The successful healing of endosseous dental implants is based on the principle of osseointegration. The traditional protocol to achieve osseointegration was developed by Brånemark and colleagues[1] and involves placing the implant below the crest of the bone, covering the implant with soft tissue, avoiding any load to the implant, and waiting 3 to 6 months to allow for uninterrupted healing at which point a second uncovering surgery is performed. The original two-stage surgical model has been the standard for implant osseointegration and success. With modern advances in implant technology and technique, traditional protocols are being reevaluated and improved upon. The concept of immediate loading of dental implants combines the surgery and the prosthetic components into 1 appointment which is undeniably beneficial to the patient.

a Department of Oral and Maxillofacial Surgery, The Brooklyn Hospital Center, 121 Dekalb Avenue, Brooklyn, NY 11201, USA; b Department of Dentistry and Oral and Maxillofacial Surgery, The Brooklyn Hospital Center, 121 Dekalb Avenue, Brooklyn, NY 11201, USA; c Private Practice, Flushing, NY, USA
1 Present address: 121 Dekalb Avenue, Brooklyn, NY 11201.
* Corresponding author. 121 Dekalb Avenue, Brooklyn, NY 11201.
E-mail address: ianmark926@gmail.com

Dent Clin N Am 68 (2024) 203–212
https://doi.org/10.1016/j.cden.2023.08.002
0011-8532/24/© 2023 Elsevier Inc. All rights reserved.

HISTORY

The first report of successful healing of immediate-load dental implants was as early as 1979 by Ledermann and colleagues[2] who immediately loaded implants in the anterior mandible. In 1990, Schnitman and colleagues[3] were the first to introduce the possibility of successful immediate loading of implants with a fixed prosthesis.

DEFINITION

Misch and colleagues[4] categorized immediate loading of implants based on 2 primary determinants: the amount of time elapsed since implant placement and whether the immediate-loaded prosthesis is in occlusion or not.

Time
- Immediate loading—restoration is inserted within 2 weeks of implant insertion
- Early—loading occurs between 2 weeks and 3 months
- Delayed or staged—loading occurs more than 3 months after insertion

Type
- Occlusal loading—prosthesis is in contact with the opposing dentition in centric occlusion
- Non-occlusal/nonfunctional loading—prosthesis has no direct occlusal load with the opposing dentition

The prosthesis can also be further classified based on whether the prosthesis is a provisional or definitive restoration.

ADVANTAGES

The advantages of immediate loading are manifold.[5] Obvious benefits to the patient include shorter overall treatment time, esthetics of having a restoration, and decreased patient morbidity due to obviating the need for a second surgery to uncover the implant. Additionally, in cases of delayed implant restorations, patients often wear a removable prosthesis which is fraught with the possibility of overloading the tissue and/or the implant. In full-arch cases, an additional benefit of an immediate prosthesis is the maintenance of muscle mass and masticatory function.

Immediate loading has soft tissue benefits as well. After placing the prosthesis, the soft tissue can heal and adapt to the prosthesis resulting in more esthetic gingival margins and papilla contours. Placing an immediate prosthesis is associated with increased psychological acceptance and patient satisfaction as well.

PREREQUISITES TO IMMEDIATE LOADING
Primary Stability

The most important factor for success for an immediately loaded endosseous implant is primary stability. Primary stability is defined as an insertion torque greater than 35 N-cm. Recent studies have even shown successful implant osseointegration in an immediately loaded implant with an insertion torque of 30 N-cm.[6] In fact, Maló and colleagues[7] found an implant success rate of 98.3% and a marginal bone loss of 1.14 ± 0.38 mm at 1 year follow-up for a maxillary All-on-4 immediate-loaded prostheses for implants inserted with a torque of less than 30 N-cm compared with 97.5% and 1.39 ± 0.49 mm for implants inserted with a torque of ≥30 N-cm. Primary stability can also be measured via resonance frequency analysis (**Fig. 1**). The standard accepted guidelines delineate an implant stability quotient of 70 or greater for immediate loading, 65 to 70 for early loading, and 60 to 65 for the traditional two-stage approach.

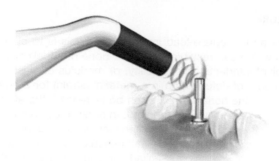

Fig. 1. Penguin resonance frequency analysis measures the resonance frequency of the Mul-tiPeg placed into the implant body and displays the implant stability quotient. (*Adapted from* Resnik, R.R. and Misch, C.E. (2021) "Immediate Load/Restoration in Implant Dentistry," in *Misch's contemporary implant dentistry.* St. Louis: Elsevier.)

If primary stability cannot be achieved, it is inadvisable to attempt an immediate or early load.

Bone Quality and Quantity

Lazzara and colleagues[8] recommend that immediate loading should only be attempted when the implants are placed in bone quality of type D1 to D3. According to Lazzara, there should also be a minimum of 6 mm of bone width and 12 mm of height (ie, for a 10-mm implant) in order to obtain adequate support. Chaushu and colleagues[9] compared immediately loaded single implants in fresh extraction sockets and immediately loaded single implants placed in healed sites and found an increased failure rate approximating 20% in fresh extraction sockets.

RATIONALE

Logically, additional load to an implant at the time of placement can cause overload resulting in implant failure. However, multiple studies have demonstrated histologically that, in fact, there is a greater bone-implant contact (BIC) in immediately loaded implants compared with traditional implants. Testori and colleagues[10] found a BIC of 64.2% for a single immediate-loaded implant compared with a BIC of 38.9% for a single submerged implant. Piattelli and colleagues[11] found that early-loaded implants in monkeys exhibited thicker lamellar cortical bone compared with unloaded implants. Apparently, early occlusal loading does not necessarily result in excess stress, but rather results in strain on the implants that actually enhances bone remodeling and increases bone density.

BONE REMODELING PROCESS

After implant osteotomy and placement, the organized and mineralized lamellar bone around the implant is replaced with an unorganized, less mineralized, woven bone. The greatest risk for implant overload and the highest chance of immediate-loaded implant failure (due to mobility and not infection) is 3 to 5 weeks after surgical insertion for at this point the bone is the most unorganized and the least mineralized.[12] In fact, the bone to implant interface has been shown to be stronger on the day of surgery compared with 3 months later.[13] At 4 months, the bone is only 60% lamellar bone; however, this has been proven to be sufficient for restoring dental implants as demonstrated by the traditional two-stage approach.

PREVENTING FAILURE

A primary goal for an immediate-load implant prosthesis is to decrease the risk of occlusal overload which can result in excessive bone remodeling and consequently weaker bone-implant interface. The flexibility, or modulus of elasticity in a material, represents the amount of deformation in a material (strain) for a given load (stress). If the strain placed on the horizontal axis can be increased, the effects of the stress positioned on the vertical axis will be reduced. In order to avoid complications or unfavorable outcomes, the clinician should aim to increase the surface area that is being immediately loaded (increase strain) and simultaneously decrease the force of the load (decrease stress) wherever possible. Similarly, it is imperative that the clinician performs the implant surgery in a manner that attentively avoids undue surgical trauma to the bone.

Increasing Surface Area

The functional surface that the occlusal load is being applied to can be increased in a number of ways including implant size, implant design, number of implants, and conditions of the implant body surface.

The greater number of implants that are being splinted together increases the percentage of survival.[14] Additionally, the increased number of implants reduces the number of pontics, which decreases the risk for fracture of the transitional prosthesis. Generally, the maxilla will require more implants than the mandible to compensate for the lower bone density and increased direction of force in the maxilla. The functional surface area of an implant can be increased by selecting a wider and longer implant. Implant width has greater overall significance in this scenario as the crest of the ridge is where the occlusal stresses are the greatest.[15] Length of the implant is still significant as it does play an important role in the initial implant stability at the time of placement. Surface area support is increased by 20% for each additional 3 mm of implant length.[16]

Implant body design is particularly relevant in immediately loaded implants as the bone does not have time to mature and grow into the undercuts or attach to the surface of an implant. In threaded implants, the bone is present in the depth of the threads at the time of insertion. This is very beneficial for an immediate-load implant. The functional surface area of the implant can be increased by increasing the number of threads. The thread depth can also be increased to further increase the functional surface area at the time of the immediate load. Additionally, chemically modified implant surfaces have been shown to have increased bone apposition and earlier formation of mature bone around the implant.[17] Nicolau and colleagues[18] demonstrated a 97.4% success rate of immediately loaded chemically modified SLActive Straumann implants in the posterior maxilla and mandible evaluated after 3 years.

Decreasing Force

A primary objective of immediately loaded implants is to minimize the risk of occlusal overload and subsequent increase in the bone remodeling rate. Patients with parafunctional habits such as bruxism and clenching have a greater risk of failure as the magnitude and duration of the occlusal force are increased and the direction of the force is more horizontal than axial.[19] Balshi and Wolfinger[20] reported that 75% of implant failures in immediately loaded implants occurs in patients with bruxism. These patients are likely not the ideal candidate that one should be considering immediate loading for. Similarly, in the postoperative period, practitioners should educate their patients on maintaining a soft diet for at least 6 weeks in order to avoid occlusal overload. Another factor to consider is the direction of the occlusal load. Posterior cantilevers are discouraged as an offset load has a greater remodeling rate and maintains less lamellar bone compared with an implant that has an axial load.[21]

Avoiding Surgical Trauma

When utilizing the immediate-loading protocol, the practitioner must be mindful to minimize all factors that would increase the risk for occlusal overload. Excess surgical trauma, including thermal injury and microfracture of bone, can lead to osteonecrosis and fibrous encapsulation of the implant. High-speed drilling should only be performed with irrigation. Cooler temperatures of saline irrigation (10°C) have been shown to produce less heat to the bone during the implant osteotomy compared with 25°C irrigation.[22] One must also be mindful to not place excessive torque on the implant as this can result in pressure necrosis resulting in bone loss and implant failure. Surgical trauma and excessive torque can result in increased bone remodeling thereby decreasing the strength of the bone-implant interface at the time of placement.

IMMEDIATE LOAD: SINGLE IMPLANTS

Successful immediate loading of single dental implants is well documented in the literature.

In a randomized clinical trial, Gjelvold and colleagues[23] demonstrated an implant survival rate of 100% and an implant success rate of 91.7% for immediate-load single-tooth implants placed in the maxillary anterior/premolar region compared with 95.8% survival and 83.3% success for delayed loading. In a meta-analysis of randomized controlled trials, Moraschini and colleagues[24] found no statistically significant difference between immediate and conventional loading of single implants placed in the posterior mandible with a survival rate ranging from 91.7% to 100% for immediate loading and from 96.6% to 100% for conventional loading at a mean follow-up of 31.2 months. In a systematic review and meta-analysis identifying more than 5000 studies, Pigozzo and colleagues[25] found no significant difference between early and immediate loading of single implants with regard to survival rate at 1 and 3 year follow-up or marginal bone loss at 1 year. The overall survival rates at 1 year were 97.5% for early loading and 97.3% for immediate loading, and at 3 years the survival rates were 97.6% and 97.3%, respectively.

A large majority of the clinical studies evaluating the immediate loading of a single-tooth implant involve a restoration that is loaded with little or no occlusion. Although there is some support in the literature for successful functional immediate loading of single dental implants,[26–28] it is the opinion of the author to avoid any occlusal load on single immediate-load implants. The rationale is that micro-movements above 150 μm can lead to fibrous formation around the implant consequently preventing osseointegration.[29] Therefore, without the cross-arch stabilization of multiple implants, all of the functional occlusal forces would be placed directly on the immediate-load single implant. In 1998, Misch[30,31] introduced a concept called N-FIT, or nonfunctional immediate teeth (**Fig. 2**). The protocol calls for a provisional prosthesis to be placed that is void of any occlusal contacts and is only for esthetics. Despite the fact that the restoration is 'nonfunctional,' the benefits of this protocol include the patient receiving an esthetic tooth replacement, no need for a second surgery, and the benefit to the developing soft tissue emergence. Most patients receiving a single dental implant have adequate remaining contact to function so it is not a challenge to have one tooth temporarily not in function. It is imperative to evaluate the occlusion in all excursions, centric and eccentric, to confirm that there is no contact at all.

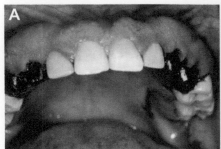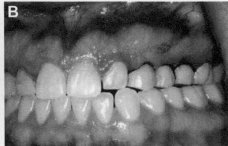

Fig. 2. (*A*) Implants were placed in the bilateral canine and second premolar area to support a three-unit fixed implant bridge. (*B*) Implants immediately loaded with a provisional nonfunctional immediate teeth bridge that is primarily for esthetics and is not in contact with the opposing teeth. (*Adapted from* Resnik, R.R. and Misch, C.E. (2021) "Immediate Load/Restoration in Implant Dentistry," in *Misch's contemporary implant dentistry*. St. Louis: Elsevier.)

IMMEDIATE LOAD: FULL ARCH

Immediate placement and loading of implants in completely edentulous arches have become exceedingly popular in implant dentistry today. Although these cases can sometimes be challenging and can be associated with a higher chance of complications, the success rate has been well documented in the literature. In a prospective four-center study, Testori and colleagues[32] evaluated 62 patients in which an interim prosthesis was immediately inserted in full-arch mandibular cases and reported a 99.4% success rate. Aalam and colleagues[33] evaluated 16 patients who received mandibular implants with screw-retained hybrid prostheses and showed a 96.6% success rate after 3 years. Tarnow and colleagues[34] followed rigidly splinted immediate-load fixed prostheses in the maxilla and mandible for 5 years. From his results and experience, Tarnow developed clinical guidelines to follow to ensure the greatest chance of success when attempting immediate load (**Table 1**).

"All-ON-4"

Malo and colleagues[35,36] first introduced the concept of All-on-4, which involves immediately loading a fixed prosthesis on 4 implants in the maxilla or mandible

Table 1 Tarnow's immediate-loading protocol	
1.	Can only attempt in edentulous arches, to utilize cross-arch stability
2.	Implants should be a minimum of 10 mm in length
3.	Diagnostic wax up should be made for template and provisional fabrication
4.	Lingual aspect of the provisional restoration should have rigid metal casting
5.	Screw-retained provisional is preferable
6.	If cement-retained, do not remove during 4–6 mo healing period
7.	Evaluate implants with Periotest and select implants with least mobility for immediate loading
8.	Use widest possible anterior-posterior distribution of implants to provide resistance to rotational forces
9.	Cantilevers should be avoided

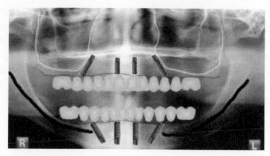

Fig. 3. All-on-4 protocol involving 2 anterior implants, two-angled posterior implants to avoid the maxillary sinus and the anterior loop of the mental nerve, and an immediately loaded fixed prosthesis. (*Adapted from* Resnik, R.R. and Misch, C.E. (2021) "Immediate Load/Restoration in Implant Dentistry," in *Misch's contemporary implant dentistry.* St. Louis: Elsevier.)

Table 2	
All-on-4 prerequisites	
1.	Insertion torque of 35 N-cm (if not achieved, then immediate loading is not recommended)
2.	Patient cannot have any parafunctional habits
3.	The minimum bone dimensions are > 5 mm width and > 8 mm height in mandible and > 10 mm height in maxilla
4.	Bone density type D1–D3

(**Fig. 3**). In general, 2 implants are placed parallel in the anterior region and 2 posterior implants are placed on an angle to increase the anterior-posterior spread, avoid the maxillary sinus or inferior alveolar nerve canal, and minimize cantilever length (see **Fig. 3**). Multi-unit abutments with varying degrees of angulation (most commonly 0°, 17°, and 30°) are placed onto the implants. The requirements for the All-on-4 immediate-load protocol are outlined in **Table 2**.

GUIDED IMMEDIATE LOAD

Various combined surgical and prosthetic protocols exist in the market (eg, nSequence) that facilitate a completely guided full-arch rehabilitation involving implant placement and an immediately loaded definitive fixed prosthesis.[37] These systems utilize 3-D precision digital implant planning using the cone-beam computerized tomography to create bone reduction guides, implant placement guides, and an immediate fixed prosthesis to be delivered on the same day.

SUMMARY

As the field of implant dentistry continues to evolve and the techniques and technologies continue to improve, new options arise which can provide great benefits to the patient. Some of the patient benefits of immediate loading include shorter treatment time, esthetics, no need for second-surgery, and soft tissue improvements. The greatest success has been demonstrated with 4 or more mandibular implants. Although there is some literature that demonstrates successful outcomes in immediate functional loading of single implants if primary stability and the aforementioned pre-requisites are achieved, the opinion of the author is to opt for a nonfunctional load that does not have any occlusal contacts when considering immediate loading of a single dental implant. With proper case selection, meticulous surgical technique, and avoidance of potential complicating factors by increasing surface area and decreasing force, immediate loading of endosseous implants can be as successful as the traditional delayed approach.

CLINICS CARE POINTS

- Immediate loading of endosseous implants is most successful when performed for full-arch rehabilitation.
- Single implants can be immediately provisionalized, but should not have any occlusal forces.
- Excessive torque and undue surgical trauma should be avoided during implant placement.
- Increasing the surface area of the load and reducing the force applied greatly enhance the bone-implant interface, increasing the likelihood of success.

DISCLOSURE

The authors have nothing to disclose.

REFERENCES

1. Brånemark PI, Hansson BO, Adell R, et al. Osseointegrated implants in the treatment of edentulous jaw: experience from a 10 year period. Scand J Plast Reconstr Surg 1977;2(10):1–132.
2. Ledermann P. Bar-prosthetic management of the edentulous mandible by means of plasma-coated implantation with titanium screws [In German]. Deutsche Zahnärztliche Zeitschrift 1979;34:907–11.
3. Schnitman PA, Wohrle PS, Rubenstein JE. Immediate fixed interim prostheses supported by two-stage threaded implants: methodology and results. Int J Oral Implantol 1990;16:96–105.
4. Misch CE, Wang HL, Misch CM, et al. Rationale for the application of immediate load in implant dentistry. I. Implant Dent 2004;13:207–15.
5. Resnik RR, Misch CE. Chapter: 33, Immediate Load/Restoration in Implant Dentistry. In: Misch's contemporary implant dentistry. St Louis (MO): Resnick, Elsevier; 2021. p. 860–89.
6. Douglas de Oliveira DW, Lages FS, Lanza LA, et al. Dental implants with immediate loading using insertion torque of 30 Ncm: a systematic review. Implant Dent 2016;25:675–83.
7. Maló P, Lopes A, de Araújo Nobre M, et al. Immediate function dental implants inserted with less than 30 N·cm of torque in full arch maxillary rehabilitations using the All-on-4 concept: retrospective study. Int J Oral Maxillofac surgery 2018;47(8):1079–85.
8. Lazzara RJ, Testori T, Meltzer A, et al. Immediate Occlusal Loading (IOL) of dental implants: predictable results through DIEM guidelines. Pract Proced Aesthet Dent: PPAD. 2004;16(4):3–15.
9. Chaushu G, Chaushu S, Tzohar A, et al. Immediate loading of single-tooth implants: immediate versus nonimmediate implantation. A clinical report. Int J Oral Maxillofac Implants 2001;16(2):267–72.

10. Testori T, Szmukler-Moncler S, Francetti L, et al. Healing of Osseotite implants under submerged and immediate loading conditions in a single patient: a case report and interface analysis after 2 months. Int J Periodontics Restorative Dent 2002;22:345–53.

11. Piattelli A, Corigliano M, Scarano A, et al. Immediate loading of titanium plasma sprayed implants: an histologic analysis in monkeys. J Periodontol 1998;69: 321–7.

12. Buchs AU, Levine L, Moy P. Preliminary report of immediately loaded Altiva Natural Tooth Replacement dental implants. Clin Implant Dent Relat Res 2001;3(2): 97–106.

13. Balshi SF, Allen FD, Wolfinger GJ, et al. A resonance frequency analysis assessment of maxillary and mandibular immediately loaded implants. Int J Oral Maxillofac Implants 2005;20(4).

14. Horiuchi K, Uchida H, Yamamoto K, et al. Immediate loading of Brånemark system implants following placement in edentulous patients: a clinical report. Int J Oral Maxillofac Implants 2000;15:824–30.

15. Strong JT, Misch CE, Bidez MW, et al. Functional surface area: thread form parameter optimization for implant body design. Compend Contin Educ Dent 1998;19:4–9.

16. Misch CE, Wang HL. Immediate occlusal loading for fixed prostheses in implant dentistry. Dent Today 2003;22:50–6.

17. Bornstein MM, Valderrama P, Jones AA, et al. Bone apposition around two different sandblasted and acid-etched titanium implant surfaces: a histomorphometric study in canine mandibles. Clin Oral Implants Res 2008;19:233–41.

18. Nicolau P, Korostoff J, Ganeles J, et al. Immediate and early loading of chemically modified implants in posterior jaws: 3-year results from a prospective randomized multicenter study. Clin Implant Dent Relat Res 2013;15:600–12.

19. Resnik R.R. and Misch C.E., Chapter: 8, Treatment Planning: Force Factors Related to Patient Conditions, In: *Misch's contemporary implant dentistry*, 2021, Resnick, Elsevier; St Louis (MO). 174-178.

20. Balshi TJ, Wolfinger GJ. Immediate loading of Brånemark implants in edentulous mandible: a preliminary report. Implant Dent 1997;6:83–8.

21. Barbier L, Schepers E. Adaptive bone remodeling around oral implants under axial and non axial loading conditions in the dog mandible. Int J Oral Maxillofac Implants 1997;12:215–23.

22. Sener BC, Dergin G, Gursoy B, et al. Effects of irrigation temperature on heat control in vitro at different drilling depths. Clin Oral Implants Res 2009;20:294–8.

23. Gjelvold B, Kisch J, Chrcanovic BR. A Randomized Clinical Trial Comparing Immediate Loading and Delayed Loading of Single-Tooth Implants: 5-Year Results. J Clin Med 2021;10:1077.

24. Moraschini V, Porto Barboza E. Immediate versus conventional loaded single implants in the posterior mandible: a meta-analysis of randomized controlled trials. Int J Oral Maxillofac Surg 2016;45(1):85–92.

25. Pigozzo MN, Rebelo da Costa T, Newton S, et al. Immediate versus early loading of single dental implants: a systematic review and meta-analysis. J Prosthet Dent 2018;120(1):25–34.

26. Calandriello R, Tomatis M. Immediate Occlusal Loading of Single Lower Molars Using Brånemark System® Wide Platform TiUnite™ Implants: A 5-Year Follow-Up Report of a Prospective Clinical Multicenter Study. Clin Implant Dent Relat Res 2011;13(4):311–8.

27. Rao W, Benzi R. Single mandibular first molar implants with flapless guided surgery and immediate function: Preliminary clinical and radiographic results of a prospective study. J Prosthet Dent 2007;97(6). https://doi.org/10.1016/s0022-3913(07)60003-1.
28. Siddiqui AA, O'Neal R, Nummikoski P, et al. Immediate loading of single-tooth restorations: one-year prospective results. J Oral Implantol 2008;34(4):208–18.
29. Pilliar RM, Lee JM, Maniatopoulos C. Observations on the effect of movement on bone in growth into porous-surfaced implants. Clin Orthop Relat Res 1986;208:108–13.
30. Misch CE. Non-functional immediate teeth in partially edentulous patients: a pilot study of 10 consecutive cases using the Maestro dental implant system. Compend Contin Educ Dent 1998;19:25–36.
31. Misch CE. Non-functional immediate teeth. Dent Today 1998;17:88–91.
32. Testori T, Szmukler-Moncler S, Francetti L, et al. Immediate loading of Osseotite implants: a case report and histologic analysis after 4 months of occlusal loading. Int J Periodontics Restorative Dent 2001;21:451–9.
33. Aalam AA, Nowzari H, Krivitsky A. Functional restoration of implants on the day of surgical placement in the fully edentulous mandible: a case series. Clin Implant Dent Relat Res 2005;7:10–6.
34. Tarnow DP, Emtiaz S, Classi A. Immediate loading of threaded implants at stage 1 surgery in edentulous arches: ten consecutive case reports with 1-to 5-year data. Int J Oral Maxillofac Implants 1997;12:319–24.
35. Malo P, Rangert B, Nobre M. "All-on-Four" immediate-function concept with Brånemark system implants for completely edentulous mandibles: a retrospective clinical study. Clin Implant Dent Relat Res 2003;5(1):2–9.
36. Malo P, Rangert B, Nobre M. All-on-4 immediate-function concept with Brånemark system implants for completely edentulous maxillae: a 1-year retrospective clinical study. Clin Implant Dent Relat Res 2005;7(1):S88–94.
37. Pikos MA, Magyar CW, Llop DR. Guided full-arch immediate function treatment modality for the edentulous and terminal dentition patient. Compend Contin Educ Dent (Jamesburg, NJ: 1995) 2015;36(2):116–9.

Post-Procedure Analgesic Management

Amanda Andre, DDS*, Michael Benichou, DMD, Harry Dym, DDS

KEYWORDS

- Dental post-operative pain management • Opioid alternatives
- Non-opioid analgesics • Dental post-procedure analgesia
- Liposomal local anesthetics

KEY POINTS

- The opioid-related increase in morbidity and mortality in the United States has led to increased efforts toward safer prescribing of opioids and the use of non-opioid analgesic alternatives for post-procedure analgesic management.
- The analgesic efficacy of maximizing the effects of non-steroidal anti-inflammatory drugs and acetaminophen through multimodal analgesia modalities is typically underestimated, although their combination has been proven to provide optimal pain control after dental and surgical procedures.
- The use of a liposomal local anesthetic allows for long-term pain relief during the initial inflammatory phase minimizing the overall analgesic drug requirements.

INTRODUCTION

Adequate prevention, assessment, and treatment of pain are fundamental in the field of dentistry. The evolution of our profession from limited emergency treatments to a broader scope including preventive and elective services may be attributed to our ability to manage intraoperative and post-operative pain. A patient's anticipation of their pain experience may influence their disposition to pursue preventive therapy, their timing in seeking emergency care, and their acceptance of elective treatments. In the acute setting, a focus on minimizing pain can lead to an enhanced patient response and have profound long-term effects. Failure to adequately treat post-operative pain may lead to negative outcomes such as tachycardia, hypertension, poor wound healing, as well as peripheral and central sensitization.[1] Post-procedure pain management models include patient optimization, the implementation of enhanced recovery protocols, the use of local anesthetics, analgesic drugs, and local wound care.

The Brooklyn Hospital Center, 121 Dekalb Avenue, Brooklyn, NY 11201, USA
* Corresponding author.
E-mail address: aafernandez@tbh.org

Dent Clin N Am 68 (2024) 213–225
https://doi.org/10.1016/j.cden.2023.07.003
0011-8532/24/© 2023 Elsevier Inc. All rights reserved.

BACKGROUND

When developing multimodal pain management protocols, practitioners should take into consideration the potential risks each treatment modality inherently carries in order to prevent or diminish harmful outcomes. As an example, the part dentists played in the early stages of the opioid epidemic in the United States of America should serve as a cautionary account. The development of the opioid crisis into a nation-wide public health emergency ought to encourage our profession to focus on the lasting impact our choices can have in the lives of our patients and communities. It is important to understand the roots of this crisis as it explains the current principles guiding pain management in our profession.

In the 1990s controlled-release opioid pain relievers, i.e. OxyContin (oxycodone), were released into the market. The promotion of these drugs by pharmaceutical companies highlighted their quality metrics of aggressive pain control and downplayed the drugs' addictive potential. Medical professionals widely adopted the use of oral opioids as an acute pain management tool and subsequently an alarming increase in the prescription frequency of opioids followed.[2,3] As we now have come to understand, opioids have potential risks including dependence, misuse, overdose, diversion, and non-medical use. Epidemiological studies have correlated the increased frequency of opioid prescriptions with an alarming rise in prescription opioid deaths.[4,5] The opioid crisis in the United States of America has had devastating consequences affecting individuals, family units, and our communities (**Fig. 1**).

Dentists have been identified as one of the top opioid analgesic prescribers.[2,6–9] The American Journal of Preventive Medicine published a study in 2016 in which the data revealed the top prescribers as internal medicine (16.4%); dentists (15.8%); nurse

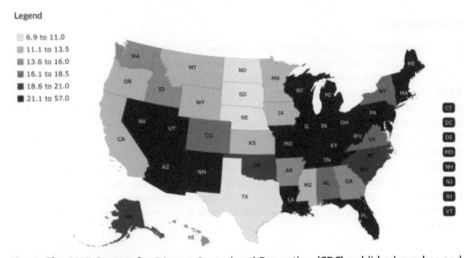

Legend

- 6.9 to 11.0
- 11.1 to 13.5
- 13.6 to 16.0
- 16.1 to 18.5
- 18.6 to 21.0
- 21.1 to 57.0

Fig. 1. The 2017 Centers for Disease Control and Prevention (CDC) published number and age-adjusted rates of drug overdose deaths by state. Number and age-adjusted rates of drug overdose deaths by state in 2017. Deaths are classified using the International Classification of Diseases, Tenth Revision (ICD–10). Drug-poisoning deaths are identified using underlying cause-of-death codes X40–X44, X60–X64, X85, and Y10–Y14. Age-adjusted death rates were calculated as deaths per 100,000 population using the direct method and the 2000 standard population. (*Courtesy of* Center for Disease Control and Prevention. Available at https://www.cdc.gov/drugoverdose/data/statedeaths.html. With permission.)

practitioners (12.3%); and family medicine (10.3%).[6] A report published by the Journal of American Medical Association (JAMA) analyzed opioid prescription patterns in the United States of America through an examination of the service delivery indicators (SDI) Health data compiling all prescriptions dispensed in the country in the year 2009. Alarmingly, dentists were the top opioid analgesics prescribers (30.8%) for patients aged 10 to 19 years old, followed by primary care (13.1%) and emergency medicine physicians (12.3%).[9] The high frequency of these high-risk prescriptions in the pediatric population was re-demonstrated in 2021 by Chua and colleagues[10] with dentists and surgeons writing 61.4% of the prescriptions. The exposure of young adults and adolescents to these narcotics has been associated with an increased lifetime risk of substance use disorders.[10]

In 2020, the Centers for Disease Control and Prevention (CDC) published an updated Opioid Prescribing Guideline and along with the development of prescription drug monitoring and public education programs awareness has been raised to improve appropriate opioid prescribing[5] (**Fig. 2**). More present data support the prescription of non-opioid analgesics as a superior pain control method. Moore and colleagues[11] performed an overview of systematic reviews of analgesic medications used in the management of acute dental pain and they concluded that non-steroidal anti-inflammatory drugs (NSAIDs), either alone or in combination with acetaminophen, were equal or superior to opioid-containing medications for the relief of post-operative dental pain. A study published by JAMA found that for dental routine procedure or surgical extractions, patients who were prescribed opioids reported greater pain compared to those who were prescribed non-opioid analgesics. In addition, opioid use was not associated with differences in patient satisfaction or telephone calls to report concerns about extraction-associated pain.[12] Safe prescribing of opioids for

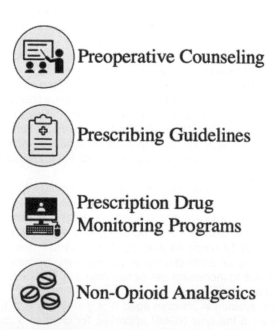

Fig. 2. Evidence-based interventions for opioid reduction. A summary of 4 practices that have the potential to minimize opioid prescribing and consumption. (*From* Upp LA, Waljee JF. The opioid epidemic. Clinics in Plastic Surgery 2020;47(2):181-90, figure 5.)

the management of dental post-procedure pain still has a role in the treatment of patients who may require management of breakthrough pain. The emphasis of this article is to explore the various non-opioid analgesic options that may be utilized for the management of dental post-operative pain.

ACETAMINOPHEN AND NON-STEROIDAL ANTI-INFLAMMATORY DRUGS
Acetaminophen

Despite being one of the most commonly used analgesics and anti-pyretics available over-the-counter, acetaminophen or paracetamol is still not entirely understood. What is known is that acetaminophen inhibits the cyclooxygenase (COX) pathways in the central nervous system. It is believed that acetaminophen reduces the activity of cyclooxygenase thus in turn inhibiting prostaglandin synthesis in the CNS.[13] Additionally, the CNS pathways also affected include production of serotonin, opioids, nitric oxide, and cannabinoids.[14] Unlike NSAIDs, acetaminophen has shown a lack of anti-inflammatory property.

The recommended maximum dosage of acetaminophen is documented to be 4 g per 24 hours, and 1 g per 4 hours. Even in patients with cirrhosis, acetaminophen is considered a safe option though reduced dosing of 2 g per 24 hours is recommended.[15] Acetaminophen is routinely administered on an around-the-clock schedule especially for early post-operative analgesia, although superiority to a schedule pro re nata pain has not been established.[16]

Non-steroidal Anti-inflammatory Drugs

NSAIDs are widely used in oral and maxillofacial surgery for their analgesic, anti-inflammatory, and anti-pyretic properties. NSAIDs are effective through their inhibitory effects on cyclooxygenases (COXs), which are involved in the synthesis of prostaglandins. Prostaglandins have an important role in the production of pain, inflammation, and fever.[17] By blocking the conversion of arachidonic acid into these eicosanoids—thromboxanes, prostaglandins, and prostacyclins, NSAIDs can be potent analgesics useful for post-operative acute pain management.[18]

There are several non-selective COX inhibitors (NSAIDs) available, including aspirin, ibuprofen, naproxen, and ketorolac. Aspirin is a non-selective NSAID that inhibits COX enzymes irreversibly, leading to a decrease in prostaglandin production. Ibuprofen and naproxen are also non-selective NSAIDs that reversibly inhibit COX enzymes. Ketorolac (Toradol) is a potent non-selective NSAID used commonly for its profound analgesic effect and most often administered via intramuscular or intravenous injection.

The maximum dosage of ibuprofen is 3,200 mg per day. A 400 mg dosage of ibuprofen has been shown to have equivalent analgesic potency as 800 mg.[19] For pain, 400 to 800 mg ibuprofen every 6 hours as needed is recommended.[20] The maximum dosage of naproxen is 1,250 mg/day and is recommended to take in 250 to 500 mg doses every 12 hours as needed. The maximum dosage of ketorolac is 120 mg per 24 hours to be administered as 30 mg every 6 hours as needed for no longer than 5 days due to increased risk of bleeding, peptic ulcers, renal failure, and cardiac thrombotic events.[21]

Aspirin should be avoided in children aged 2 or younger due to the risk of Reye's syndrome. Ibuprofen is the only NSAID approved for children 3 months and older. Ibuprofen is also shown to be less likely to cause gastrointestinal injury compared to naproxen.[22] When there is concern for a patient's heightened risk for vascular complications, the safest option among NSAIDs is naproxen.[23] Due to the various potential side effects of NSAIDs, it is critical to use the least dosage necessary for desired effect and to prescribe the appropriate drug for each particular patient.

Cyclooxygenase-2-specific inhibitors

Cyclooxygenase-2 (COX-2)-specific inhibitors influence central nervous system nociception while limiting the potential for adverse side effects seen with non-selective NSAIDs. In the oral and maxillofacial surgery model, administering 200 mg pre-op celecoxib, a COX-2 inhibitor, limited the inflammatory response of prostaglandin E2 in local tissues at 80 to 240 minutes post-mandibular third molar removal.[24] In another study by Akinbade and colleagues[25] comparing analgesic efficacy of celecoxib and tramadol on post-operative third molar extraction pain, patients taking celecoxib reported significantly lower visual analog scale (VAS) scores over the course of 48 hours post-operation.

The maximum recommended dosage of celecoxib is 400 mg a day. Compared to non-selective NSAIDs, celecoxib has a favorable profile of gastrointestinal (GI) side effects and a comparable risk of cardiovascular events. A meta-analysis by Bally and colleagues[26] also confirmed there was no significant difference in the rate of myocardial infarction between celecoxib and non-selective NSAIDs. A study by Nissen and colleagues noted that cardiovascular event rates were similar among celecoxib, naproxen, and ibuprofen. Additionally, the report noted that GI tolerability was better for celecoxib. It noted that celecoxib had decreased rates of renal events compared to ibuprofen, but not compared to naproxen.[27] However, celecoxib is contraindicated in patients having undergone coronary artery bypass graft surgery because of an increased risk of cardiovascular events. Also, since celecoxib contains a sulfonamide moiety, it should be avoided in patients with a documented sulfonamide allergy.[28]

Combination of Non-steroidal Anti-inflammatory Drugs and Acetaminophen

A multitude of studies have shown the combination of NSAIDs and acetaminophen to be a potent analgesic strategy in post-op acute pain management, certainly better than either medication alone.[29] Combining NSAIDs and acetaminophen provides a synergistic effect.[29] Another study had concluded that adding 60 mg codeine to a regimen already consisting of 1000 mg acetaminophen and 400 mg ibuprofen taken every 6 hours does not add any additional analgesia during recovery from third molar extraction.[30] A combination of acetaminophen and ibuprofen was found to be more effective for managing acute pain than the combination of acetaminophen and opioids, and associated with less adverse side effects.[31]

LOCAL ANESTHETICS AND LIPOSOMAL FORMULATIONS
Local Anesthetics

The use of peripheral nerve blocks and local anesthetic techniques can improve post-operative pain management and reduce the need for opioid-containing analgesics post-operatively. A small number of well-controlled clinical studies support the use of pre-incisional local anesthesia may prevent the establishment of central sensitization by preemptively blocking the N-methyl-D-aspartate (NMDA)-induced hyperexcitability and subsequent release of inflammatory mediators.[32,33] For immediate post-operative analgesia, local anesthetics can be highly effective until patients retrieve rescue analgesia medications. Long-lasting anesthetics like bupivacaine have proven effective for this reason. Bupivacaine, or Marcaine, can provide anesthesia for 6 to 8 hours following administration. In a 2017 study by Olmedo-Gaya and colleagues, patients taking no rescue medication and given bupivacaine during the removal of impacted third molars reported significantly lower VAS scores at all times during the first 48 hours post-operative except for hour 8 compared to when articaine was used.[34] Patients taking rescue medication and given bupivacaine reported significantly lower VAS scores within the first 8 hours post-operatively compared to those given articaine, but no difference in VAS scores between the 2 groups were reported after 8 hours. The maximum recommended dosage of bupivacaine in the literature ranges from 2.5 to 3 mg per kg with epinephrine, or 2 to 2.5 mg per kg without epinephrine.[35]

Liposomal Local Anesthetic

Liposomal bupivacaine (trade name Exparel) is a long-acting formulation of bupivacaine approved by the United States Food and Drug Administration (FDA) for infiltration in adults to produce post-surgical local analgesia.[36,37] Exparel is the only extended release local analgesic currently approved by the FDA. Liposomal bupivacaine is an amide local anesthetic within a multilamellar liposome of triglycerides, cholesterol, and phospholipids. The drug is released by systemic absorption of plain bupivacaine from the liposomal bupivacaine solution followed by a gradual sustained release from the multilamellar vesicles. The drug has a long half-life with peak plasma concentration up to 96 hours post-injection.[38] It is metabolized by the glucuronide conjugation and dealkylation and it is then excreted by the kidney. It is recommended that care be taken in patients who are administered Exparel with severe liver disease. According to Saraghi and Hersh, there are no recommended dose adjustments in patients with renal impairment.[39]

Lipsomal bupivacaine can be administered via infiltration up to a maximum dose of 266 mg.[38] Exparel should not be used in pregnant women or in patients under the age of 18 and those allergic to bupivicaine. It is recommended to wait at least 20 minutes after administering a non-bupivicaine local anesthetic such as lidocaine because co-administration may cause an immediate release of bupivicaine from the liposomes.[39] Exparel can cause systemic toxicity with effects on both the central nervous system (seizures, dizziness) and the cardiovascular system (chest pain, palpations, bradycardia) if it enters the bloodstream. That is why it is only used for oral infiltration and aspiration prior to injection is highly recommended.

The most frequently reported adverse events after Exparel administration for third molar extractions were oral hypoesthesia, dysgevsia, and nausea.[36] Lieblich's[36] study published in the Journal of Oral and Maxillofacial Surgery came to the conclusion that patients who received local liposomal bupivacaine after third molar extractions received significantly less prescriptions for morphine and had a significant reduction in the proportion of patients requiring opioid prescription refills. In a comparison study by Davidson and colleagues, the administration of subcutaneous 20 mL of 2% bupivacaine liposome vs. 20 mL of 0.5% plain bupivacaine in humans showed no difference in peak plasma concentration between the 2 groups and the prolonged pharmacodynamic effect of the liposomal preparation was confirmed.[39,40] The study demonstrated the long-lasting analgesic effect of liposomal local anesthetics without an increase in systemic side effects. Unfortunately, the cost per single use of Exparel is approximately $250.00, which has prevented its widespread use in private practice.

KETAMINE AND DEXMEDETOMIDINE

Ketamine is a non-competitive N-methyl-D-aspartate (NMDA) receptor antagonist, introduced over 30 years ago, with a wide safety margin. Several publications in the clinical literature have concluded the use of ketamine in subanesthetic doses has analgesic effects. The drug has been used to manage post-operative pain, acute and chronic pain, including cancer pain and neuropathic pain. In the field of dentistry, ketamine is more commonly used by oral surgeons to provide moderate and deep sedation. The intranasal and submucosal formulations have recently been studied in the dental surgery setting. A randomized control trial by Christensen and colleagues[41] evaluated the efficacy and safety of intranasal ketamine (10, 30, and 50 mg) vs. placebo for the management of post-operative pain following molar extractions. Statistically significant analgesia was observed with the 50 mg dose over a 3-hour period without dissociative effects. The evidence supported a single dose of approximately 0.5 mg/kg intranasal ketamine as an analgesic.

Dexmedetomidine is classified as an alpha-2 adrenergic receptor agonist with sedative, analgesic, and anxiolytic effects. Similarly to ketamine, lower doses of dexmedetomidine have more recently been investigated for its analgesic effects when combined with local anesthetics. A randomized double-blinded study by Gursoytrak and colleagues[42] published in the Journal of Oral and Maxillofacial Surgery explored the pain, swelling, and trismus outcomes of submucosal administration of ketamine compared to dexmedetomidine. Pain was measured using a 100-point VAS. While the study did not find a significant difference in terms of swelling and trismus, ketamine demonstrated to have superior effects for the management of post-operative pain during the first 12 hours after third molar surgery.

MULTIMODAL ANALGESIA AND ENHANCED RECOVERY AFTER SURGERY PROTOCOL

Acute post-operative pain is complex and multifactorial with various mechanisms contributing to the patient's pain experience. The use of a multimodal pain therapies aims to target each mechanism and contribute to the overall improvement of the pain experience.[1] Multimodal analgesia (MMA) focuses on the additive or synergistic combinations of analgesics to achieve analgesia while minimizing side effects (**Table 1**). Generally, MMA practices utilize an optimal combination of non-opioid and non-pharmacologic interventions as first-line treatments and higher doses or opioids for breakthrough pain.[18,43] Furthermore, enhanced recovery after surgery (ERAS) protocols utilize MMA components to optimize patients in the pre-operative period with the goal of standardizing pain management efforts, minimizing side effects, expediting the return of patient to baseline function, and improving patient outcomes. While no single protocol has been agreed upon in the literature for the management of post-procedure dental and surgical pain, these methods have been more widely explored for operating room procedures such as orthognathic surgery (**Table 2**) and head and neck surgery.[44,45]

Corticosteroids

The origin of odontogenic and acute post-operative pain is mainly inflammatory in nature. The concept of reducing inflammation and swelling to allow for pain relief is intuitive. Two meta-analyses published in 2018 demonstrated the use of corticosteroids had a significant impact on post-operative pain reduction for endodontic treatment.[46,47] The evidence presented by Shamszadeh et al[46] concluded that corticosteroids might reduce the incidence of post-operative pain up to 24 hours after root canal therapy. A systematic review and meta-analysis published in the International Journal of Oral and Maxillofacial Surgery by Almeida and colleagues investigated the effectiveness of corticosteroids in the post-operative control of pain, edema, and trismus after extraction of their molars. Corticosteroids proved to be satisfactory for post-operative control in the most critical period of the inflammatory process, and as expected this effect diminished by post-operative day 7. Maintenance use of corticosteroids was

Table 1
Side effects of commonly used treatments for post-procedural dental and surgical pain[7,41–43,48,50,55,56]

Opioids analgesics	Respiratory and cardiovascular depression Nausea, vomiting, ileus Urinary retention Pruritus and skin rash Sedation/dizziness Tolerance and dependence Misuse and diversion
Local anesthetics	Cardiac arrhythmias Motor and sensory changes Allergic reaction Respiratory arrest
Non-steroidal anti-inflammatory drugs (NSAIDS) and COX-2 inhibitors	Operative site and gastrointestinal bleeding Renal tubular dysfunction Allergic reactions Hepatorenal syndrome Pre-term delivery, congenital malformations
Acetaminophen	Hepatotoxicity Agranulocytosis Sweating Gastrointestinal upset
Ketamine/NDMA antagonists	Hypertension Psychomimetic reactions "Ketamine terrors" Diplopia/nystagmus Dizziness/confusion Nausea/vomiting
Alpha-2 adrenergic receptor agonist	Sedation Dizziness Hypotension at low doses, hypertension at high doses Bradycardia
Adjunctive drugs	Corticosteroids: Adrenal suppression, reduction in secretion of endogenous cortisol Gabapentinoids (gabapentin and pregabalin): weight gain, somnolence, dizziness, and peripheral edema,
Non-pharmacological techniques	Skin irritation

not associated with an increased benefit and thus a single dose is sufficient and may reduce side effects including adrenal suppression.[48] Overall, the use of corticosteroids can have a positive impact for pain control in the post-operative period in dental and surgical procedures.

Gabapentin

Gabapentin (GBP) is an anti-epileptic drug that binds and inhibits the alpha-2 delta subunit of the pre-synaptic voltage-gated calcium channels involved in the release of excitatory neurotransmitters involved in pain pathways.[1]

GBP has demonstrated analgesic effects for post-operative pain management. Recent reviews and meta-analyses concur that perioperative gabapentin improves post-operative pain score and minimizes the amount of opioids needed relative to

Table 2
Example of an enhanced recovery after surgery protocol for orthognathic surgery by Stratton et al with permission

Perioperative Phase	Medications
Night before surgery	8 mg dexamethasone, 0.5 mg clonazepam, scopolamine patch
Preoperative	2 mg IV midazolam
Intraoperative	100 μg fentanyl at induction, 10 mg/kg IV tranexamic acid after induction, dexmedetomidine (0.4 mcg/kg/min) and propofol (25–100 mcg/kg/min) intraoperatively, 30 mg ketorolac at closure, 0.5% bupivacaine with 1:200,000 epinephrine local injection at closure Note: total fluids were generally limited to less than 1800 mL
Post-operative	300 mg gabapentin in PACU, 600 mg ibuprofen scheduled every 6 hours, 0.5 mg lorazepam as needed Note: opioids were given as needed and varied by provider but consisted of morphine, hydrocodone/acetaminophen, and dilaudid

Abbreviations: IV, intravenous; PACU, post-anesthesia care unit.

control groups.[49] A double-blinded randomized clinical published in The Journal of Dental Anesthesia and Pain Medicine analyzed the effects of administering GBP and pregabalin (PGB) compared with placebo prior to endodontic therapy. Patients were separated into 3 groups: 300 mg GBP, 75 mg PGB, and placebo. Using the numerical rating scale, patients were asked to rate their pain after the completion of the root canal therapy. The study showed that a single dose of GBP and PGB administered prior to treatment had a greater analgesic effect than placebo in single-visit root canal treatment.[50]

Lyrica

PGB, or Lyrica, is a medication belonging to the drug class of gabapentinoids often used for chronic neuropathic pain, but also shown to be effective for acute post-operative pain. Gabapentinoids work by inhibiting voltage-gated calcium channels, in turn suppressing neuronal excitability.[51] The use of gabapentinoids for perioperative pain control has been controversial due to the possible adverse side effects such as sedation, visual disturbance, or dizziness. Caution should be used when prescribing for patients at high risk of respiratory depression (eg, elderly, severe obstructive sleep apnea).

PGB is more rapidly and predictably absorbed after ingestion and more potent than gabapentin.[52] The recommended dosing strategy when using PGB is 75 to 150 mg orally preoperatively and 75 mg every 12 hours post-operatively.[28] Though other sources have recommended 150 to 300 mg 1 to 2 hours preoperatively.[53] Dose reductions should be considered for patients with renal impairment. Gabapentinoids have also shown to decrease requirement for opioids, though these are typically used as a component of a MMA strategy. A 2017 meta-analysis found that perioperative PGB reduced the first post-operative day opioid usage by 5.8 milligram morphine equivalents (MME). When used as part of a MMA strategy, PGB reduced the first post-operative day opioid usage by 3.7 MME.[54] Due to the possible adverse events with gabapentinoids, these are typically reserved for moderate-severe post-operative pain procedures.[53]

NON-PHARMACOLOGIC THERAPIES

Various non-pharmacologic therapies may be utilized for the enhancement of patient recovery after dental procedures including acupuncture, laser therapy, and local wound care techniques. Of note, low-level laser therapy (LLLT) has been utilized in the field aiming to promote analgesia, reduce inflammation, and enhance tissue healing. LLLT achieves its effects via vasodilation, an increase of adenosine triphosphate and cortisol levels and thus inhibiting the production of inflammatory factors. There are conflicting data regarding the efficacy of this treatment, and although recent studies show improved pain results compared to mock lasers, the overall data lack heterogeneity and standardization of laser protocols indicating a need for further research in this field to achieve a consensus.[55]

CLINICS CARE POINTS

- Multimodal pain management methods can be employed to achieve optimal post-operative analgesia while simultaneously diminishing potential side effects.
- The combination of NSAIDs and acetaminophen is underestimated and underutilized but can provide powerful pain relief when used in combination.
- Opioids are no longer recommended as first-line therapy for the treatment of mild to moderate dental post-procedure pain but can be considered to manage breakthrough pain.
- NDMA receptor antagonists and alpha-2 adrenergic receptor agonists are more recently being administered in lower doses for the prevention of pain after dental procedures.
- Adjunct drugs such as corticosteroids and anti-convulsants may be prescribed to enhance patient recovery.

SUMMARY

With a greater understanding of the opioid epidemic and its grave consequences on our communities, it is ever more important to explore all means of post-operative pain control to best aid our patients. A principal rule of safe prescribing is to anticipate the level of post-operative pain and prescribe the minimum dosage appropriate to control the pain, whether opioid or otherwise. Such a rule is sure to minimize adverse side effects while treating the acute post-operative pain. Of note, multimodal regimens for pain control have even been found to be more effective than opioids alone. The most effective non-opioid regimen is the synergistic combination of NSAID and acetaminophen. Celecoxib, a Cox-2–specific inhibitor, has also been shown to provide analgesia while limiting adverse gastrointestinal side effects. Gabapentinoids, including pregabalin and gabapentin, have been shown to be effective especially when used in a multimodal regimen, and most noteworthy for chronic opioid users experiencing breakthrough pain. In addition to medication per os, particularly effective for post-operative pain management has been the advent of Exparel, a long-acting liposomal bupivacaine anesthetic. With the many modalities for pain control, it is especially important a post-operative pain control regimen be individualized to the needs of each patient to ensure safe, yet effective analgesia.

DISCLOSURE

All images and tables are from Elsevier publications. The authors of this article have received no external funding or grants or any remuneration regarding any commercial items mentioned within the article.

REFERENCES

1. Vadivelu N, Mitra S, Narayan D. Recent advances in postoperative pain management. Yale J Biol Med 2010;83(1):11–25.
2. Thornhill MH, Suda KJ, Durkin MJ, et al. Is it time US dentistry ended its opioid dependence? J Am Dent Assoc 2019;150(10):883–9.
3. Timeline of Selected FDA Activities and Significant Events Addressing Substance Use and Overdose Prevention. Department of Health and Human Services Food and Drug Administration 2023. Available at: https://www.fda.gov/drugs/information-drug-class/timeline-selected-fda-activities-and-significant-events-addressing-substance-use-and-overdose.
4. Wide-ranging online data for epidemiologic research (WONDER). Atlanta (GA): CDC, National Center for Health Statistics; 2021. Available at: http://wonder.cdc.gov.
5. Upp LA, Waljee JF. The opioid epidemic. Clin Plast Surg 2020;47(2):181–90.
6. Guy GP Jr, Zhang K. Opioid Prescribing by Specialty and Volume in the U.S. Am J Prev Med 2018;55(5):e153–5.
7. Becker DB, Schwartz AI. The opioid crisis and dentistry. J Massachusetts Dent Soc 2015;64(3):7.
8. Eliav E. The role of dentistry in the opioids crisis. Quintessence Int 2017;48(4):271–2.
9. Volkow ND, McLellan TA, Cotto JH, et al. Characteristics of opioid prescriptions in 2009. JAMA 2011;305(13):1299–301.
10. Chua KP, Brummett CM, Conti RM, Bohnert AS. Opioid Prescribing to US Children and Young Adults in 2019. Pediatrics 2021;148(3):1–12.
11. Moore PA, Ziegler KM, Lipman RD, et al. Benefits and harms associated with analgesic medications used in the management of acute dental pain: an overview of systematic reviews. J Am Dent Assoc 2018;149(4):256–65.e3.
12. Nalliah RP, Sloss KR, Kenney BC, et al. Association of opioid use with pain and satisfaction after dental extraction. JAMA Netw Open 2020;3(3):1–11.
13. Ghanem CI, Pérez MJ, Manautou JE, et al. Acetaminophen from liver to brain: New insights into drug pharmacological action and toxicity. Pharmacol Res 2016;109:119–31.
14. Lachiewicz PF. The role of intravenous acetaminophen in multimodal pain protocols for perioperative orthopedic patients. Orthopedics 2013;36(2):15–9.
15. Chandok N, Watt KD. Pain management in the cirrhotic patient: the clinical challenge. Paper presented at: Mayo Clinic Proceedings, 2010.
16. Riddell RRP, Craig KD. Time-contingent schedules for postoperative analgesia: a review of the literature. J Pain 2003;4(4):169–75.
17. Bushra R, Aslam N. An overview of clinical pharmacology of Ibuprofen. Oman Med J 2010;25(3):155.
18. Bhatia A, Buvanendran A. Anesthesia and postoperative pain control-multimodal anesthesia protocol. J Spine Surg 2019;5(Suppl 2):S160–5.
19. Motov S, Masoudi A, Drapkin J, et al. Comparison of oral ibuprofen at three single-dose regimens for treating acute pain in the emergency department: a randomized controlled trial. Ann Emerg Med 2019;74(4). 530-537.
20. Scott LJ. Intravenous ibuprofen: in adults for pain and fever. Drugs 2012;72:1099–109.
21. Vacha ME, Huang W, Mando-Vandrick J. The role of subcutaneous ketorolac for pain management. Hosp Pharm 2015;50(2):108–12.

22. Tai FWD, McAlindon ME. Non-steroidal anti-inflammatory drugs and the gastrointestinal tract. Clin Med 2021;21(2):131.

23. Coxib, traditional NTC, Bhala N, et al. Vascular and upper gastrointestinal effects of non-steroidal anti-inflammatory drugs: meta-analyses of individual participant data from randomised trials. Lancet 2013;382(9894):769–79.

24. Xie L, Yang R-T, Lv K, et al. Comparison of low pre-emptive oral doses of celecoxib versus acetaminophen for postoperative pain management after third molar surgery: a randomized controlled study. J Oral Maxillofac Surg 2020; 78(1):75.e1–6.

25. Akinbade A, Ndukwe K, Owotade F. A comparative analgesic efficacy and tolerability of celecoxib and tramadol after mandibular third molar extraction: a double blind randomized controlled trial. Int J Oral Maxillofac Surg 2015;44:e22–3.

26. Bally M, Dendukuri N, Rich B, et al. Risk of acute myocardial infarction with NSAIDs in real world use: bayesian meta-analysis of individual patient data. BMJ 2017;357:j1909.

27. Nissen SE, Yeomans ND, Solomon DH, et al. Cardiovascular safety of celecoxib, naproxen, or ibuprofen for arthritis. N Engl J Med 2016;375:2519–29.

28. Schwenk ES Nonopioid pharmacotherapy for acute pain in adults.: UpToDate 2023. Available at: "https://www.uptodate.com/contents/nonopioid-pharmac otherapy-for-acute-pain-in-adults?search=gralise&source=search_result&sele ctedTitle=1~150&usage_type=default&display_rank=1". Accessed February 9, 2023.

29. Hersh EV, Moore PA. Combination analgesics for pain management. Drugs 2013; 73(9):963–74.

30. Best AD, De Silva R, Thomson W, et al. Efficacy of codeine when added to paracetamol (acetaminophen) and ibuprofen for relief of postoperative pain after surgical removal of impacted third molars: a double-blinded randomized control trial. J Oral Maxillofac Surg 2017;75(10):2063–9.

31. Chang AK, Bijur PE, Esses D, et al. Effect of a single dose of oral opioid and nonopioid analgesics on acute extremity pain in the emergency department: a randomized clinical trial. JAMA 2017;318(17):1661–7.

32. White PF. The changing role of non-opioid analgesic techniques in the management of postoperative pain. Anesth Analg 2005;101(5 Suppl):S5–22.

33. Woolf CJ, Chong MS. Preemptive analgesia–treating postoperative pain by preventing the establishment of central sensitization. Anesth Analg 1993;77(2): 362–79.

34. Olmedo-Gaya MV, Manzano-Moreno FJ, Muñoz-López JL, et al. Double-blind, randomized controlled clinical trial on analgesic efficacy of local anesthetics articaine and bupivacaine after impacted third molar extraction. Clin Oral Investig 2018;22:2981–8.

35. Williams D, Walker J. A nomogram for calculating the maximum dose of local anaesthetic. Anaesthesia 2014;69(8):847–53.

36. Lieblich SE, Misiek D, Olczak J, et al. A retrospective cross-sectional study of the effect of liposomal bupivacaine on postoperative opioid prescribing after third molar extraction. J Oral Maxillofac Surg 2021;79(7):1401–8.e1.

37. Bulbake U, Doppalapudi S, Kommineni N, et al. Liposomal formulations in clinical use: an updated review. Pharmaceutics 2017;9(2).

38. Kaye AD, Armstead-Williams C, Hyatali F, et al. Exparel for postoperative pain management: a comprehensive review. Curr Pain Headache Rep 2020; 24(11):73.

39. Saraghi M, Hersh EV. Three newly approved analgesics: an update. Anesth Prog 2013;60(4):178–87.
40. Manchikanti L, Fellows SHB, Janata JW, et al. Opioid epidemic in the United States. Pain Physician 2012;15(3S):ES9.
41. Christensen K, Rogers E, Green GA, et al. Safety and efficacy of intranasal ketamine for acute postoperative pain. Acute Pain 2007;9(4):183–92.
42. Gursoytrak B, Kocaturk Ö, Koparal M, et al. Comparison of dexmedetomidine and ketamine for managing postoperative symptoms after third-molar surgery. J Oral Maxillofac Surg 2021;79(3):532–6.
43. Mehlisch DR. The efficacy of combination analgesic therapy in relieving dental pain. J Am Dent Assoc 2002;133(7):861–71.
44. Coyle M, Main B, Hughes C, et al. Enhanced recovery after surgery (ERAS) for head and neck oncology patients. Clin Otolaryngol 2016;41(2):118–26.
45. Stratton M, Waite P, Powell K, et al. Benefits of the enhanced recovery after surgery pathway for orthognathic surgery. Int J Oral Maxillofac Surg 2022;51(2):214–8.
46. Shamszadeh S, Shirvani A, Eghbal MJ, et al. Efficacy of corticosteroids on postoperative endodontic pain: a systematic review and meta-analysis. J Endod 2018;44(7):1057–65.
47. Nath R, Daneshmand A, Sizemore D, et al. Efficacy of corticosteroids for postoperative endodontic pain: A systematic review and meta-analysis. J Dent Anesth Pain Med 2018;18(4):205–21.
48. de AC Almeida R, Lemos C, De Moraes S, et al. Efficacy of corticosteroids versus placebo in impacted third molar surgery: systematic review and meta-analysis of randomized controlled trials. Int J Oral Maxillofac Surg 2019;48(1):118–31.
49. Mathiesen O, Møiniche S, Dahl JB. Gabapentin and postoperative pain: a qualitative and quantitative systematic review, with focus on procedure. BMC Anesthesiol 2007;7:1–15.
50. Verma J, Verma S, Margasahayam SV. Comparison of pretreatment gabapentin and pregabalin to control postoperative endodontic pain - a double-blind, randomized clinical trial. J Dent Anesth Pain Med 2022;22(5):377–85.
51. Alles SR, Cain SM, Snutch TP. Pregabalin as a pain therapeutic: beyond calcium channels. Front Cell Neurosci 2020;14:83.
52. Bockbrader HN, Wesche D, Miller R, et al. A comparison of the pharmacokinetics and pharmacodynamics of pregabalin and gabapentin. Clin Pharmacokinet 2010;49:661–9.
53. Dowell D, Ragan KR, Jones CM, et al. CDC clinical practice guideline for prescribing opioids for pain—United States, 2022. MMWR Recomm Rep (Morb Mortal Wkly Rep) 2022;71(3):1–95.
54. Fabritius M, Strøm C, Koyuncu S, et al. Benefit and harm of pregabalin in acute pain treatment: a systematic review with meta-analyses and trial sequential analyses. Br J Addiction: Br J Anaesth 2017;119(4):775–91.
55. Guerreiro MYR, Monteiro LPB, de Castro RF, et al. Effect of low-level laser therapy on postoperative endodontic pain: an updated systematic review. Complement Ther Med 2021;57:102638.
56. Deshpande AA, Hemavathy OR, Krishnan S, et al. Comparison of effect of intra socket ketamine and tramadol on postoperative pain after mandibular third molar surgery. Natl J Maxillofac Surg 2022;13(1):95–8.

Moving?

Make sure your subscription moves with you!

To notify us of your new address, find your **Clinics Account Number** (located on your mailing label above your name), and contact customer service at:

Email: journalscustomerservice-usa@elsevier.com

800-654-2452 (subscribers in the U.S. & Canada)
314-447-8871 (subscribers outside of the U.S. & Canada)

Fax number: 314-447-8029

Elsevier Health Sciences Division
Subscription Customer Service
3251 Riverport Lane
Maryland Heights, MO 63043

*To ensure uninterrupted delivery of your subscription, please notify us at least 4 weeks in advance of move.

Printed and bound by CPI Group (UK) Ltd, Croydon, CR0 4YY

03/10/2024

01040471-0004